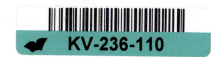

S. Krall
R. Peveling
D. Ba Diallo

New Strategies
in Locust Control

Birkhäuser Verlag
Basel · Boston · Berlin

Authors

S. Krall
R. Peveling
Gesellschaft für
Technische Zusammenarbeit GTZ
P.O. Box 5180
D-65726 Eschborn
Germany

D. Ba Diallo
CILSS-UCTR/PV
P.O. Box 1530
Bamako
Mali

A CIP catalogue record for this book is available from the Library of Congress, Washington D.C., USA

Deutsche Bibliothek Cataloging-in-Publication Data
New strategies in locust control / S. Krall... - Basel ; Boston ;
Berlin : Birkhäuser, 1997
    ISBN 3-7643-5442-9 (Basel...)
    ISBN 0-8176-5442-9 (Boston)

The publisher and editor can give no guarantee for the information on drug dosage and administration contained in this publication. The respective user must check its accuracy by consulting other sources of reference in each individual case.

© 1997 Birkhäuser Verlag, P.O.Box 133, CH-4010 Basel, Switzerland
Cover design: Micha Lotrovsky, Therwil, Switzerland
Printed on acid-free paper produced from chlorine-free pulp. TCF ∞
Printed in Germany
ISBN 3-7643-5442-9
ISBN 0-8176-5442-9

9 8 7 6 5 4 3 2 1

Table of contents

Biology of desert locust and research priorities

Forecasting and modelling

Control agents and methods: Working groups

Chemoecology and semiochemicals

Chemoecology and semiochemicals: Poster contribution

Environmental impact

Management strategies

Management strategies: Poster contribution

Management strategies: Working groups

Acknowledgements

We are grateful to ten anonymous experts for reviewing the articles in this book. Our special thanks go to Mrs Carolin Bothe (GTZ) and Mr Heimo Posamentier for their technical and organisational assistance.

The editors

Foreword

Locust swarms' ability to devastate agricultural crops has been feared for tousands of years. And for just as long, people have been trying out different ways of preventing these insects from inflicting damage. One crucial breakthrough came with the development of synthetic insecticides, which have been used in locust control for about 50 years. For decades, these were mainly chlorinated hydrocarbons. Owing to their negative environmental impact, however, they gave way to less persistent insecticides some ten years ago. Yet the new products also have considerable repercussions on the environment, especially when sprayed on a large scale.

The last major locust plague – in the late 1980s – triggered an intensive international research effort to develop environmentally sound alternatives to synthetic insecticides. At the same time, control strategies and early warning systems began to be discussed. The last ten years have yielded wide-ranging results, reflecting the intensity of the research work and discussions. But despite the successes achieved, it is also becoming apparent that, particularly in the area of strategy, a great deal of work remains to be done before we arrive at a truly practicable concept of integrated locust control.

This book reflects the work done in recent years, providing an overview of the current state of research. The articles and working group results were presented at a conference in Bamako, Mali on April 3–8, 1995, organized by the Comité Permanent Inter-Etats de Lutte contre la Sècheresse dans le Sahel (CILSS) and the Deutsche Gesellschaft für Technische Zusammenarbeit (GTZ) GmbH.

On behalf of the German Federal Ministry for Economic Cooperation and Development (BMZ), the GTZ is conducting a project to study new early warning techniques and environmentally sound methods for controlling locusts. This project, along with other projects, institutions and organisations, presented the results of its work at a conference. Workshops were also organised to discuss the future of locust control and possibilities for applying new strategies to achieve greater effectiveness, reduce costs, and minimize negative impacts on the environment. It is essential to continue and promote this process of intense sharing of knowledge and experience. The close international cooperation practiced to date shows that this path has been the right one, and that we should pursue it further.

Johannes Christenn (BMZ)
Dr. Rolf Link (GTZ)

Biology of desert locust and research priorities

New Strategies in Locust Control
S. Krall, R. Peveling and D. Ba Diallo (eds)
© 1997 Birkhäuser Verlag Basel/Switzerland

Evaluating recent locust research

P. Symmons

Brooklands, Bishops Frome, Worcestershire WR6 5BT, UK

Summary. The purpose of the Conference is to assess the practical value of recent locust research, especially research related to the desert locust. Desert locust plagues follow upsurges in which an initially non-gregariously behaving population increases in size and becomes gregarious to a progressively greater degree, over a number of generations. Control is attempted by the ultra low volume application of contact pesticides. Successful locust control is technically possible with current methods; the problems are logistical, organisational, financial and political. The practical implementation of the results of research must be assessed in the light of those constraints.

Résumé. La Conférence a pour objet l'évaluation de la valeur pratique des recherches récentes sur les locustes en général et sur le Criquet pèlerin en particulier. Les fléaux de criquets pèlerins surviennent à la suite de périodes d'invasion dans lesquelles des populations initialement non grégarigestes augmentent de taille et deviennent progressivement grégaires dans l'espace de plusieurs générations. La principale stratégie de lutte employée consiste en applications en ULV de pesticides agissant par contact. Il est techniquement possible de lutter efficacement contre les locustes avec les méthodes actuelles, les problèmes sont d'ordre logistique, organizationnel, financier et politique. La mise en oeuvre pratique des résultats de la recherche doit être évaluée dans l'optique de ces contraintes.

Introduction

During the last major desert locust upsurge somewhere between $US200 and $US300 million was provided in aid and about 15 million litres of concentrated pesticide was donated. What did this achieve? No one knows, but I am not alone in thinking "not much". There was then, a widespread and understandable wish to do better, more cheaply and with less potential environmental hazard. Donors have spent a great deal over the last four or five years in the hope of getting more reliable and cheaper locust control, specifically desert locust control. The main purpose of the Conference is to try to estimate what they have got for their money.

That may seem a simple question, but it is not. Desert locust control involves many disciplines. A scientist is reluctant to criticise work outside his field when the scientific validity of the research is not the issue. Scientists are sanguine about the benefits of research when funding depends on practical use. Funding agencies like to think their decisions have been wise. There is a convergence of interest in being "economical with the truth".

Nor is it easy to measure practical value. Many share the responsibility for combating the desert locust, so no one can be held to account. In the words of the late Sir Boris Uvarov,

"Swarms never leave countries; they only invade countries". This lack of accountability makes objective evaluation, whether of current control or of innovations, very difficult and often very suspect.

The technical problem

Technically we can combat locust outbreaks successfully without using vast quantities of pesticides and without great environmental damage. That has been demonstrated repeatedly in Australia with a difficult locust. But in Australia there are good roads and good technical facilities, and security is not a problem. The Australia Plague Locust Commission (APLC), which is responsible for control, does not have a large budget, but the budget is certain. On the other hand, the APLC must deliver, especially since part of the budget comes directly from a levy on farmers.

The problems of locust control are organisational, logistical, financial; ones of training and security; and of course, problems of politics. There is good evidence that where those can be solved, the locust problem can be solved as well. So to be useful, new methods must avoid these logistical, financial and related difficulties or at least mitigate them.

Research has indeed transformed locust control, but it is essentially modern pesticides, the transistor, light aircraft and recently global positioning devices that have brought about the change, not primarily research on locusts.

How plagues develop

In order to evaluate recent desert locust research, it is necessary to understand how plagues arise and how locusts are killed.

It is now generally accepted that desert locust plagues follow a sequence of successful breedings starting with a non-gregariously-behaving population (Fig. 1). That requires a series of unusual widespread and heavy rains, in areas to which the locust migrate in successive generations. The size of the gregariously behaving units increases progressively, and the proportion of the population that is "scattered" decreases. It is convenient to call the breeding where gregarisation first occurs an outbreak, and the whole sequence leading to a plague an upsurge. A plague is characterised by many swarms and very many nymphal (hopper) bands, and some of these are large.

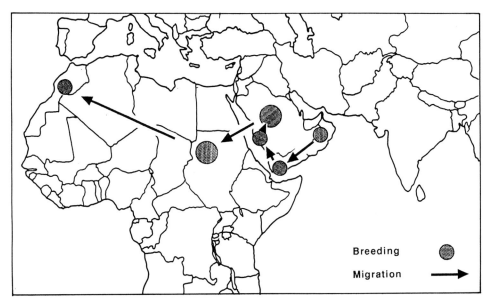

Figure 1. Simplified 1967–68 desert locust upsurge sequence.

The outbreak targets are mostly "patches" of hoppers covering a few square metres, each made up of a few thousand middle instar individuals. There are likely to be many tens of thousands of patches in an outbreak population. That is the type of population against which an innovatory outbreak suppression technique must be deployed.

Ultra low volume (ULV) spraying

Most desert locust control is now attempted by "incremental" spraying of concentrated pesticides which act mainly by contact. Large areas can be treated quickly, and the volumes to be transported are greatly reduced by not having to dilute the formulation.

The technique requires a spinning disc or spinning cage atomiser. It involves spraying cross-wind runs and relying on the wind to spread small, essentially involatile drops of pesticide over a wide swath. The tracks must be close enough for the swaths to overlap and so build up the deposit "incrementally", and there must be enough swaths to create a deposit "plateau" (Fig. 2). The swath width is largely determined by the height of the spray head. Very roughly, the peak deposit occurs about 10 times the spray head height downwind. If spray blocks are

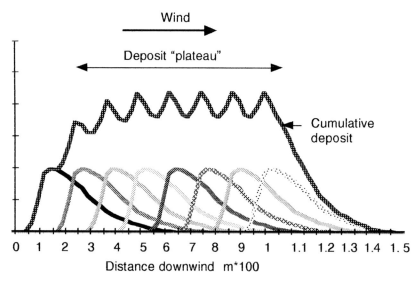

Figure 2. Diagrammatic representation of incremental spraying. Deposit (vertical scale) in arbitrary units. Distance downwind appropriate to aircraft treatment at a height of ca. 10 m.

approximately square, the minimum target size for a vehicle sprayer will be about 4 ha and for an aircraft, 1 km^2. This means the ULV hopper targets must, in general, be groups of infestations, not single bands, and certainly not individual patches.

Incremental spraying does not apply with flying locusts, but ULV pesticides are still necessary. Flying desert locust swarms were sprayed in the past but are now rarely attacked.

The research evaluation criteria

Any system of combating the desert locust must take account of the nature of the populations we have to deal with and their behaviour. Any alternative to spraying pesticides that uses the same application technique will face the same difficulties as pesticide treatment. If an alternative avoids those application problems, the feasibility of the new method must be compared with the difficulties of spraying pesticides. A new method will be likely to be a non starter if it is logistically more difficult, more risky or more expensive than spraying pesticides.

Some questions

There are a number of questions which the Conference should attempt to answer. These should include the following:
- Are locusts, in particular the desert locust, an important economic problem? How much damage would the desert locust cause if left uncontrolled?
- What use are forecasts? If future events depend on future rain and future winds, are we likely to be able to forecast either reliably enough or far enough ahead to be useful? For the same reason, can comprehensive population models ever be of practical use? Can analogy forecasts be of more value? Specific forecasts should trigger specific actions. Can these situations be identified?
- If key events require widespread, heavy rains that will not be missed, why do we need remote sensing? If we survey regularly, we will know the state of the habitat by direct observation. If we rely on remote sensing to trigger survey, what are the Locust Units supposed to do between times? This is a point that is commonly completely ignored. It is precisely the problem of maintaining an effective army in times of peace.
- Can any pesticide, however persistent, replace dieldrin if it is not cumulative?
- Do ecological breeding classifications help the experienced field officer or would a straightforward habitat map be more useful?
- Can "preventative control" by attacking outbreaks or the early stages of upsurges work with the desert locust, either in theory, that is assuming reasonable security, adequate funding, improved training and so on, or in practice, that is assuming the funding, security and logistics situation continues much as at present?
- Does current practice have a long-term harmful effect on the environment? Could alternative strategies or target choice or improved spray application methods using pesticides, substantially reduce the harmful effect?
- Do any pesticide alternatives pose fewer organisational, logistical, target detection and delimitation, and application problems than contact pesticides?

I fear it will prove impossible to determine the economic and sociological importance of the desert locust, although theoretical estimates might show that the importance is likely to be less than is commonly supposed. Most probably when swarms form, money will always be found and control attempted.

Forecasting, remote sensing, models do not kill locusts. So it is not enough to decide they are in some way a "good thing". We must show specifically how their use would help, that is what control actions follow, or might follow, specific outputs.

Alternatives to pesticides have great appeal, but do we need them? Pesticides kill; that is not the problem. So alternatives need to be easier to deploy, not more difficult, and perhaps less risky.

Current practice

If innovations are to overcome some of our current difficulties, it is important to know what those difficulties are. Currently some pilots use normal crop spray methods. Some ground spraying is carried out without any attempt to control the track spacing. Some of those responsible for spraying both in the field and at head quarters, do not know how to treat a block, how to calibrate equipment, what track spacings to use. Some targets are sprayed that contain very few locusts. Organisation in some countries is cumbersome and inadequate.

I know these problems exist with the desert locust, and I suspect they are widespread. For example, I know of no single case where a target block has been sampled to find out what it contained and sampled again after spraying to find the effect of treatment. There are numerous estimates of area treated. But these are obtained simply by dividing the pesticide sprayed and missing in other ways by the recommended volume application. That practice is justified only if there is tight control of emission rate, sprayer speed and track spacing; there seldom is. So the "area treated" is really just the "pesticide used" in different units.

These comments are not intended as criticisms. Locust control is a very difficult business. It is a pseudo military operation; public services – departments of agriculture, plant protection departments and so on – are not structured to allow the freedom of action and operational independence locust control requires. Facilities for desert locust training are generally inadequate. Staff tend not to stay. There is in most countries a lack of cash, especially of hard currency, for equipment and operations. Infrastructure is often poor. There are security problems in a number of areas.

But these difficulties are unlikely to be overcome readily. So unless a new method requires less operational independence, is simpler to organise, simpler to apply, more reliable and cheaper than pesticides, it is not likely to be viable. Any aids to existing methods must similarly be simpler to apply, not more difficult.

It is, I believe, the task of the Conference to evaluate recent research findings with those constraints in mind.

New Strategies in Locust Control
S. Krall, R. Peveling and D. Ba Diallo (eds)
© 1997 Birkhäuser Verlag Basel/Switzerland

Ecology of *Schistocerca gregaria* (Forskål): observations in West Africa from 1990 to 1994

H. Wilps

GTZ Eschborn, P.O. Box 5180, D-65726 Eschborn, Germany

Summary. In recent decades extensive research has been carried out on the biology and ecology of *Schistocerca gregaria* (Forskål) and its behaviour in the field and laboratory. In this chapter an outline is given of key findings in the field compared to the author's own observations conducted in West Africa in recent years. The results obtained with respect to phase change and polymorphism of *S. gregaria* contradicted laboratory findings. The phase change takes much more time in the field than in the laboratory. Similar differences were also detected regarding the time period necessary to reach sexual maturity. Investigations of the impact of predators on hopper bands indicate that these can eliminate bands of some 100,000 hoppers. It is, therefore, discussed to what extent natural predation should be considered in future locust control.

Résumé. Au cours des dernières décennies, un nombre considérable de travaux de recherche ont été réalisés tant sur le terrain qu'en laboratoire sur la biologie, l'écologie et le comportement de *Schistocerca gregaria* (Forskål). Ce chapitre expose succinctement les résultats des recherches propres menées sur le terrain et les compare aux observations faites ces dernières années en Afrique de l'Ouest. En ce qui concerne la transformation et le polymorphisme phasaires de *S. gregaria*, les résultats obtenus diffèrent des constatations faites en laboratoire. Des divergences ont pu également être relevées au niveau de la période de temps nécessaire pour que le criquet pèlerin atteigne sa maturité sexuelle. Quant aux études portant sur l'influence des prédateurs sur les bandes larvaires, elles semblent indiquer que les prédateurs sont capables d'exterminer des bandes de quelque 100,000 individus. Ce chapitre s'interroge donc sur l'opportunité de prendre en compte les prédateurs dans la mise au point de stratégies de lutte antiacridienne.

Introduction

Of all orthopteran species, *Schistocerca gregaria* (Forskål) has the largest distribution area. This extends from West Africa through the Middle East to South-West Asia. These regions are characterised by seasonal rainfall averaging between 80 and 400 mm annually, which can vary dramatically from year-to-year with annual rainfall being up to 70% above or below the average (Magor 1994). Precipitation can be extremely heterogeneous in frequency and intensity, and can differ regionally as well as locally. This rainfall determines whether there is sufficient growth of vegetation to provide an adequate food supply for *S. gregaria*. Although such vegetation islands can be as big as several square kilometres in size, the overall degree of vegetation coverage in the breeding and recession areas is never more than 10 to 30% after substantial rainfall. In dry years, however, it is well below 10%. This means that *S. gregaria* must not only locate scarce and seasonally variable habitats, but also exploit them optimally.

Adapted utilisation may perhaps be explained by the two-phase theory first proposed by Uvarov (1921) and further developed by Roffey (1982). According to this theory, during dry periods *S. gregaria* occurs primarily or exclusively in the less mobile solitary phase. When environmental conditions change, gregarisation may set in. This process depends on biotic and abiotic factors which are not completely understood. In general, the presence of favourable environmental conditions and an increasing number of locusts can lead to local outbreaks, regional upsurges and, in more favourable conditions, to plagues. In a first approach, this hypothesis can be contrasted to the theory of swarm continuity put forward by Rainey and Betts (1979) who argue that swarms are born from swarms. However, during some periods in the seventies there was no confirmed evidence at all of migrating swarms. Therefore, the hypothesis was based on the assumption that large, but undetected, gregarious populations must be present even during recession periods.

Gregarious *S. gregaria* can migrate up to 3000 or 4000 km according to Rainey (1963) and Pedgley (1981). These migrations are more or less downwind, although a swarm migrating this way generally spreads slower than the mean speed of the wind (Johnson 1969). Even solitary locusts show local migration, and it is suggested that they travel distances of up to 1000 km. These distances are normally covered when solitary locusts follow their seasonal migration (Rao 1942). In contrast to gregarious swarms, however, solitary locusts fly during the night in order to search for more favourable habitats.

The marching behaviour of hopper bands was investigated in various cases and was correlated to the size of the hopper band, biotic and abiotic factors as well as to the different instars (Kennedy 1945; Ellis and Ashall 1957). The daily marching time and the distances covered differed according to temperature and instar and varied between 100 m and 1000 m per day.

In the limited data published so far on reproductive success, Roffey and Popov (1968) determined a multiplication rate of 16. That means that the population they observed increased from 5 million to 80 million in one generation. But in relation to the total egg production of the initial population, they found that 92% of the nymphs died during development, even though there was little evidence of notable parasitisation of eggs or predation on nymphs. Ashall and Ellis (1962) established multiplication rates between 9 and 36 in a two-season investigation. In contrast to Roffey and Popov's findings, the authors found that up to 50% of the eggs were parasitised by larvae of *Stomorhina lunata* (Diptera: Calliphoridae). The same authors as well as Hudleston (1958) reported reductions of up to 100% in hopper bands due to the activity of predators like birds, jackals, rodents, reptiles and arthropods.

The observations presented here reflect the occurrence and behaviour of solitary and gregarious populations with regard to different environmental conditions in West Africa from 1990 to

1994. Furthermore, the importance of predation on hoppers is demonstrated, with particular reference to birds and sphecoid wasps.

Observations in West Africa

During recent years, observations were conducted in the Tamesna desert, the Aïr mountains (Republic of Niger), Boumdeid and Inchiri (Mauritania). Climate and biotope conditions differed particularly with respect to rainfall, vegetation cover and floral composition. In 1990 and 1992, rainfall was below the annual average, while in 1991 and since 1993 the amount was above average (see Tab. 1). Breeding and recession sites in the Tamesna were vegetation islands of up to several square kilometres in size, covered up to 80% with annual plants like *Schouwia thebaica, Aerva javanica, Tribulus terrestris, Citrullus colocyntis* and some grass species. Similar habitats were found in the Aïr mountains, but these were mostly surrounded by sandy and/or stony areas. Around Boumdeid, however, the situation was quite different. The vegetation occurred in scattered spots of several square metres in size, and overall coverage reached only 30 to 50%. The vegetation was composed of *Panicum turgidum, T. terrestris, C. colocyntis* and various annual grasses such as *Aristida* spp. In Inchiri again, the type of vegetation was somewhat similar to the Tamesna. Apart from *S. thebaica* vegetation of several hectares, plots were densely covered (up to 90%) with species such as *Fagonia olivieri, Boerhavia* sp., *C. colocyntis*

Table 1. *S. gregaria* populations 1990–1994

Year	Country	Rainfall [1]	Swarms [2]	Solitary populations [3]		
				Area infested (km^2)	Density: hoppers and adults/ha	Dominant plant species [4]
1990	Niger	less	3 [A]	6.5	2000 [B]	*S. thebaica*
1991	Niger	somewhat less	6 [A]	4	5000 [B]	*S. thebaica* *T. terrestris*
1992	Mauritania	much less	4 [A]	1.5–2	600–1000 [B]	*H. muticus*
1993	Mauritania	double	> 50 [A+B]	0.5	40,000[5] [B]	*F. olivieri*
				0.3	50,000 [B] mostly adults	*H. muticus*
1994	Mauritania	< double	> 10 [A+B]	3–4	60,000 [B]–80,000 [5] [B]	*F. olivieri*
1995	Mauritania	< double	> 10 [A+B]	0.5–1	30,000 [B]	*F. olivieri*

A: Reports from plant protection services. B: Own observations. (1) Data from Agrhymet Niamey and Nouakchott; the average rainfall calculated on the basis of data from 1972 onwards. (2) Swarm sightings reported by nomads are sometimes difficult to verify, since no geographical data are provided; therefore, double counting cannot be excluded. (3) Nymphs and adults. (4) Species covering more than 60% of the total vegetation cited. (5) These populations contained up to 80% transiens hoppers.

Table 2. Polymorphism of *S. gregaria* in field cages

Year	Locusts/cage (size: 2×2×2 m)		Observation time	Shift of
	gregarious	solitary	(days)	phase
1990	-	3000–5000 adults	90	no
1990	50 adults	2000 adults	40	no
1991	200 hoppers instar 2–4	200 hoppers instar 1–4	15	no
1993	4000–6000 hoppers instar 2 and 3	30 hoppers instar 2 and 3	25	no
1993	-	1000 [A] adults	60	no
1994	-	1000–2000 [B] instar 2–6	25	no

A: Two cages, each containing 2000 to 3000 gregarious adults, were placed next to this cage (distance 80 cm). B: Two cages, each containing about 3000 gregarious hoppers of the same instar, were placed to the right and left of this cage. Phase was determined according to the following criteria: (1) Adults: coloration and social behaviour; during the whole observation time solitary locusts did not change their light brown colour, except with increasing age, when the back side of males became light yellow. When basking in the morning, gregarious adults aggregated on the ground, whereas solitary locusts were spread over the whole cage. (2) Nymphs: Coloration, eye stripes and colour; 6th instar aggregation behaviour as described for adults. Solitary hoppers always underwent a sixth moult and had six eye stripes. The body colour varied between green and light brown with more or less distinct black spots (transiens phase).

and scattered *T. terrestris*. North and north-west of Akjoujt, in a seasonally inundated zone of approximately 300 ha, dense *Hyoscyamus muticus* vegetation (up to 90% cover) hosted a permanent population of solitary desert locusts.

In various laboratory trials, phase modification of *S. gregaria* could be triggered by changing the social environment (reared in crowds or in isolation). A shift to the gregarious phase took

Table 3. Polymorphism of *S. gregaria* in the field

Year	Solitary population			Gregarious population		
	Area	Density	Instar	No. of hoppers	Instar	Behaviour
1993	4 ha	20–80/m²	Nymphs and adults	≈120,000	4th–5th	stayed until adult moult
1993	0.5 ha	60–120/m²	Nymphs and adults	≈70,000	5th	stayed
1993	0.1 ha	90–150/m²	Nymphs	30,000–40,000	4th	dispersed as 5th instar
1994	120 ha	3–10/m²	Nymphs and adults	8–10 bands [A]	1st–5th	stayed until adult moult

A: The assessment of the number of hoppers per band proved difficult, because bands mixed up or separated several times during the observation period of 16 days; fledglings dispersed 8–10 days after the adult moult (beginning of December). The solitary population dispersed by mid-January 1995. Similar observations were made in 1993. Eight to 10 days after the adult moult gregarious locusts left the area, while solitary populations stayed until the vegetation started to dry out (mid to end of January).

Table 4. Winter breeding of gregarious and solitary *S. gregaria*

| Month | period | Solitary adults | | | | | | Gregarious adults | | | | | |
| | | Field | | | Field cages | | | Field | | | Field cages | | |
		m	ov	ha	m	ov	ha	m	ov	ha	m	ov	ha
Nov.	1–15	+	+	+	+	+	+	+	+	+	+	+	+
	16–30	+	+	+	+	+	+	n.o.	n.o.	n.o.	+	–	–
Dec.	1–15	+	+	+	+	+	+	n.o.	n.o.	n.o.	+	–	–
	16–31	+	+	+	+	+	+	–	–	–	–	–	–
Jan.	1–15	+	+	+	+	+	+	–	–	–	–	–	–
	16–31	+	+	+	+	+	+	–	–	–	–	–	–
Feb.	1–15	+	n.o.	+	+	+	+	–	–	–	–	–	–
	16–28	+	n.o.	n.o.	+	+	+	–	–	–	–	–	–

+ = yes; – = no; n.o. = not observed; m = sexually mature; ov = oviposition; ha = hatching

Observations were made in Akjoujt from 1993–1995. Starting from mid-November, daily temperatures dropped from 35–25 °C; at night, temperatures ranged from 10–16 °C. Although daily temperatures were > 30 °C, sexual maturity could neither be observed in locusts captured in the field nor reared in cages. This is attributed to the fact that temperatures exceeded 30 °C for 3–5 h only. However, when the same locusts were transferred to laboratory cages maintained at 28–30 °C for 12–14 h daily, they reached maturity within 3–5 days. It should be mentioned that these locusts had already completed their somatic growth.

place very rapidly in nymphs (Ellis 1953, 1963). It has been suggested that airborne chemical factors (pheromones) affect aggregation behaviour (Gillet 1968, 1988). Preliminary investigations under semi-field conditions contradicted these results. Gregarisation was neither induced when solitary adults were maintained at high density nor when solitary nymphs were maintained together with or in close proximity to gregarious hoppers (Tab. 2). These observations were confirmed in the field, where solitary and gregarious hoppers occupied the same area, with no indications of phase shift during the monitoring period (Tab. 3).

In laboratory investigations, female *S. gregaria* fledglings reached maturity under optimal breeding conditions within 6 to 8 days after the adult moult (Muschenich, unpublished data). This does not conform with field and semi-field observations as summarised in Table 4. Breeding of solitary locusts continued throughout the winter, while gregarious adults did not become sexually mature at lower temperatures, and breeding ceased by the middle of December. It should be noted that field-caged locusts were provided the same food, consisting of older *S. thebaica, H. muticus* and *Boerhavia* sp. leaves. Therefore, both groups must have received the same amount of the plant growth hormone giberellin A3, which is considered to stimulate the maturation of *S. gregaria* (Ellis et al. 1965). This was not true for free-living hoppers, whose diet varied depending on the local vegetation. Surprisingly, when males which had matured

Table 5. Predation on hopper bands by birds

Year	Initial hopper band size	Instar	Bird species	Time of attack (days)	Hoppers left
1993	130,000 [A]	4th	*Cursoris cursor*	6	<1000
1994	180,000 [A]	4th	various	4	<5000
1995	190,000 [A]	2nd	various	10	<500
1995	250,000	2nd	various	11	<5000
1995	1,100,000 [A]	2nd–3rd	various	9	<50,000
1995	500,000 [A]	4th	various	10	<5000

Various: *Passer luteus, Lanius* sp. and others

A: Hoppers had been treated with sub-lethal dosages of neem oil (content of active ingredient <300 ppm/l) 3 to 5 days before the end of observations. The mortality rate caused by neem oil was <40% (cage control), but hopper mobility was reduced; i.e., the distances covered daily decreased from nearly 1000 m to less than 250 m.

indoor at higher temperatures were returned to field cages, they immediately copulated with sexually immature females.

The movement of hopper bands and the distances covered daily depend on the instar, the kind, density and distribution of vegetation, and on climatic factors. The average distance covered daily was below 300 m in dense and homogeneously distributed vegetation composed of, for example, *S. thebaica* or *F. olivieri*. In contrast, hopper bands in sandy areas with isolated vegetation walked up to 2000 m per day. In this case, they had to cross plain sandy areas and were more heavily pursued by predators like birds, lizards, wind scorpions (Solifugae) and wasps. The impact of bird predation on hoppers is summarised in Table 5. Birds are particularly important as a natural control factor, and hoppers were sometimes reduced to 1% of the initial population. However, no details can be given as to what extent other predators like scorpions, beetles and ant lions had contributed to the overall reduction. It is possible that their impact was just as important.

The consumption rate of the desert sparrow, *Passer simplex saharae*, a common predator of all instars of desert locust in the Inchiri region of Mauritania, was estimated in a simple experimental design. Third and fourth instar nymphs were maintained in a field cage ($2 \times 2 \times 2$ m) which had small holes at the bottom. The holes were big enough for hoppers to escape, but too small for birds to enter. This controlled release of hoppers allowed quantification of the number killed by desert sparrows (Tab. 6).

Among insects, a sphecoid wasp, as yet unidentified, was a particularly effective predator of hoppers. Several hundred wasps followed hopper bands, paralysed and buried their prey in holes in burrows which were grouped in so-called wasps fields up to 100 m² in size (Tab. 7). Predation continued until hoppers moulted into third instars and decreased thereafter.

Table 6. Consumption of hoppers by *Passer simplex saharae*

Trial	Time (min)	No. of birds	No. of hoppers killed	Hoppers/bird
1	30	4	63	15.8
2	30	4	49	12.3
3	30	5	61	12.2
4	30	4	55	13.8
5	30	4	48	12.0
6	30	5	51	10.2

The trials were conducted on two days between 9.00 and 12.00 a.m. Temperatures ranged from 23 °C to 27 °C. Most hoppers (nearly two-thirds) were consumed immediately. Others were killed, left on the ground and consumed within 3 h after the end of the trial.

Table 7. Predation on hoppers by sphecoid wasps

Field no.	Estimated number of hoppers per band (m²)	Size of wasp field per m²	Mean no. of burrows	Total no. of burrows (n = 6)	Mean no. of hoppers/burrow
1	80 000–150 000	36	40	1440	
2	80 000–150 000	33.8	52.7	1778	11.3
3	>300 000	108	52.3	5652	13.1
4	10 000–15 000	10.5	28	294	
5	80 000–150 000	72	50	3600	
6	>500 000	107.3	55.3	5931	10.6
7	600 000–700 000	112.5	49	5513	

The number of burrows is the average of three quadrate counts (1 m²) in each wasp field associated with hopper bands 1 to 7. On the average, each burrow contained 11 paralysed hoppers (n = 50). Assuming that predation continued for 10 to 12 days, all hopper bands would have been reduced to <20% of their original size.

Discussion and conclusions

In 1993, numerous swarms invaded Mauritania (FAO 1994) and started breeding. Following intensive rainfall, favourable vegetation conditions developed, and locust upsurges were reported from all over the country. Despite heavy rainfall in the following two years, no further increase in population density was noted except for scattered local outbreaks. This was more than astonishing, because additional winter breeding was reported from northern Mauritania. This suggests that upsurges do not necessarily develop into plagues even under favourable conditions. However, an increase in solitary/transiens populations was observed. Whether these will increase further and create new upsurges will be answered in the near future.

A phase change between two or three instars or even one hopper generation could not be confirmed. This holds true for dense populations in the field, crowded rearing conditions in field cages and even when gregarious and solitary populations were mixed up. These findings contrast sharply with laboratory results and indicate that phase change in the field requires more time and that there are possibly additional factors which influence polymorphism of *S. gregaria*.

Solitary and gregarious females require a different temperature regime to become sexually mature. For gregarious locusts the temperature must not only exceed a certain threshold, it also has to be maintained above this threshold for a certain period of time. In Mauritania, therefore, swarms which undergo the adult moult in the beginning of December are unlikely to start breeding before the end of February. Moreover, it is not known to what extent adults which are three months old are able to reproduce successfully, where breeding takes place and which temperature regime is necessary.

The observations of and experiments with predators demonstrate that they can heavily decimate or even totally eliminate bands of up to some 100,000 hoppers, which is in line with former findings (Ashall and Ellis 1962; Kooyman and Godonou 1994). In the case of plagues, the importance of predators is doubtful and requires further investigations, especially when predator populations increase in response to growing desert locust populations.

Even if preventive locust control is recognized as a useful and necessary control strategy, the following questions arise: In general, is it worthwhile to combat locusts wherever and whenever they are found, for example, when sexually immature small swarms occur in the beginning of December with low temperatures and an advancing dryness? Should bands of up to 100,000 hoppers scattered over large areas be treated with toxic chemicals? Would it not make more sense to leave them simply to predators, perhaps immobilising them using neem oil (cf. Diop and Wilps, this volume). Or, if the mortality rates of 92% observed by Roffey and Popov (1968) are right, is it worthwhile to combat bands of fewer than 100,000 hoppers? In this case only 8000 insects will survive anyway. These questions raise even more questions: What will these surviving adults do? Will they form swarms by joining other small groups of fledglings or will they disperse and return to solitary populations? In conclusion, despite all the research done so far, we are faced with a substantial lack of knowledge about the biology, ecology and behaviour of *S. gregaria* in the field, which is a prerequisite for the development of economically viable and environmentally friendly control strategies.

References

Ashall C, Ellis PE (1962) Studies on numbers and mortality in field populations of the desert locust, *S. gregaria* Forsk. Anti-Locust Bull 38: 1–59

Ellis PE (1953) Social aggregation and gregarious behaviour in hoppers of *Locusta migratoria migratorioides* (R. et F.). Behaviour 5: 225–260

Ellis PE, Ashall C (1957) Field studies on diurnal behaviour movements and aggregation in the desert locust, *S. gregaria* Forsk. Anti-Locust Bull 25: 1–94

Ellis PE (1963) Changes in the social aggregation of locust hoppers with changes in rearing conditions. Ann Behav 11, 152–160

Ellis PE, Carlisle DB, Osborne DJ (1965) Desert locusts: sexual maturation delayed by feeding on senescent vegetation. Science 149: 546–547

FAO (1994) The desert locust situation to date. Meeting of donor countries and institutions and affected countries on the desert locust emergency 1993–94, 1–3

Gillett SD (1968) Airborne factors affecting the grouping behaviour of locusts. Nature 218: 782–783

Gillett SD (1988) Solitarisation in the desert locust *Schistocerca gregaria* (Forsk.) (Orthoptera: Acrididae) Bull Ent Res 78: 623–631

Hudleston JA (1958) Some notes on the effects of bird predators on hopper bands of the desert locust (*Schistocerca gregaria* Forskål). Ent Mon Mag 94: 210–214

Johnson CG (1969) Migration and dispersal of insects by flight. Bungay Guffolk: Richard Clay Ltd., 550–573

Kennedy JS (1945) Observations on the mass migration of desert locust hoppers. Trans R Ent Soc Lond 95: 247–262

Kooyman C, Godonou I (1994) Infection of *Schistocerca gregaria* (Orthoptera, Acrididae) hopper by *Metarhizium flavoviride* (Deuteromycotina, Hyphomycetes) conidia in an oil formulation applied under desert conditions. Bulletin of Entomological Research; in press

Magor JI (1994) Desert locust population dynamics. In: van Huis A (ed) Desert locust control with existing techniques. Proceedings of the seminar held in Wageningen, The Netherlands 6–11 December 1993, Wageningen Agricultural University, 31–54

Pedgley DE (ed) (1981) Desert locust forecasting manual. Vol. 1. London: HMSO, 268 pp

Popov GB (1954) Notes on the behaviour of swarms of the desert locust (*Schistocerca gregaria* Forskål) during oviposition in Iran. Trans R Ent Soc Lond 195: 65–77

Rainey RC (1963) Meteorology and the migration of desert locusts: applications of synoptic meteorology in locust control. Anti-Locust Memoir no 7. Also as WMO Technical Notes 54: same as WMO no 138, TP 64

Rainey RC, Betts E (1979) Problems of alternative hypotheses. Continuity in major populations of migrant pests: the desert locusts and the African army worm. Phil Trans R Soc Lond B 287: 359–374

Rao YR (1942) Some results on studies of the desert locust (*Schistocerca gregaria* Forskål) in India. Bull Entomol Res 33: 241–265

Roffey J (1982) The desert locu st upsurge and its termination 1977–79. In: Field Research Stations – Technical Series. FAO Report no AGP/DL/TS/23, iii–iv + 1–74

Roffey J, Popov GB (1968) Environmental and behavioural processes in a desert locust outbreak. Nature 219: 446–450

Uvarov BP (1921) A revision of the genus *Locusta* L. (= *Pachytylus* Fieb.), with a new theory as to the periodicity and migrations of locusts. Bull Entomol Res 12: 135–163

Forecasting and modelling

New Strategies in Locust Control
S. Krall, R. Peveling and D. Ba Diallo (eds)
© 1997 Birkhäuser Verlag Basel/Switzerland

Desert locust forecasters' GIS: a researchers' view

J.I. Magor and J. Pender

Natural Resources Institute, Central Avenue, Chatham Maritime, Chatham, Kent ME4 4TB, UK

Summary. The geographic information system (GIS) SWARMS (*Schistocerca* WARning Management System) offers researchers and decision makers improved facilities for studying population dynamics and for displaying and testing alternative control strategies. A brief description is given of the information collected and archived by locust organisations and the subset of detailed and summarised data transferred to SWARMS. Detailed locust weather and habitat data will be stored by the date and site of observation and will be input from 1996 when the system becomes operational. Data for 1985–1989 plague will be added and researchers may enter data for other periods from archived maps and reports. The 'read only' historical dataset is currently for 1930 to 1984 and has a spatial resolution of 1° latitude by 1° longitude and a temporal resolution of one month. This is suitable for risk analyses but not for migration studies. The latter require daily data at a finer spatial resolution to be found in the detailed dataset.

Résumé. Le SIG SWARMS (*Schistocerca* WARning Management System) fournit aux chercheurs et décideurs des moyens améliorés pour l'étude de la dynamique des populations de Criquet pèlerin, la visualisation et la mise à l'essai de stratégies de lutte. Cette étude décrit succinctement les types d'informations recueillies et archivées par les organizations de lutte contre le Criquet pèlerin, ainsi que les données détaillées et résumées transmises vers SWARMS. Des données détaillées sur les conditions climatiques favorables au Criquet pèlerin et sur son habitat seront mémorisées d'après la date et le lieu d'observation et seront entrées à partir de 1996 lorsque le système sera opérationnel. Les informations recueillies concernant les infestations de 1985–1989 seront ajoutées au système de traitement et les chercheurs pourront entrer des données sur d'autres périodes à partir d'archives de cartes et de rapports. Les ensembles de données historiques 'read only' (à lecture seulement) concernent actuellement les années 1930 à 1984 et ont une résolution spatiale de 1° de latitude sur 1° de longitude et une résolution temporelle de un mois. Ces données se prêtent certes à l'analyse des risques, mais pas à l'étude des migrations qui requiert la saisie quotidienne de données avec une résolution spatiale plus fine et que l'on trouvera dans les ensembles de données détaillées.

Introduction

The desert locust early warning system described by Pedgley (1981) was made possible by cartographic analysis of systematically collected locust information (Uvarov 1951). The lack of serious damage in recent plagues has called into doubt major expenditure (approaching $US 400 million in 1986–94) on large-scale pesticide campaigns to control the desert locust and concurrent grasshopper outbreaks. Three studies (The US Congress, Office of Technology Assessment 1990; van Huis 1994; Joffe 1995) advocated a need to reexamine control strategies, to develop tactics using environmentally safer pesticides, to assess the risk of attack and to establish the economic impact of desert locusts.

This paper suggests that a geographic information system (GIS) SWARMS (*Schistocerca* WARning Management System) can help researchers and decision makers study population dynamics and test alternative control strategies on a regional and interregional scale. It describes the information collected and archived by locust organisations and the subset already in SWARMS. Finally, it discusses data required for risk analysis, population and migration studies.

Desert locust archives

Reports from all affected countries were mapped, analysed and archived, initially (1930–1978) at the Anti-Locust Research Centre (now the Natural Resources Institute (NRI)) and subsequently at the Food and Agriculture Organisation of the United Nations, Rome (FAO). Earlier data are less complete, except in India and Algeria where reliable records of invasions exist from the 1860s (Waloff 1976). NRI archived maps at three scales. Large-scale maps (1:500,000 to 1:5 million) show the location and date of all reported desert locust infestations for each month from 1926 to 1973 and in Africa and Arabia from 1985 to 1989. From 1974, information was plotted on 1:5 million wall charts which were not archived. Each month's data (1926–1978) were condensed onto medium-scale maps (1:11 million to 1:12 million) to show the full range of locust stages and observation dates on a single sheet. Small-scale maps (1:45 million) of the most important locust population in a degree square (1° latitude × 1° longitude) have accompanied desert locust Bulletins since 1958. They proved useful for reviewing developments and identifying analogous locust events, and a series of monthly maps (1942–1987) was prepared.

SWARMS GIS and its datasets

At FAO, SWARMS runs on a SUN SPARC 10 workstation and uses the GIS software ARC/INFO and the relational database management system INGRES. The user interface and user-specified tasks were developed using ARC MACRO language. Programs in this language will not run on a PC, but datasets can be exported in ARC/INFO format and transferred to PC-based GIS. ARCEDIT is used to input and edit data, ARCPLOT to query and display data, and GRID executes and displays the results of arithmetic and spatial operations on gridded data subsets. GRID cells may be degree squares or other user-defined units. GRID results are stored as map covers and are retrieved and displayed with details of the query which generated them.

SWARMS is linked to two models. The development period model (Reus and Symmons 1992) was programmed into the system, and an interface exists for importing trajectory datasets from a migration model developed for FAO by Meteo Consult. Interfaces are planned to capture and display rainfall and vegetation imagery and to display population model outputs. Machine readable datasets were acquired to replace topographical maps, gazetteers, thematic maps, weather charts and climate statistics used in the previous manual system.

SWARMS was designed to contain both the detailed and summarised datasets used by desert locust forecasters. Detailed locust, weather and habitat data are stored by date and site of observation. Inferred events are tagged and stored with reported events making inferences easily available during analyses. NRI will enter data used in an analysis of the 1985–1989 plague. FAO will input reports into this detailed dataset from 1996, when the system becomes operational. No firm plans exist for entering the intervening 1990–1995 dataset, which consists of reports and Bulletin maps archived at FAO, or the pre-1985 data archived at FAO and NRI. The database design allows researchers to enter these data and any supplementary information held in affected country archives.

SWARMS also contains "read only" historical locust data to replace the archived small-scale maps. This dataset summarises monthly data for each degree square and currently covers the period 1930 to 1984. The period up to 1978 was extracted from large-scale maps (1930, 1931), and from medium-scale maps (1932–1978). This part of the dataset records which of 15 population categories were present and if they were recorded 1–4 or 5 or more times. The 15 categories, also used on current FAO Bulletin maps, are a matrix of three phase types (swarming, groups and low or unspecified density) and five life stages (hoppers, immature, mature or maturing, laying adults or eggs and adults of unknown maturity). For 1979–1984, only small-scale maps were archived. These recorded the most gregarious of the 15 types present. Hoppers and adults were both shown if they were in the same phase and adults were selected in the order laying < mature < immature unless immature adults indicated a new generation.

The GIS functions of SWARMS will provide researchers with an improved working environment, since spatial data from different sources can be displayed over a range of background maps, including remote sensing products of habitat quality. Queries can be made on reported and inferred events so that researchers can examine the relation between weather events and locust distribution and the time lapse between them. Researchers considering intervention strategies can display monthly distribution maps in quick succession to produce an animation-like effect of successive developments. The system can produce frequency-of-incidence maps for different periods quickly and easily.

Quality of source material

Spatial and temporal gaps exist in locust data because they were collected by mobile teams who could sample only part of the infested area. Even large swarming populations sometimes remained undetected. In addition, relevant information was sometimes either not recorded or transmitted and few survey notebooks have survived. Transcripts of radio messages from field teams provide the most complete set of data regularly archived. They are stored at national head-quarters, and their content varies according to local procedures. Reports archived at NRI and FAO were summarised from the radio messages. Common omissions from internationally exchanged reports were the latitude and longitude of observation sites, precise dates of observa-tion and details of life stages. Errors, such as transposing letters and numbers, could usually be corrected during mapping, but substituting the date of a radio message for the date of observa-tion could not.

For many studies, errors and lack of precision in reporting observations may be unimportant. Rainey (1963, 1989) concluded that archived data were valuable for year-to-year or season-to-season studies but were usually too incomplete to reveal day-to-day changes. The full range of dates for each life stage is also needed to estimate missing laying and fledging dates for popula-tion studies. An accurate observation date is also essential for estimating migration trajectories, since the winds used to model downwind displacement vary between days.

The geographical extent of populations often cannot be estimated from archived material. First, it is seldom clear if reports refer to the gross infested area, to particularly heavily infested parts of the gross area or to the net infested area. These distinctions are significant, since even during a heavy invasion swarms may infest as little as 1% of the gross infested area (Rainey 1963) and hopper bands 1–5% of the band zones which together form the gross infested area (Roffey 1965). Secondly, although quantitative and qualitative hopper band and swarm sizes can be obtained from reports, they are difficult to interpret. No correlation exists between the number of reports and the number of swarms present (Rainey 1963; Venkatesh et al. 1982). Swarm sizes, unless estimated by aircraft or radar, may be unreliable (Roffey 1965). In addition, FAO recently changed the number of qualitative categories used to report hopper band and swarm sizes, from three (Pedgley 1981) to five (FAO 1994).

Three facts suggest that researchers undertaking detailed studies of early plague upsurges will find early records sparse and may need to remap non-swarming locust population reports. First, regular surveys for non-swarming populations did not exist before the late 1950s. Secondly, symbols before 1956 did not enable "grouped" locusts to be mapped. Thirdly, reports often provide areal densities or transect counts rather than stating if locusts are scattered or grouping, and conventions for converting these counts and densities for mapping have changed.

Discussion

Despite imperfections, desert locust records are among the most complete which exist for an insect pest. Changes in data collection and map conventions were outlined here. They will be described more fully in SWARMS manuals to help users to interpret computer-generated results correctly. Case studies of locust events such as those included in the *Desert Locust Forecasting Manual* (Pedgley 1981) will require researchers to use the detailed dataset and sometimes to supplement it with daily records from affected country archives. The inclusion in SWARMS of a representative 60-year gridded dataset of infestations and of climate records for the whole invasion area offers researchers many opportunities for further studies, such as locust response to climate variability.

The 60-year historical dataset has the same spatial and temporal resolution as the degree square frequency maps (Steedman 1990). These were used as indicators of risk to develop control policy (Waloff 1960) and, with additional information on cropping systems, to assess the potential economic impact of desert locusts (Bullen 1969; Herok and Krall 1995). Researchers may wish to use the gridded historical dataset to reexamine these issues.

To date, frequencies based on data from 1939 to 1963 have been used to represent risk during plagues and those based on data from 1964 to 1985 omitting 1968, to indicate risk during recessions. However, both were derived from populations against which concerted and increasingly effective control campaigns were being mounted. The two sets of maps were also based on different criteria. The former counted cells containing bands and swarms, whilst the latter counted any sighting of desert locusts and omitted 1968, a plague year. SWARMS makes it feasible to reexamine risk. Frequencies can be easily and quickly calculated for differing periods, and previously omitted data can be included. Calculations might also include inferred events to offset control and unreported events. Frequency of infestation, also exist for countries and user-defined territories (Lean 1960; Waloff and Connors 1964; Waloff 1976). Frontiers between territories pass through some cells. Consequently, users will require rules for assigning values in cells shared by two or more territories when reassessing these frequencies.

The climate records examined in conjunction with the historical dataset during recessions, upsurges and plagues supplemented by selected examples of detailed data may shed new light on whether the relatively plague free period since the 1960s was caused by improved control, drier weather or a combination of the two.

Acknowledgements
SWARMS was developed for FAO by NRI and Edinburgh University within the United Nations Development
Programme (UNDP): Development of Environmentally Acceptable Alternative Strategies for Desert Locust
Control.

References

Bullen (1969) The distribution of the damage potential of the desert locust (*Schistocerca gregaria*
 Forsk). Anti-Locust Mem no 10. London: Anti-Locust Research Centre, 44 pp
FAO (1994) Desert locust guidelines 2. Survey. Rome: Food and Agriculture Organization, 49 pp
Herok C, Krall S (1995) Economics of desert locust control. Rossdorf: TZ-Verl-Ges, 70 pp
Joffe S (1995) Desert locust management: a time for change. World Bank Discussion Paper no 284.
 Washington DC: World Bank, 58 pp
Lean OB (1960) Annual and monthly frequencies of desert locust infestations. FAO Plant Prot Bull
 8(7): 82–85
Pedgley DE (ed) (1981) Desert locust forecasting manual. Vol 1 text, vol 2 maps. London: Centre for
 Overseas Pest Research, 268 and 142 pp
Rainey RC (1963) Meteorology and the migration of desert locusts. Applications of synoptic meteoro-
 logy in desert locust control. Anti-Locust Mem no 7. London: Anti-Locust Research Centre, 115 pp
Rainey RC (1989) Migration and meteorology: flight behaviour and the atmospheric environment of
 locusts and other migrant pests. Oxford: Clarendon Press, 314 pp
Reus JAWA, Symmons PM (1992) A model to predict the incubation and nymphal development peri-
 ods of the desert locust, *Schistocerca gregaria* (Orthoptera: Acrididae). Bull Ent Res 82: 517–520
Roffey J (1965) Nature and scale of the desert locust problem and survey costs. Pages 173–205 and
 General references. Pages 284–285 in Final report of the Operational Research Team of the United
 Nations Special Fund Desert Locust Project. Vol 1. Rome: Food and Agriculture Organization
Steedman A (ed) (1990) Locust Handbook. 3rd ed. Chatham: Natural Resources Institute, 204 pp
US Congress Office of Technology Assessment (1990) A plague of locusts. US Congress, Office of
 Technology Assessment Special Report, OTA-F-450. Washington DC: US Government Printing
 Office, 129 pp
Uvarov BP (1951) Locust research and control 1929–1950. Colonial Res Publ no 10. London: His
 Majesty's Stationery Office, 67 pp
van Huis A (ed) (1994) Desert locust control with existing techniques: an evaluation of strategies.
 Wageningen The Netherlands: Wageningen Agricultural University, 132 pp
Venkatesh MV, Chaudan A, Srinivas MV, Chandra R (1982) Some aspects of the desert locust swarm
 infestation in the year 1962 – the terminal year of the last plague in India. Plant Prot Bull (India)
 34(34): 27–29
Waloff Z (1960) The fluctuating distributions of the desert locust in relation to the strategy of control.
 Pages 132–140 in Report of the Seventh Commonwealth Entomological Congress, London, July
 1960. London: Commonwealth Institute of Entomology
Waloff Z (1976) Some temporal characteristics of desert locust plagues. With a statistical analysis by
 SM Green. Anti-Locust Mem no 13. London: Centre for Overseas Pest Research, 36 pp
Waloff Z and Connors JM (1964) The frequencies of infestations by the desert locust in different terri-
 tories. FAO Plant Prot Bull 12(5): 3–11

New Strategies in Locust Control
S. Krall, R. Peveling and D. Ba Diallo (eds)
© 1997 Birkhäuser Verlag Basel/Switzerland

SWARMS: A geographic information system for desert locust forecasting

K. Cressman

Food and Agriculture Organisation of the United Nations, AGP Division, Rome 00100, Italy

Summary. The Food and Agriculture Organisation of the United Nations operates a centralised Desert Locust Information Service. Similar to most early warning systems, it relies on accurate information received in a timely manner, in this case, from countries affected by locusts, regional centres and meteorological services. Until recently, this information was managed manually at FAO Headquarters. However, this has changed with the introduction of a computer-based geographic information system. This system operates on a UNIX workstation and uses ARC/INFO and INGRES software. It is connected to a satellite receiving station and to the Internet. The system will allow forecasters to manage locust and environmental data better, and it may encourage more precise data collection in the field. As locust forecasters become more proficient in the use of SWARMS, as field data improve and as remote sensing imagery become validated, FAO should be able to provide more accurate forecasts and early warnings to affected countries. FAO should also be able to provide better advice to the international donor community, which in turn could contribute to improved planning and decision making.

Résumé. L'Organization des Nations-Unies pour l'Alimentation et l'Agriculture, la FAO, a mis en place un service d'information sur le Criquet pèlerin. Comme pour la plupart des systèmes d'alerte précoce, son efficience dépend de l'exactitude des informations qui lui parviennent et de leur réception en temps opportun. Celles-ci lui sont transmises par les services nationaux des pays concernés par ce locuste, par des services régionaux et météorologiques. Encore récemment, ces informations étaient gérées manuellement au siège de la FAO. Aujourd'hui, l'organization dispose d'un système d'information géographique. Ce système fonctionne sur une station de travail UNIX et utilise les logiciels ARC/INFO et INGRES. Il est relié à une station de réception satellite et à Internet. Il permettra aux services prévisions de mieux gérer les informations sur les criquets et l'environnement et devrait inciter les observateurs sur le terrain à fournir des renseignements plus précis. Lorsque les services prévisions auront acquis une bonne maîtrise de l'emploi de SWARMS, que la qualité des informations recueillies sur le terrain se sera améliorée et que les données de télédétection pourront être validées, la FAO devrait être en mesure de fournir aux pays concernés des bulletins de prévision et d'alerte précoce plus précis. Elle sera alors également mieux à même de conseiller la communauté des bailleurs de fonds internationaux –, ce qui devrait se traduire par une amélioration au niveau de la planification des mesures et de la prise de décisions.

Introduction

Information used as early warning for outbreaks and plagues of the desert locust (*Schistocerca gregaria*, Forskål) varies in source, format and quality. National Locust Units (NLUs) collect data on locust infestations, vegetation and rainfall by undertaking ground surveys in desert and semi-desert areas. These surveys generally last from one day to several weeks. They involve interviewing local residents and checking areas of green vegetation and other places where locusts have been seen in the past. Survey results are radioed, posted or hand-carried to the headquarters of the NLU, where they are collated and reviewed. A copy of this data or a summary is transmitted to FAO Headquarters.

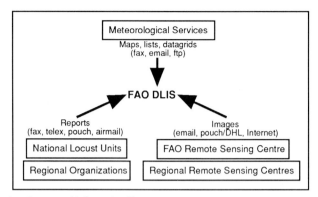

Figure 1. Locust and environmental information flow.

A centralised system of reports, mapping and analysis of data on the changing distribution of the desert locust was first set up in 1929 at the Anti-Locust Research Centre in London (Uvarov 1951). By 1979, FAO had assumed this responsibility and since then, the organisation has operated a centralised Desert Locust Information Service (DLIS) in Rome. A centralised system offers the following advantages: (1) a worldwide view of the desert locust and weather situation over the entire invasion area, (2) access to environmental information not easily available at the national or regional level, (3) an objective interpretation of the data, (4) the ability to provide affected countries with information and forecasts that countries themselves would not produce or otherwise obtain, and (5) a reliable telecommunications system that can transmit information directly by electronic mail, facsimile, telex and through the Internet.

FAO receives locust and environmental data from national, regional and international organisations by facsimile, telex, electronic mail, the Internet, pouch and airmail (Fig. 1). Environmental data consist of daily synoptic charts and rainfall totals received by facsimile from several meteorological organisations, and PC-based remote sensing imagery from various regional centres and the FAO Africa Real Time Environmental Monitoring Information System (ARTEMIS). These products indicate possible areas of rainfall and green vegetation.

Locust forecasters at FAO plot locust reports on maps of various scales to compare with current environmental data in order to estimate the scale and distribution of current locust infestations. These reports are compared with historical locust frequencies and long-term rainfall averages to determine if they represent unusual events for that particular time of year. Previous breeding, rainfall, prevailing winds and recent atmospheric disturbances are examined to try to understand how the current situation came about. Historical locust data and case studies are reviewed to find instances in the past that are similar to the current situation. From this information, forecasters attempt to estimate the scale, distribution and timing of locust breeding and the scale, direction and timing of locust migration in the future. A monthly bulletin is prepared summarising the current locust situation, ecological conditions and the forecasted breeding and movements for the next six weeks. This bulletin is distributed to countries affected by locusts, donors and other international organisations by facsimile and electronic mail usually within one day.

Until recently the majority of the work within the DLIS was done manually. Computer equipment was used primarily for viewing remote sensing products and producing the monthly bulletin. With the explosion in the use of electronic mail, the Internet and mobile satellite communications equipment, more data is being transferred electronically. This allows easier access and the possibility of processing and storing data electronically. In the last few years, geographic information systems have been developed to cope with the increase in the availability of data in electronic format and its management. These new technologies are being introduced in the DLIS at FAO.

Geographic information systems

The 1986–89 desert locust plague prompted research to improve monitoring and forecasting, and to review control strategies for the desert locust. The FAO Scientific Advisory Committee identified geographic information systems (GIS) as the most appropriate technology to aid locust forecasters and researchers achieve these objectives. It was hoped that GIS would improve their ability to access and interpret current and historical data on locusts and the environment (FAO 1989; Healey et al., 1996).

A GIS is a computer-based program consisting of software tools that operate on a database (Fig. 2a). It is more than simply a computer program for making maps; it is a powerful tool for

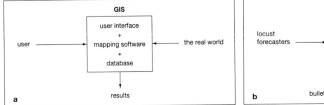
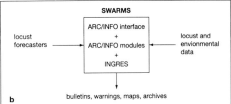

Figure 2. (a) Components of a typical GIS (after ESRI 1992); (b) components of SWARMS.

data interpretation. Data can be entered and displayed geographically, as is possible with many other computer programs. The difference, however, lies in the fact that GIS allows the user to interrogate databases by latitude and longitude, continually refine the desired data and perform spatial operations on them (ESRI 1992).

SWARMS

The University of Edinburgh in collaboration with the Natural Resources Institute (NRI UK) and FAO developed a geographic information system for the administration, mapping and analysis of locust and environmental data for operational forecasting within the DLIS at FAO. The system, known as SWARMS (*Schistocerca* WARning Management System), was developed over a three-year period with funding from the United Nations Development Programme.

SWARMS operates on a UNIX-based SUN workstation. The workstation is located within the DLIS at FAO Headquarters. It consists of two terminals and a colour printer. This system was chosen because the quantity, diversity and complexity of the data used for forecasting requires a computer with a considerable amount of processing power and speed, full-function relational databases and large quantities of disk storage. SWARMS uses ARC/INFO software in which the user interface has been extensively customized (Fig. 2b). INGRES software is used for database purposes. The system is connected to a Meteosat receiving station, to the FAO network and to the Internet (Fig. 3). SWARMS cannot operate on a personal computer.

SWARMS consists of three modules that manage locust and environmental data received from countries affected by locusts and various organisations. ARCEDIT, the first module, allows rapid and accurate input of locust and weather data (Fig. 4). Data can also be refined and corrected. The second module, ARCPLOT, allows for general database browsing and map production, including remote sensing images and weather data received by electronic mail and through the Internet (Fig. 5). The last module, GRID, provides Boolean functions for interpre

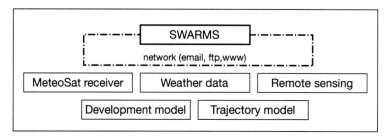

Figure 3. Schematic of SWARMS connectivity.

Time Period

	Day	Month	Year	Hr	Min	Exact period
From:	12	12	1994			✓
To:	13	4	1994			

Month part: | n/a | early | mid | late | 1st fortnight | 2nd fortnight |

Locusts

Confirmation: | confirmed | species query | unconfirmed |

Locusts present: | y | n |

Control?: | y | n | unknown | Breeding: | y | n | unknown |

Comment: ▲

Adults

Present: | y | n | No./ha (<25) (25–500) (>500)

✓ SOLITARIOUS 90 | isolated | scattered | group | unknown |

✓ GREGARIOUS Swarm sizes: ☐ very small _____ (<1 sq.km)

No. swarms: _____ ☐ small _____ (1 – <10 sq.km)

✓ immature Copulating ✓ medium _____ (10 – <100 sq.km)

☐ maturing | y | n | unknown | ☐ large _____ (100– <500 sq.km)

✓ mature Laying ✓ very large 650 (500+ sq.km)

☐ unknown | y | n | unknown | ☐ unknown

Flight from 225 | n/a | N | NE | E | SE | S | SW | W | NW |

(deg) to 0 | n/a | N | NE | E | SE | S | SW | W | NW |

Hoppers

Present: | y | n | No. (at site) (per sq.m)

✓ SOLITARIOUS min: 5 _____ | isolated | scattered | group | unknown |

max: 10 _____ (<10/site) (10+/site)

✓ GREGARIOUS

No. bands: _____ Band sizes: ☐ very small _____ (1 – <25 sq.m)

☐ egg fields ✓ 4th instar ✓ small 28 (25 – <2500 sq.m)

✓ hatching ☐ 5th instar ☐ medium _____ (0.25 – <10 ha)

☐ 1st instar ☐ 6th instar ✓ large 40 (10 – <50 ha)

☐ 2nd instar ✓ fledgling ☐ very large _____ (50+ ha)

✓ 3rd instar ☐ unknown

Figure 4. The locust data input from ARCEDIT.

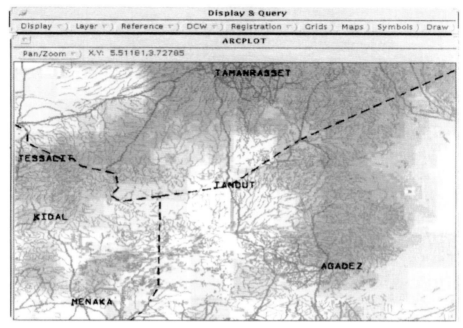

Figure 5. Example of a background map displayed in ARCPLOT.

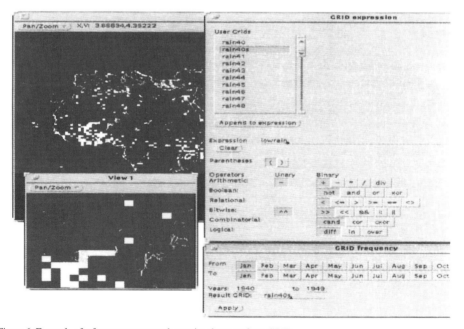

Figure 6. Example of a frequency map and associated menus from GRID.

Table 1. Databases and software in SWARMS

Type	Description	Source	Size
1. Background	• digital chart of the world[1]	DCW (USA)	500 Mb
	• soils	FAO	75 Mb
	• topography – 5' resolution	US Navy	2 Mb
	• world database II[2]	CIA (USA)	2 Mb
2. Locusts	• historical locusts (1929–1989)	NRI (UK)	2 Mb
	• new reports[3]	FAO	300 Mb
3. Historical weather	• weather stations	GHCN (USA)	30 Mb
4. Remote sensing	• meteosat[3]	EUMETSAT	200 Mb
	• tokar delta[4]	GTZ	6 Mb
5. Other software	• operating system	SUN (USA)	350 Mb
	• ARC/INFO	ESRI (USA)	220 Mb
	• INGRES	INGRES (USA)	100 Mb

[1]Includes aeronautical, cultural landmarks, drainage, political, railroads, roads, towns, transportation; [2]includes borders, coastlines and rivers; [3]buffer area; [4]example of a single potential desert locust biotope image.

tation which the forecaster can define. This allows the forecaster to ask an initial question of the GIS (e.g. display swarms in West Africa in August 1945 and rainfall during June 1945) followed by further refinement as more information is revealed (e.g. show only those swarms that are immature and rains greater than 20 mm). Frequency maps can be generated and viewed using animation (Fig. 6).

SWARMS contains a number of databases that include historical locust data from 1929 to the present, weather data and background information (Tab. 1). Before SWARMS, forecasters did not have easy access to historical locust data as it was only available at NRI in the UK.

Information contained in the databases is displayed as a series of maps overlaid on top of each other. SWARMS allows the forecaster to construct an infinite number of maps. For example, SWARMS can display locusts of a specific maturity for a certain period on a map with country boundaries, topography, rivers, towns, weather stations, roads, railroads, clouds, vegetation and so on.

Models and future developments

Models and model output can be incorporated into SWARMS. Currently, a locust trajectory model and a development model are part of SWARMS. The system has been designed to allow incorporation of future plug-in modules that are developed for SWARMS as technology increases, information improves and funds become available.

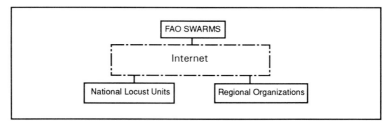

Figure 7. Example of an integrated desert locust information network, LocustNet.

It is anticipated that the open architecture design of SWARMS could stimulate development of geographic information systems at the national level. Due to the global level of forecasting at FAO, SWARMS is both larger and more complex than systems that NLUs would require or could maintain. National systems would probably be a smaller version of SWARMS that would meet national needs and could operate on personal computers yet be compatible with SWARMS (Healey 1995). However this requires further study and the experience of using SWARMS.

Healey (1995) has identified four probable benefits from national GIS:

- a more structured approach to data collection;
- improved checking and monitoring procedures;
- enhanced ability to map the locations of reported locust sightings;
- access to historical data on locusts, weather and habitat.

As telecommunications improve in countries affected by locusts, an international desert locust Information Network (LocustNet) could be established consisting of national and regional geographic information systems integrated with SWARMS to allow data sharing between affected countries and FAO (Fig. 7).

Conclusion

At the international level, GIS technology can be applied to improve the management of locust and environment data. There is also potential for GIS technology to be used at the national level linked by an international network, but that requires further study. A GIS is not a substitute for data. Field surveys to collect locust and other information are as essential as before. Every locust early warning system, whether a large centralised system like SWARMS or a smaller national GIS, will rely on data gathered during locust surveys, supplemented by remote sensing imagery. A concentrated effort is needed to improve these inputs. Thus far, one such effort has resulted in the adoption of a standard form for collecting information during surveys. As locust forecasters become more proficient in the use of SWARMS, as field data improve and as remote sensing imagery becomes validated, FAO should be able to provide more accurate forecasts and early warnings to affected countries. FAO should also be able to provide better advice to the international donor community, which in turn could contribute to improved planning and decision making.

References

ESRI (1992) ArcView user's guide. Redlands, California: Environmental Systems Research Institute
FAO (1989) Desert locust research priorities. Report of the FAO Research Advisory panel, 2–5 May 1989. Rome: FAO
Healey RG (1995) Issues in the development of GIS for national and regional locust organisations. In: FAO (ed) Report of the 33rd session of the FAO Desert Locust Control Committee, 16–20 January 1995. Rome: FAO
Healey RG, Robertson SG, Magor JI, Pender J, Cressman K (1996) A GIS for desert locust forecasting and monitoring. Intl J GIS 10(1): 117–136
Uvarov BP (1951) Locust research and control. Colonial Research Publication, No 10: 67 pp, London

New Strategies in Locust Control
S. Krall, R. Peveling and D. Ba Diallo (eds)
© 1997 Birkhäuser Verlag Basel/Switzerland

Mapping of desert locust habitats using remote sensing techniques

F. Voss and U. Dreiser

Technical University Berlin, Institute of Geography, Budapester Strasse 44–46, D-10787 Berlin, Germany

Summary. The results of research on the Sudan Red Sea coast, which was part of the project "integrated biological control of grasshoppers and locusts" of the GTZ (Gesellschaft für Technische Zusammenarbeit, Germany), will be shown. For detecting desert locust biotopes, multitemporal digital Landsat Thematic Mapper (TM) data and ground truth information were used. The information about the reported oviposition sites came from the local plant protection directorates. The Normalised Difference Vegetation Index of the satellite image shows the areas covered with vegetation. These areas were separated and then classified based on their spectral characteristics. Rectification and ground truthing was done by using a global positioning system. The result of the classification was merged with an enhanced satellite scene. The resulting map shows the main vegetation units together with relevant geographical information. The estimated suitability value based on the field studies and local desert locust information is added to the legend to identify the potential desert locust biotopes. The actual desert locust breeding areas, which are dependent on rainfall and flooding, can be determined by using National Oceanic and Atmospheric Administration Advanced Very High Resolution Radiometer (NOAA AVHRR) in combination with actual meteorological data. Further maps of the desert locust recession areas in the northern Tilemsi/Adrar des Iforhas (Mali) and the Akjoujt/Atar area (Mauritania) were produced with this method.

Résumé. Cette étude présente les résultats des recherches menées sur la côte de la Mer Rouge au Soudan dans le cadre du projet de la GTZ «Lutte biologique intégrée contre les sauteriaux et les locustes». Pour détecter les biotopes des criquets pèlerins, on a utilisé les données numérisées Landsat de cartographie thématique multidate et des informations recueillies sur le terrain. Les renseignements sur les champs de ponte ont été fournis par les directorats locaux de protection des végétaux. Le «Normalised Difference Vegetation Index» des images satellites montre les zones couvertes par la végétation. Ces zones ont été délimitées et classifiées selon leurs caractéristiques spectrales. Les rectifications et vérifications sur le terrain ont été réalisées au moyen d'un GPS («Global Positioning System»). Les résultats de la classification ont été intégrés à une scène satellite agrandie. La carte dressée ensuite montre les principales unités végétales accompagnées de données géographiques correspondantes. La valeur estimée d'adéquation basée sur les études sur le terrain et les informations sur les criquets pèlerins recueillies localement ont été ajoutées saux légendes afin d'identifier les biotopes potentiels du Criquet pèlerin. Les zones exactes où se multiplient les criquet pèlerins et qui dépendent des pluies et des inondations peuvent être déterminées en utilisant les données NOAA AVHRR et les données météorologiques disponibles. Cette méthode à permis l'établissement d'autres cartes des aires de rémission du Criquet pèlerin dans le Nord du Tilemsi/dans l'Adrar des Iforhas (Mali) et dans la région Akjoujt-Atar (Mauritanie).

Introduction

Spurred on by the desert locust plague of 1988, there have been urgent and repeated requests to international bodies such as Food and Agriculture Organisation of the United Nations (FAO), the European Community and the African Development Bank for remote sensing techniques to be applied and installed. Satellite data provide information for detecting areas where rainfall and vegetation conditions are suitable for desert locust breeding and development (FAO 1993). The reasons for using satellite images covering large areas are obvious from the continental scale of the problem alone.

Some initial studies have been made through the initiative of FAO Rome. These were pilot studies that basically applied remote sensing techniques to making biotope inventories related to quelea control in East Africa (Voss 1986; Meinzingen 1993; Dreiser 1993) and migratory locust control in Madagascar (Voss 1989).

Generally, habitat monitoring with remote sensing techniques is based on vegetation mapping. The vegetation influences swarm settlement and egg laying (Pedgley 1981). Popov (1984) and Roffey (1994) reported that in the area of Tamesna in northern Niger, selective settling in *Tribulus* and *Schouwia* habitats induced very rapid sexual maturation. The density of desert locust in these plant communities was thousands of times greater than the average density.

Tucker et al. (1985) evaluated the potential of satellite data for desert locust forecasting. They found that spatial distribution and density of plant cover agree with satellite data. Bryceson (1989) used Landsat Multispectral Scanner (MSS) data to determine the distribution of breeding areas of the Australian plague locust (*Chortoicetes terminefera*).

The FAO Remote Sensing Centre in Rome has been using the imagery from a series of permanent satellites for several years now to monitor the state of vegetation (undifferentiated) and the distribution of precipitation as part of the Global Food and Feed Security and Surveillance Programme. FAO has been working with a spatial resolution of between 1.7 and 16 km^2. A pilot study in Niger demonstrated the integration of field surveys, and high and low resolution satellite data for desert locust habitat monitoring (FAO 1993).

In 1990 the GTZ (Gesellschaft für Technische Zusammenarbeit, Germany) started the project "Integrated Biological Control of Grasshoppers and Locusts". One part of the project has concentrated on the mapping of potential desert locust breeding habitats using remote sensing techniques. The intention of the project is to support desert locust control in recession areas before they start gregarisation and swarming (Hielkema et al. 1981, 1986).

The GTZ project started with the Tokar delta, a recession area on the Sudan Red Sea coast (Pedgley 1981). To investigate the main desert locust breeding areas in northern Africa, the northern Tilemsi and Adrar des Iforhas area in Mali and the Akjoujt/Atar area in Mauritania were selected for studies. The principal methods for mapping the potential desert locust biotopes are described briefly using the Tokar delta as an example.

Research area

On the advice of FAO, the Tokar delta (18°30'N, 37°30'E) was selected as the pilot area. Normally, locust breeding extends from November to February. The Tokar delta is an inland delta, which is flooded in autumn by floods from the Khor Baraka. The main catchment is in the Asmara area of the highlands of Eritrea; there annual rainfall is some 500 mm. Additional soil moisture is provided by the winter rains. The mean annual rainfall in Tokar is about 100 mm, but there are great variations from year-to-year. The main land use of the area is confined to government-controlled cotton and millet production. The research area encloses the main delta structure and covers around 70×70 km (Voss and Dreiser 1994).

In the Red Sea coastal areas the important desert locust biotopes can be found principally within the wadi and the cropping areas. The practice of shifting cultivation created many habitats within the wadi areas (Steedman 1988). Abandoned fields were invaded by weeds which are favoured by locusts. The patchiness of the vegetation cover leads to concentration of desert locusts. In the Tokar delta most of the desert locust breeding was reported within the cropping areas.

Technical equipment

For mapping desert locust habitats data from the Landsat Thematic Mapper (TM) were used. One satellite scene covers an area 185 km × 170 km. The TM sensor of the Landsat satellite is a multispectral scanner with seven spectral channels and a spatial resolution of 30 m (band 6 = 120 m). The TM sensor can detect different vegetation communities especially by their reflection in the infrared electromagnetic spectrum (Mather 1987). This makes it an ideal instrument for landscape monitoring at scales up to 1:100,000.

During the field surveys a global positioning system (GPS) was used to support navigation and localisation of relevant test sites. For the transformation of the satellite image to the map projection, the geometric correction, significant points were located with an accuracy of 30 m.

Biotope mapping of desert locust breeding areas was handled by processing and interpretation of satellite scenes and other digitized data applying the digital image processing system ERDAS (Earth Resources Data Analysis System).

Field studies

The satellite scene was the basis for the field studies. The scene was enhanced using digital image-processing methods. Hereby the distribution of vegetation is of main interest. During the field trip, the available maps, a hard copy of the satellite scene on photographic paper at the approximate scale 1:100,000 and a GPS were used. The ground truthing in Sudan was carried out during four weeks in December 1990 in co-operation with G.B. Popov and the local plant protection directorates. During the survey the following studies were carried out:

- comparison of interpreted Landsat-TM scenes with the natural features;
- mapping of vegetation units;
- evaluation of ecological parameters, soil type, soil moisture, salinity and vegetation patterns at the oviposition sites of the desert locust;
- definition of test sites for the classification of satellite data;
- precise location of test sites with GPS for ground truth and geometric correction of satellite data;
- collection of desert locust reports and additional information, such as extension of flooding.

The study was based on the desert locust information from the plant protection directorates (PPD) in Suakin and Tokar. Guided by H. Shamseldin of the PPD in Tokar, the geomorphologic, soil and vegetation patterns were recorded at the reported oviposition sites within the delta. To cover the full range of ecological habitats, selected areas outside the delta structure, which showed up as green vegetation in the satellite image, were visited. The evaluation of these areas is mainly based on the appearance of specific vegetation, such as *Salvadora persica*, and the patchiness of the vegetation within the sandy wadis.

During the survey the environmental conditions were very unfavourable because of the extremely low level of flood and the disappearance of rainfall. The description of the annual vegetation was based on the identification of dry remains and the information given by the staff of the PPD in Tokar. Cropping was possible within only a small part of the delta. The evaluation of the desert locust potential of the habitats was therefore less objective than under good vegetation conditions.

Interpretation of the preliminary images and the results of the field studies allowed the exclusion of large areas that are of no interest for desert locust studies. At the Tokar delta these areas are mainly the salt flats (sebkhas), the areas dominated by *Suaeda monoica* (adleeb) and the stony plains. The habitats in the Tokar delta most favourable for desert locusts are associated with the millet fields together with communities of weeds like *Dipterigium glaucum*, *Heliotropium bacciferum*, *Solanum dubium*, *Aerva javanica* and *Tribulus longipelatus*. Other habitats are the sandy planes and wadis adjacent to the delta with scrubs and weeds, mostly *Panicum turgidum* and *Dipterigium* sp., which may become important in years with above average amounts of rainfall.

Image processing

It is always advisable to use multitemporal satellite scenes because of variations in vegetation conditions. In the case of the Tokar delta a multitemporal interpretation is necessary due to the high variations of flooding. Three Landsat-TM quarter scenes from 22.12.1988, 27.5.1989 and 6.11.1990 were interpreted. The first ones overlap with the locust plague of 1988. According to the field survey from November 1990 the scene from the same date was acquired.

The Normalised Difference Vegetation Index (NDVI) was used for masking the images. The classification of only the area which had a high vegetation index improved the accuracy of the results. To produce the map, the following steps were carried out:

- overlay of the image histograms using a grey value less than 0.01%;
- separation of water and bare sands, such as dunes, from the areas of interest using TM channel 5 of the scene with the highest quality;
- calculation of the NDVI for each scene;
- separation of vegetation and bare soils using the NDVI;
- transformation of the GPS co-ordinates to ERDAS or ARC/INFO format;
- determination of the test fields in the image;
- classification of the vegetation units for each scene;
- interactive logical combination of the classification results;
- geometric correction using the GPS points;
- enhancement of the highest quality scene using histogram equalisation and edge en-hancement filtering to illustrate the physiographic background;
- combination of the multitemporal classification with the enhanced image.

For detecting potential desert locust biotopes, the vegetation coverage was classified in each of the multitemporal satellite images. The interpretation of the satellite data was carried out using supervised classification techniques. The test sites, which were defined during the field studies, were used as training samples. The statistical characteristics of the digital multispectral satellite data were determined for each sample. Using TM channels 5, 4 and 2, which allow good visual interpretation of the data, each sample consisted of three dimensions, so the training samples could be described as a cloud of points representing a class of interest. For each point in the satellite image the probability of belonging to one of the defined classes was calculated. Then each point was assigned to a specific class.

The map shows the main vegetation units and soil types. For each class of vegetation an ecological potential value was estimated by G. Popov based on the field studies and the information of the oviposition sites given by the PPD. Although this value is subjective, it helps to evaluate the potential of the defined vegetation units under different rainfall and flooding conditions. The multitemporal interpretation allowed us to estimate the principal and marginal flooding areas in December 1988 by comparing the classification results of the images from December 1988 and May 1989. This led to the definition of two classes within the cropping area. Depending on flooding, the cropping area varies from year-to-year. Therefore, additional information about variations of rainfall and flooding is added in form of small maps. Photographs at the margin of the map show a selection of typical biotopes in the research area.

Further research in West Africa

The northern Tilemsi (Mali) and the Tamesna/Air area (Niger) are also typical desert locust breeding areas (Pedgley 1981). Hielkema et al. (1986) consider the areas in the region of the borders between Mali and Niger, and Algeria, as containing the main ecological units in West Africa with high frequencies of desert locust breeding and gregarisation.

To increase the range of desert locust habitats with different vegetation type studies, the Akjoujt/Atar area (19°45–20°45N, 13°00–14°30E) in Mauritania was selected as a second pilot area. This region is a typical summer breeding area. The area receives 100–200 mm average annual rainfall, mainly in August and September. The desert locust breeding areas are associated with the drainage areas and the depressions bordering the highlands. The sand coverage of the silty and clay soils causes slow desiccation. The most important plants for desert locust *Schouwia thebaica, Tribulus* sp., *Citrullus colocyntis* and *Hyoscyamus muticus* keep some greenness up to four months after a period of heavy rainfall (Steedman 1988).

The research area is defined by Akjoujt in the south-west and Atar in the north-east and measures about 160 km × 110 km. In the Akjoujt/Atar area only one satellite scene from 19.9.1988 was used due to limited financial resources, assuming that the good vegetation conditions in September 1988 would show the main potential breeding habitats in this area. Also, more recent data were not available. The field survey was carried out by U. Dreiser and G.B. Popov in October 1992.

Advantage was taken of the good vegetation condition in 1991 in Mali to produce two map sheets of the potential desert locust breeding habitats of an area measuring 200 km × 100 km in the Northern Tilemsi/Adrar des Iforhas area in Mali (19–21°N, 0–2°E). Because of safety problems in Mali and Niger in the years 1991 and 1992 a field survey was impossible. The selection of test sites for image classification was carried out in co-operation with G.B. Popov, using data collected during field surveys by OCLALAV (Organization Commune de Lutte Antiacridienne et de Lutte Antiaviare) and G.B. Popov in the 1980s. The data were used to illustrate the vegetation condition and the distribution of potential habitats.

The image processing methods were the same as those used in the Tokar delta. But only one satellite scene for each area was used. It was found that in the Akjoujt/Atar area (Mauritania) and in northern Tilemsi (Mali), the large dune fields with bare sands can be excluded from interpretation using the high backscattering values of sands in the infrared spectrum. Thus these areas can be masked using the highest digital value of Landsat TM channel 5.

Based on the field studies and the information of the oviposition sites given by the plant protection services and OCLALAV, an ecological potential value for desert locust surveillance, breeding and gregarisation was estimated by G.B. Popov for the maps of Mali and Mauritania. As in the Tokar delta, the values are subjective. But they will help to evaluate the potential of the defined vegetation units as desert locust habitats.

The inventory and monitoring of variable parameters

The present study showed the mapping possibilities of permanent parameters. Variable data from monitoring satellites with a high temporal resolution, like NOAA and Meteosat, as provided through the ARTEMIS (African Real Time Environmental Monitoring Information System) of FAO have been analysed by C. Dreiser (1994).

According to the findings of his doctoral thesis it is possible to monitor precipitation and vegetation dynamics in various quelea breeding habitats of East Africa. These results can be used to forecast the migration patterns of quelea and the time of establishment of breeding colonies. The results need to be tested on their applicability on desert locust habitats.

Conclusion

To produce a potential desert locust biotope map of the Tokar delta, the results of field studies, classified satellite scenes, desert locust reports and other ecological data were integrated.

Masking regions with low potential for desert locust breeding, such as water, bare sands or areas with low vegetation index, favours the classification of the satellite data. The printed result is a base map that considers the yearly variations of flooding and vegetation. The actual biotopes can be determined using meteorological and NOAA AVHRR data.

Further maps of the desert locust recession areas in Mali, Mauritania and Niger can be produced using this method. A minimum of two satellite scenes from years with good vegetation conditions should be used to cover the main desert locust biotopes. The maps should be printed at scale 1 : 200,000. In 1995 the GTZ team in Akjoujt reported vegetation coverage, mainly *Tribulus* sp., in the southern part of the mapped area in Akjoujt/Atar (Mauritania), which was not visible on the satellite image from September 1988. The differences can be explained by different distributions of rainfall and demonstrate the necessity of the multitemporal approach in arid areas.

Acknowledgements
G.B. Popov provided invaluable help and advice during this study. We also thank the Plant Protection Department in the Sudan, the desert locust Control Organisation of East Africa and the Tokar delta Agricultural Corporation, especially Shaban Shehara and Haider Shamseldin. In Mauritania we thank Mohammad Abdoullahi o. Mohammad Mahmoud from Plant Protection Headquarters, Baba Diop and Amadou Sy from the Plant Protection Service in Akjoujt. The experience and the helpful co-operation of the national plant protection services and desert locust control organisations helped to make the present studies possible. We wish to express our appreciation of the excellence and efficiency of all the arrangements made by the GTZ, initially through S. Krall in Germany, G. Hanrieder in Sudan and V. Leffler, O. Nasseh and H. Wilps in Mauritania. Special thanks are due to FAO manager W. Meinzingen for his kind assistance in this project.

References

Bryceson KP (1989) The use of Landsat MSS data to determine the distribution of locust eggbeds in the riverine region of New South Wales, Australia. Int J Rem Sens 11: 1749–1762
Dreiser C (1993) Mapping and monitoring of quelea pest habitats in East Africa. Berliner Geographische Studien 37, Berlin
FAO (1993) Calibration and integrated modelling of remote sensing data for desert locust habitat monitoring. RSC-Series 64, Rome
Hielkema JU, Ayyangar RS, Sinha PP (1981) Satellite remote sensing: a new dimension in international desert locust survey and control. Plant Protection Bulletin (New Delhi): 3–4: 165–173
Hielkema JU, Roffey J, Tucker CJ (1986) Assessment of ecological conditions associated with the 1980/81 desert locust plague upsurge in West Africa using environmental satellite data. Int J Rem Sens 7: 1609–1622
Mather PM (1987) Computer processing of remotely-sensed images: an Introduction. Wiley, Chichester
Meinzingen W (ed) (1993) A guide to migrant pest management in Africa. Rome: FAO
Pedgley D (ed) (1981) Desert locust forecasting manual. London: Centre of Overseas Pest Research
Popov GB, Wood TG, Haggis MJ (1984) Insect pests of the Sahara. Pages 145–171 in Cloudsley-Thompson, JL (ed) Key environments. Sahara Desert. Oxford
Roffey J (1994) The characteristics of early desert locust upsurges. Pages 55–61 in: van Huis A (ed) Desert locust control with existing techniques: an evaluation of strategies. Proceedings of the seminar held in Wageningen, The Netherlands, 6–11 December 1993. Wageningen Agricultural University

Steedman A (ed) (1988) Locust handbook. 2nd ed, London: Overseas Development Natural Resources Institute

Tucker CJ, Hielkema JU, Roffey J (1985) The potential of satellite remote sensing of ecological conditions for surveying and forecasting desert locust activity. Int J Rem Sens 6: 127–138

Voss F (1986) Quelea habitats in East Africa. Rome: FAO

Voss F (1989) Biotopes acridiens dans le Sud-Ouest de Madagascar. Rome: FAO

Voss F, Dreiser U (1994) Mapping of desert locust and other migratory pests habitats using remote sensing techniques. Pages 23–39 in Krall S, Wilps H (eds) New trends in locust control. Schriftenreihe der GTZ 245. Rossdorf: TZ-Verlagsgesellschaft

The following locust habitat maps are available at the author or the GTZ-Locust-Project

Dreiser U, Voss F, Popov G (1992) Potential desert locust biotopes – Tokar delta (Sudan). Map sheet. Eschborn: GTZ

Dreiser U, Voss F, Popov G (1993a) Principaux biotopes du criquet pèlerin dans le Nord du Tilemsi (Mali). Map sheet. Eschborn: GTZ

Dreiser U, Voss F, Popov G (1993b) Principaux biotopes du criquet pèlerin dans l'Adrar des Iforhas (Mali). Map sheet. Eschborn: GTZ

Dreiser U, Voss F, Popov G (1994) Principaux biotopes du criquet pèlerin dans la région Akjoujt – Atar (Mauritanie). Map sheet. Eschborn: GTZ

New Strategies in Locust Control
S. Krall, R. Peveling and D. Ba Diallo (eds)
© 1997 Birkhäuser Verlag Basel/Switzerland

Vertical-looking radar as a means to improve forecasting and control of desert locusts

J.R. Riley and D.R. Reynolds

Natural Resources Institute, Radar Entomology Unit, North Site, Leigh Sinton Road, Malvern, Worcestershire WR14 1LL, UK

Summary. Outbreaks of desert locusts are believed to start when solitarious phase locusts encounter favourable conditions and breed prolifically. The current method used to obtain the earliest warning of outbreaks is therefore to combine survey information on the distribution and abundance of solitarious phase populations with data on the distribution of concurrently favourable habitats. This paper introduces the idea that it may now be practicable to routinely supplement conventional survey data with information about the abundance of solitarious phase locusts flying at high altitude, i.e., above 100 m. The objective would be to detect moving solitarious phase populations, and so enhance the accuracy and reliability of outbreak forecasts. Routine aerial monitoring has recently been made possible by the advent of a new technique which uses inexpensive, vertical-looking radar (VLR) to detect the presence of insects flying overhead. The radar runs automatically for long periods, analyses its own data and produces plots of the density, altitude and direction of the insects' migration, and of their size and hence of their probable identity. VLRs are based on standard marine radar transmitters, which are mass produced, and reliable, and the systems are designed to be run by non-specialist personnel.

Résumé. Il est généralement admis qu'une invasion de Criquets pèlerins se déclenche lorsque les locustes en phase solitaire rencontrent des conditions qui leur sont favorables pour se multiplier. La méthode couramment utilisée pour détecter le plus tôt possible une invasion est donc de combiner des informations générales sur la distribution et l'abondance des populations en phase solitaire à des données sur la distribution d'habitats susceptibles d'être simultanément favorables. Cette étude se propose de montrer qu'il devrait être maintenant possible de compléter systématiquement les informations générales par des renseignements sur l'abondance des locustes en phase solitaire volant à haute altitude, c'est-à-dire à plus de 100 mètres. L'objectif serait de détecter des populations de solitaires en déplacement afin d'accroître la précision et la fiabilité des prévisions. Une surveillance aérienne régulière est devenue depuis peu possible grâce à l'adoption d'une nouvelle technique peu onéreuse utilisant un radar à visée verticale (vertical-looking radar – VLR) pour détecter la présence d'insectes volant au-dessus de ces radars. Le radar fonctionne de façon automatique sur de longues périodes, analyse ses propres données et fournit des informations et des graphiques sur la densité, l'altitude et la direction de vol des insectes, ainsi que sur leur taille et donc sur leur probable identité. Les radars à visée verticale sont basés sur la technologie des radars standard de la marine qui sont fabriqués en série, peu onéreux et fiables. Leur fonctionnement ne requiert pas un personnel spécialisé.

Introduction

Most authorities now accept that during periods of recession the desert locust exists at low densities, behaving in a solitary manner (Hemming et al. 1979; Magor 1994a). Such locusts are found mainly in the normally arid recession area, but if they encounter exceptionally favourable conditions (i.e., areas where widespread and heavy rains have fallen), they breed successfully and generate the gregarising populations which give rise to local outbreaks (Roffey 1994). Heavy rain within the recession area does not, however, automatically lead to outbreaks. One explanation of this is that not enough locusts always reach the newly favourable locality (Roffey 1994). If this is correct, solitarious phase locusts would appear not to be ubiquitous, and their windborne movement from place to place within the recession area must therefore be a factor (and probably a critical one) in starting outbreaks. If an outbreak is followed by two or more successive generations of transiens to gregarious reproduction in complementary breeding areas connected by migration, there will be an enormous increase in numbers of locusts (Waloff 1966; Magor 1994a). When this process continues for six or more generations, it constitutes an upsurge (Magor 1994b) which may in turn lead to a full plague.

In summary, the nocturnal migration of behaviourally solitarious phase locust populations is probably a determinant in the onset of outbreaks, and it is also of particular significance in the early stages of upsurges (Pedgley 1981). The purpose of this paper is to show that it may now be practicable to monitor this movement using a new and inexpensive vertical-looking radar (VLR), and that this should lead to an improved understanding of the role which these locusts play in starting outbreaks. The ultimate objective of using VLRs would be more accurate, reliable and quicker detection of outbreaks in key areas.

Radar and the study of locust flight

Desert locusts showing solitary behaviour fly at night. They therefore cannot be tracked by eye, and so most of our knowledge of their migration has been inferred from studies of changes in their distribution on the ground, which suggests that their movements may be somewhat similar to those of the highly visible day-flying swarms (Pedgley 1981). In order to gain more reliable information about the flight behaviour of solitary locusts, the Anti-Locust Research Centre (a precursor of the Natural Resources Institute) sponsored a pioneering attempt in 1968 to use radar to observe locust flight over the Sahara. This was the first time that radar had been used specifically for an entomological experiment, and the study was a great success (Roffey 1969; Schaefer 1969, 1972, 1976), providing novel measurements of aerial density, orientation, direction and speed of migration, and demonstrating for the first time that locusts showing solitary behaviour migrated at altitudes of several hundred metres. These results led to early speculation by Schaefer (1972) that chains of strategically placed locust monitoring radar stations would facilitate cheaper and more effective locust control operations; a proposal which was probably impracticable at the time. In any event, although radar found wide application in entomology over the following decades (Reynolds 1988; Riley 1989), the complexity of the equipment, and especially the time-consuming nature of the data analysis, meant that it was impractical to use the technique for routine monitoring of migratory flight.

Radar as a migration monitor

In addition to the drawback of being labour intensive, conventional scanning entomological radars suffered from the serious limitation that their capability to identify the species of the insects which they detected was very limited. During rotational scanning, targets appeared simply as anonymous dots on the radar screen, with clues to their identity being limited to their maximum detectable range and to their air speed. Supplementary information on identity could sometimes be gained by parking the radar beam so that passing insects remained in it for long enough for their wing-beat frequencies to be recorded. Wing-beat frequency can be a powerful aid to identification in certain cases (Schaefer 1976; Riley and Reynolds 1983), but in other situations, spread within species, and overlap between them, makes identification impractical.

Over recent years, the dramatic and continuing fall in the cost of computing equipment made it possible to envisage novel methods of improving the target identification capacity of entomological radars, and also to automate both their operation and the analysis of radar data. We therefore attempted to develop a radar specifically for routine monitoring of locust movement, and capable of long-term operation by non-specialists (Riley 1993; Riley and Reynolds 1993). The system which we adopted uses a nutating, vertical-looking beam in which the plane of (linear) polarisation is rotated, because this arrangement allows extraction of insect body mass and shape data, as well as displacement velocity and orientation (Smith et al. 1993). It is the body size and shape data, plus measurements of wing-beat frequency, which were intended to allow the radar to perform the key task of distinguishing desert locusts from other high-flying insects. The radar monitors the passage of any insects of mass above about 2 mg flying through a column approximately 30 m in diameter, and extending from about 100 m up to 1500 m directly above the radar. Some idea of the area "surveyed" by a VLR during a night's operation may be obtained if one notes that windborne locusts might well move over the radar at about 10 ms^{-1} for six hours in a night. This is equivalent to a sampling area of about $10 \times 6 \times 3600 \times 30$ m^2, or about 650 ha.

Field trials of locust-monitoring radar in Mauritania

Field trials of a prototype VLR were held in Mauritania in the autumn of 1993 and 1994. They were conducted in collaboration with the Mauritanian Direction du Développement des Ressources Agro-Pastorales, and with the logistic support of the Deutsche Gesellschaft für Technische Zusammenarbeit (GTZ).

The trials were carried out in three widely separated localities: Akjoujt and Achram (in 1993) and Aioun-el-Atrouss (in 1994) (Fig. 1), so that we could evaluate the radar's capacity to cope with different densities and types of aerial fauna typical of Mauritania. Thus, if the normal density of the aerial fauna was such that, on average, more than one insect occupied the beam within each 45-m altitude interval (i.e., more than about one insect per 8×10^3 m^3), the analysis procedures would break down, and we obviously needed to know if this was likely to occur. Equally, if other insects of comparable mass but different shape from desert locusts were found to be present, we required evidence that VLR could, in fact, distinguish between them.

Each trial lasted two to three weeks, and in the 1993 experiments, desert locusts were fairly common in the vicinity of both experimental sites. At Akjoujt, a conventional scanning entomo-logical radar (Riley and Reynolds 1983) was used to check the accuracy of the VLR flight tra-jectory and aerial density measurements. The trials were primarily intended to evaluate the capa-

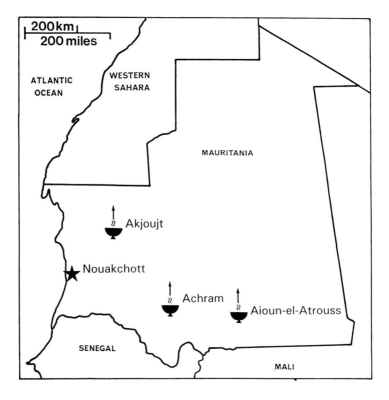

Figure 1. Map showing the location of the three radar trial sites in Mauritania. Akjoujt, in the north, is in the desert zone; Achram and Aioun are in the northern Sahel.

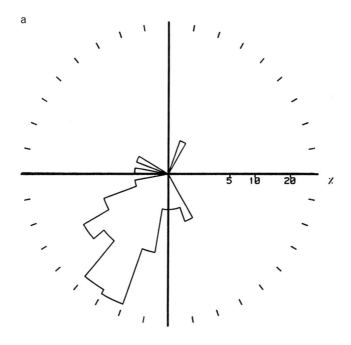

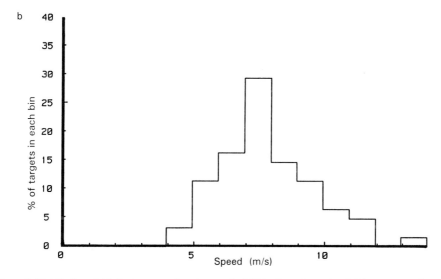

Figure 2. Distribution of (a) displacement directions, and of (b) horizontal speeds of airborne targets detected at Aioun-el-Atrouss on 27 September 1994, during the 5 min period 22:18 to 22:23, in the altitude range between 150 m and 1000 m above the radar. In (a), north is vertical, and the radial axis is scaled to produce an equi-areal plot. Number of targets = 61.

city of VLR to monitor nocturnal flight by non-swarming locusts, so the radars were operated each day from dusk until flight activity declined to a low level, usually around midnight. Occasionally the VLR was set to run automatically until dawn.

Detailed analysis of the data from the field trials has not yet been completed, and in particular we have not assessed the degree to which shape-factor and mass estimates can be combined to confidently identify desert locusts in the presence of the aerial fauna which we encountered in Mauritania. We have therefore included in this paper only a typical example of the output produced by VLR, which shows the detection of targets in the size range predicted for desert locusts.

Figure 2 shows plots of the distribution of displacement directions and speeds of insects overflying the radar in 1994, during a period of five minutes. Figure 3 gives the distribution of the radar cross-section term σ_{xx} of these insects, from which estimates of their mass can be derived (Smith et al. 1993). Desert locusts might typically have values of σ_{xx} in the region of 7 cm^2, i.e., ≈ 8 dB relative to 1 cm^2 (Riley 1985), and so could have accounted for about 3% of the total in Figure 2. For much of the time, the percentage of targets in the locust cross-section range was much lower than this, demonstrating that desert locusts comprised at most only a small minority of the aerial fauna. This pattern was repeated at Achram, and also at Akjoujt,

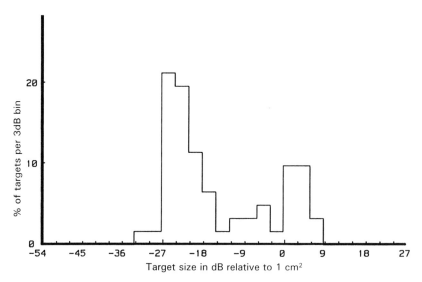

Figure 3. Distribution of the radar cross-section parameter σ_{xx} for the targets in Figure 2. Desert locusts have values of σ_{xx} of ≈ 8 dB relative to 1 cm^2.

where the scanning radar data confirmed that the aerial density of locust-sized targets was very low (typically fewer than five locusts per 10^6 m^3). This aerial density would result in the interception of only one or two desert locust-sized targets per hour by VLR. Nevertheless, given the significance which is attached in forecasting work to the sighting, in certain circumstance, of small numbers of desert locusts, the data acquired by VLR would appear to be potentially very valuable.

Conclusions

There is good reason to believe that nocturnal migration of solitarious phase desert locusts may play an important role in determining whether rainfall in suitable areas will trigger the initial outbreaks in a locust upsurge. Little attention has been paid to this possibility up to now, for the very good reason that using conventional entomological techniques to monitor solitarious migration would be prohibitively expensive, and probably quite impracticable. The provisional results of our trials in Mauritania indicate that VLR may have the potential to provide an inexpensive and effective means to investigate this hitherto intractable problem.

References

Hemming CF, Popov GB, Roffey J, Waloff Z (1979) Characteristics of desert locust plague upsurges. Phil Trans R Soc Lond B 287: 375–386

Magor J (1994a) Desert locust population dynamics. Pages 31–54 in van Huis A (ed) Desert locust control with existing techniques: an evaluation of strategies. Wageningen: Wageningen Agricultural University

Magor J (1994b) Appendix II. Locust glossary. Pages 119–127 in van Huis A (ed) Desert locust control with existing techniques: an evaluation of strategies. Wageningen: Wageningen Agricultural University

Pedgley DE (ed) (1981) Desert locust forecasting manual. Vol 1. London: Centre for Overseas Pest Research, viii + 268 pp

Reynolds DR (1988) Twenty years of radar entomology. Antenna 12: 44–49

Riley JR (1985) Radar cross-section of insects. Proc IEEE 73: 228–232

Riley JR (1989) Remote sensing in entomology. Ann Rev Ent 34: 247–271

Riley JR (1993) Long-term monitoring of insect aerial migration. Pages 28–32 in Isard SA (ed) Alliance for Aerobiology Workshop Report. Champaign, Illinois: Alliance for Aerobiology Workshop Writing Committee

Riley JR, Reynolds DR (1983) A long-range migration of grasshoppers observed in the Sahelian zone of Mali by two radars. J Animal Ecol 52: 167–183

Riley JR, Reynolds DR (1993) Radar monitoring of locusts and other migratory insects. Pages 51–53 in Cartwright A (ed) World Agriculture 1993. London: Sterling Publications

Roffey J (1969) Report on radar studies on the desert locust, Schistocerca gregaria (Forskål), in the Niger Republic, September–October 1968. Anti-locust Research Centre Occasional Report no 17, 16 pp

Roffey J (1994) The characteristics of early desert locust upsurges. Pages 55–61 in van Huis A (ed) Desert locust control with existing techniques: an evaluation of strategies. Wageningen: Wageningen Agricultural University

Schaefer GW (1969) Radar studies of locust, moth and butterfly migration in the Sahara. Proc R Ent Soc Lond C 34: 33 and 39–40

Schaefer GW (1972) Radar detection of individual locusts and swarms. Pages 379–380 in Hemming CF, Taylor THC (eds) Proceedings of the International Study Conference on the Current and Future Problems of Acridology, London 1970. London: Centre for Overseas Pest Research

Schaefer GW (1976) Radar observations of insect flight. Pages 157–197 in Rainey RC (ed) Insect Flight. Symposia of the Royal Entomological Society no 7. Oxford: Blackwell

Smith AD, Riley JR, Gregory RD (1993) A method for routine monitoring of the aerial migration of insects by using a vertical-looking radar. Phil Trans R Soc Lond B 340: 393–404

Waloff Z (1966) The upsurges and recessions of the desert locust plague: an historical survey. Anti-Locust Memoir no 8. London: Anti-locust Research Centre, 111 pp

New Strategies in Locust Control
S. Krall, R. Peveling and D. Ba Diallo (eds)
© 1997 Birkhäuser Verlag Basel/Switzerland

Forecasting the early-season eclosion of *Oedaleus senegalensis* in the Sahel: the role of remotely sensed rainfall data

P.J.A. Burt, J. Colvin and S.M. Smith

Natural Resources Institute, Central Avenue, Chatham Maritime, Chatham, Kent ME4 4TB, UK

Summary. *Oedaleus senegalensis* (Krauss) (Acrididae: Oedipodinae) is a serious grasshopper pest in the Sahel. This species passes the dry season as eggs in the soil and emergence is triggered by the onset of rain in May/June. Satellite imagery enables the monitoring of rainfall over much wider areas than those possible by ground-based observers. Although this has been investigated for some areas of the Sahel, any relationship between cloud temperature and the rainfall measured at the surface has never been quantified for Mali. Such rainfall information will lead to more effective identification of areas where grasshopper hatching may occur and enable ground control teams to target such areas more efficiently than at present. The results of a four-year field investigation into the use of satellite imagery to assess rainfall in Mali are presented, as well as the findings of an investigation into the influence of rainfall on eclosion. The effects of rain-gauge spacing for reliable point measurements of rainfall are discussed, and a possible relationship between cloud temperature and the amount of rain received at the surface is presented. Implications for improved pest control are summarised.

Résumé. *Oedaleus senegalensis* (Krauss) (Acrididae: Oedipodinae) est un ravageur provoquant des dégâts considérables dans le Sahel. Ce criquet passe la saison sèche sous la forme d'oeufs déposés dans le sol. L'émergence est déclenchée par le début des pluies en mai/juin. Les images satellitaires permettent d'évaluer les précipitations sur des étendues beaucoup plus vastes que les postes d'observation terrestres. Aucune étude quantitative sur la relation entre la température des nuages et la quantité des précipitations mesurées à la surface du sol n'a encore été réalisée au Mali, contrairement à ce qui a été fait dans d'autres régions du Sahel. Ces données pluviométriques permettraient une meilleure identification des zones d'éclosion des oeufs du criquet sénégalais et un ciblage plus précis de ces zones par les équipes de lutte terrestre contre les âcridiens. Cette étude présente les résultats de quatre années d'utilisation sur le terrain d'images satellitaires pour évaluer les précipitations au Mali, ainsi que les conclusions d'une enquête sur l'influence des pluies sur l'éclosion des oeufs. Les effets de l'écartement des pluviomètres sur la qualité des mesures ponctuelles des pluies seront discutés et le rapport possible entre température des nuages et la quantité de pluie tombée sera exposé. Les implications qui en découlent pour améliorer la lutte anti-acridienne seront récapitulées.

Introduction

The Senegalese grasshopper, *Oedaleus senegalensis*, is a major grasshopper pest of subsistence crops in the West African Sahel, and its importance is increasing (Maiga 1992). In northern Mali, *O. senegalensis* spends the dry season (normally late October to early May) as eggs in the soil. Eclosion is triggered by the first rains of the following year, which usually occur in May and June (Popov 1980). Although it is well established that rainfall triggers eclosion, and that egg pod survey data collected at the end of the dry season can be used to estimate hopper numbers at the start of the next rainy season (Popov 1988), a major constraint on the success of early season control is the problem of obtaining rainfall data rapidly from extremely remote sites.

Such data, if linked with a reliable method of assessing rainfall, would greatly improve the management and control of this pest, enabling ground control teams to target likely outbreak areas more efficiently. This paper presents the results of a study investigating the feasibility of monitoring rainfall over larger areas than would normally be possible using ground-based information alone.

Rainfall estimation by satellite imagery is the only feasible way of monitoring the large geographical areas involved. Previous studies attempting to forecast grasshopper and locust outbreaks assessed rainfall indirectly by locating new vegetation growth (Bryceson 1989; Kogan 1990), but this approach may not be ideal because new vegetation in arid and semi-arid environments only becomes detectable by satellite several weeks after rainfall (Justice et al. 1991). By this time, emerging *O. senegalensis* populations would probably be well established and already have caused substantial damage.

Most precipitation in the Sahel falls from local convective systems, including squall lines, (Hoepffner et al. 1989), and it is known that convective clouds with cloud-top temperatures below a certain threshold, usually around –50 °C, have a higher probability of producing rain (Barrett and Martin 1981), although the distribution of rainfall from such systems is usually patchy.

Studies in Niger and Burkina Faso have indicated that a statistical relationship exists between cloud temperature and rainfall, which can provide reasonable rainfall estimates for remote regions (Hoepffner et al. 1989; Turpeinen and Diallo 1989; Milford and Dugdale 1990), although the statistical relationship needs to be verified for each new geographical area examined. Accordingly, in the first part of this study the amounts of rain received from convective rainstorms passing over the Mourdiah area, northern Mali (7° 28'N, 14° 28'W) were investigated through the use of a network of rain-gauges, and the relationship between cloud-top minimum temperature and the amount of rain received was established. The variation between rainfall amounts over distances of several kilometres was also investigated, in order to determine the reliability of point measurements of rainfall. The results of these investigations were then related to a study of the amount of water required to trigger early season eclosion of *O. senegalensis* in the field.

Materials and methods

Fieldwork was conducted in the Mourdiah area between 1990 and 1994 (Fig. 1). Hourly Meteosat infrared images were collected at the Natural Resources Institute, UK, from early June to the end of October in 1990 and 1991. Cloud-top temperatures of storms with tracks over the study area were extracted, and relationships between these and rainfall were investigated.

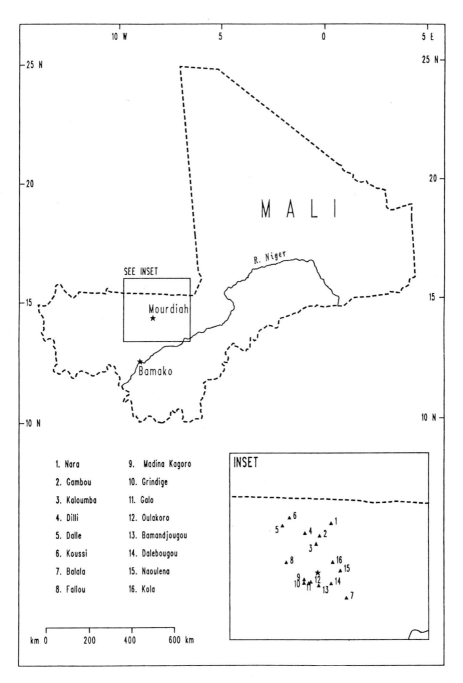

Figure 1. The location of villages equipped with rain-gauges in the Mourdiah area of northern Mali.

In order to investigate how representative a single measure of rainfall is for a given area, in 1990 rainfall data were collected in a series of rain-gauges arranged in a cross. The gauges covered an array of about 17 km north to south and 15 km east to west. Gauges were read daily between 8.30 and 9.00, local time. In order to assess the effect of greater separation between gauges, rainfall was also collected at 16 surrounding villages, located within a 98-km radius of Mourdiah. In 1991, a simplified rain-gauge system was used at Mourdiah, with 8 rain-gauges, 100 m apart, positioned in a line running north-east to south-west. Correlation coefficients were calculated for all combinations of rain-gauges in the cross and in the villages.

Before the beginning of the rains in May 1993, viable egg pods were taken from the field and reburied at two different sites, one with predominantly sandy soil and one with clay soil. The egg pods at each site were subjected to six different treatments of simulated rainfall, applied by watering can: volumes of 10 and 20 mm were applied to the egg pods once every 3, 5 or 10 days. Sites were monitored daily for evidence of eclosion. Eclosion was also monitored at a 25-m^2 plot located in a field used to grow millet the previous year, which was given 10 mm of simulated rainfall every day for 21 days.

In 1994, daily surveys for *O. senegalensis* were made in a 2-km radius of Mourdiah, between the first (7 May) and second (18 May) rainfalls of the season.

Results and discussion

Correlations between the 1990 raingauges were highly significant ($P<0.0001$, $r >= 0.68$). The village rain-gauge pairs were less well correlated, and none of the correlation coefficients were above 0.9, a lower limit suggested by McConkey et al. (1990) for obtaining accurate point measurements of rainfall. No rain-gauge pair in the 1991 investigation had a correlation coefficient <0.98 ($P<0.0001$).

Since all the rain-gauge data in both years were highly correlated with those of the central gauge (at the axis of the cross), ($r = 0.974$ and $r = 0.991$ in 1990 and 1991 respectively, $P<0.0001$ in both cases), the central gauge rainfall data were used for rainfall assessment in relation to minimum cloud temperatures. There was a tendency for colder clouds to produce more rainfall, especially when clouds with minimum temperatures below $-50\ °C$ were considered (Fig. 2).

The relationship between minimum cloud temperature and log(rainfall + 1) over the period June to August in both years was highly significant ($r = -0.6$, $P<0.0001$). In addition, there were instances when late season rains produced relatively large quantities of rainfall (see

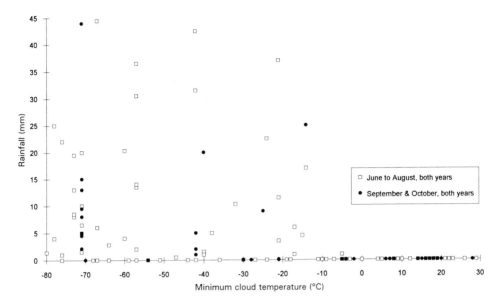

Figure 2. The relationship between cloud minimum temperature and rainfall in 1990 and 1991.

September and October data in Fig. 2). This is of less importance than may at first be imagined, since these instances lie well outside the early-season eclosion period. They are, however, of importance when using the satellite imagery to assess rainfall later in the season.

Soil type and watering regime influenced the length of time between first wetting and eclosion. The shortest interval (8 days) between first wetting and eclosion was found for the 20-mm water treatments in the clay, on the 5-day rewetting regime and in the sand with 3-day rewettings. The 10-day watering regimes, for both types of soil, contained eggs that failed to hatch after 30 days. In the second experiment, eclosion was observed from all (17) egg pods in the site, between 9 and 13 days after first wetting.

In 1994 the first rainfall of the season yielded 8 mm of rain, and the first instar *O. senega-lensis* nymphs were found throughout the survey area nine days afterwards (i.e., before the next rains).

Conclusions

1. The results from Mourdiah, suggesting an optimum rain-gauge separation of 6–8 km for reliable point measurements of rainfall, are similar to those found by other workers in diffe-

rent parts of the Sahel, and a maximum separation of about 8 km should be aimed for in future studies in this area.

2. It would be useful to provide villages with their own rain-gauges, providing rainfall reports to plant protection staff as part of an early warning system.

3. The results from this investigation support the conclusions of previous studies for other areas of the Sahel, that colder cloud is more likely to produce rain, particularly in the early part of the rainy season.

4. Field observations show that as little as 8 mm of rainfall is sufficient to trigger eclosion at the start of the rainy season.

5. The relationship between cloud temperature and rain amount is less clear. Rainwater runoff caused increases in local rain amounts over egg pod areas, resulting in *O. senegalensis* eclosion with very light rain.

6. Satellite imagery is clearly of use in giving an indication of where rain is likely to have fallen. Cloud temperature data, in conjunction with rain-gauge and egg pod survey data, could help to target more clearly the areas covered by ground control teams at the start of the rainy season.

Acknowledgements
We are very grateful to Drs M. Sanghata, B. Maiga and M. Sissoko of the Service de la Protection des Végétaux., Mali, for their assistance at all stages of this study. The assistance of J. Williams, P. Navarro and R. Loftie from the NRI LARST (Local Applications of Remote Sensing Techniques) team is also gratefully acknowledged.

References

Barrett EC, Martin DW (1981) The use of satellite data in rainfall monitoring. Academic Press: London, 340 pp
Bryceson KP (1989) The use of Landsat MSS data to determine the distribution of locust eggbeds in the riverine region of New South Wales, Australia. Int J Remote Sensing 10: 1749–1762
Hoepffner M, Lebel T, Sauvagest H (1989) EPSAT Niger: a pilot experiment for rainfall estimation over West Africa. Pages 251–258 in WMO/IAHS/ETH International Workshop on Precipitation Measurement, St Moritz
Justice CO, Dugdale G, Townsend JRG, Narracott AS, Kumar M (1991) Synergism between NOAA-AVHRR and Meteosat data for studying vegetation development in semi-arid West Africa. Int J Remote Sensing 12: 1349–1468
Kogan FN (1990) Remote sensing of weather impacts on vegetation in non-homogeneous areas. Int J Remote Sensing 11: 1405–1419
McConkey BG, Nicholaichuk W, Cutforth HW (1990) Small area variability of warm-season precipitation in a semiarid climate. Agric For Meteorol 49: 225–242
Maiga B (1992) Mali: notes on the acridid problem in Mali. Pages 82–85 in Lomer CJ, Prior C (eds) Biological control of locusts and grasshoppers. Wallingford, UK, CAB International
Milford JR, Dugdale G (1990) Monitoring of rainfall in relation to the control of migrant pests. Phil Trans R Soc Lond B 328: 689–704

Popov GB (1980) Studies on oviposition, egg development and mortality in *Oedaleus senegalensis* (Krauss) (Orthoptera: Acridoidea) in the Sahel. Centre for Overseas Pest Research Miscellaneous Report 53, 48 pp

Popov GB (1988) Sahelian grasshoppers. Overseas Development Natural Resources Bulletin no 5, vi + 87 pp, London

Turpeinen OM, Diallo AA (1989) Estimation of rainfall in Burkina Faso using ESOC precipitation index. J Climate 2: 121–130

New Strategies in Locust Control
S. Krall, R. Peveling and D. Ba Diallo (eds)
© 1997 Birkhäuser Verlag Basel/Switzerland

Biotic and abiotic factors affecting the population dynamics of the Senegalese grasshopper, *Oedaleus senegalensis*

J. Colvin

Natural Resources Institute, Central Avenue, Chatham Maritime, Chatham ME4 4TB, UK

Summary. The Senegalese grasshopper, *Oedaleus senegalensis* (Krauss), is an important pest of graminaceous crops such as millet and sorghum. Evidence is presented to show that this species has an egg diapause, the induction of which is regulated both by the photoperiod and temperature experienced by females. In northern Mali, 97–100% of eggs have broken diapause ca. seven months after oviposition and remain quiescent in the soil until post-diapause embryonic development is triggered by rain. Several egg-predator species prey on *O. senegalensis*, the most important one in northern Mali being the bombyliid *Xeramoeba* nr. *oophaga* (Zakhvatkin). The dry season survival strategy of this species differs from that of *O. senegalensis* in that emergence occurs after diapause termination, irrespective of soil moisture conditions. A population model based on the results of this study is described, illustrating a potential mechanism operating behind major *O. senegalensis* outbreaks. The model's conclusions and predictions are discussed in relation to *O. senegalensis* outbreak forecasting.

Résumé. Le criquet sénégalais, *Oedaleus senegalensis* (Krauss), cause de graves dégâts sur les cultures de graminées telles que le mil et le sorgho. Cette étude montre que le développement des oeufs de cet insecte est interrompu par une diapause, induite chez les femelles par la photopériode et la température auxquelles elles sont exposées. Dans le nord du Mali, 97 à 100% des oeufs subissent une diapause d'environ sept mois après l'oviposition et demeurent en quiescence dans le sol jusqu'à ce que la diapause soit levée avec le retour des pluies. Le développement embryonnaire peut alors reprendre. De nombreux prédateurs s'attaquent aux oeufs d'*O. senegalensis*, le plus important étant au nord du Mali *Keramoeba* nr. *oophaga* (Zakhvatkin) (*Bombylidae*). La stratégie de survie en saison sèche de cette espèce diffère de celle d'*O. senegalensis*, l'émergence se produisant après la levée de la diapause quel que soit le degré d'humidité du sol. L'article décrit un modèle de population basé sur les résultats de cette étude et qui illustre un mécanisme potentiel influant sur les pullulations majeures d'*O. senegalensis*. Les conclusions et prévisions du modèle sont discutées par rapport aux prévisions sur les infestations d'*O. senegalensis*.

Introduction

The Senegalese grasshopper, *Oedaleus senegalensis* (Krauss) (Orthoptera: Acrididae), is periodically an important pest of graminaceous crops such as millet and sorghum (Cheke 1990). This species inhabits the drier, highly seasonal, savannah areas of Africa and India, and in order to cope with the vagaries of its habitat, its life history has evolved to include both migration and an egg diapause (Launois 1978; Riley and Reynolds 1983; Colvin and Cooter 1995).

Damage caused by *O. senegalensis* is most serious when it occurs at the seedling crop stage, often necessitating multiple resowing. Due to the short duration of the rainy season in areas such as the West African Sahel, damage of this type can result in there being insufficient time left during the rainy season for the crops to reach maturity (Popov 1988).

In common with control strategies designed to combat other migratory pest species, forecasting outbreaks of *O. senegalensis* is probably the most cost-efficient way of reducing crop damage. Accurate methods of forecasting *O. senegalensis* outbreaks, however, can only be developed through a more complete understanding of the physiology, ecology and behaviour of both *O. senegalensis* and its major predators. In this article, the results of a recent investigation into several important biotic and abiotic factors influencing the population dynamics of West African *O. senegalensis* are presented and discussed in relation to outbreak forecasting.

Diapause induction, duration and egg survival

Before the end of the rainy season which occurs in September to October in northern Mali, *O. senegalensis* females begin to oviposit diapausing eggs, which spend the following dry season in pods approximately six centimetres beneath the surface of the soil. Diapause induction is caused by the short days ($<$L:D 12:12 h) and relatively cool temperatures (ca. 30$\pm$5 °C) which occur during this period (Diop 1993; Colvin and Cooter 1995).

Various estimates exist for the length of time that *O. senegalensis* eggs can remain in diapause. Saraiva (1962) provides anecdotal evidence that *O. senegalensis* eggs can survive in the soil for up to five years, although whether the eggs were in diapause or quiescent was not determined. Under laboratory conditions, Fishpool and Cheke (1983) found that roughly 2.6% of viable eggs remained in diapause for 2.7–3.6 years. Under field conditions in Niger, Popov (1980) found that by mid-March 90% of eggs had broken diapause and that it was merely the lack of adequate soil moisture which prevented the eggs from completing development. As a part of this study, egg-diapause duration was examined both in the laboratory and the field.

At the end of the rainy season in Mali, diapausing egg pods were collected and brought back to the Natural Resources Institute, UK, where they were maintained either at a constant 30 °C or an alternating temperature of 23 and 35 °C for 10 h and 14 h respectively. Over a 24-h period, therefore, both treatments had a mean temperature of 30 °C. Each month for the duration of the experiment, samples of ca. 30 egg pods from each treatment were wetted, and percentage eclosion was recorded.

Before the beginning of the rains in April and May of 1993 and 1994, fields were selected which had been ploughed at the start of the previous rainy season and egg pods were collected from them. These egg pods, therefore, had not been in the soil for longer than one year. Egg pods were wetted, and nymph emergence was recorded as above.

In both of these experiments, diapause in 90–100% of egg pods had broken by May, at the beginning of the following rainy season.

Rainfall and eclosion

Experiments at 30 °C in the laboratory have shown that, provided viable quiescent eggs receive sufficient water, embryonic development is continuous, leading to nymph emergence ca. 9 and 18 days later, respectively, from eggs that have broken diapause and those that were originally non-diapausing (Colvin and Cooter 1995).

Simulated rainfall experiments and grasshopper surveys in the field (see Burt et al. 1995) showed that *O. senegalensis* is adapted to resume development after a rainfall of as little as 8 mm. With quantities of rain lower than this, hopper emergence is likely to be less synchronous and in some pods may be delayed until the next rainstorm.

Egg pod predation

O. senegalensis eggs are attacked by several predatory spp. including larvae of the bombyliid fly, *Xeramoeba* nr. *oophaga* (Zakhvatkin); the meloid beetle, *Mylabris vicinalis* Marseul; and various tenebrionid spp. (Popov 1988). The level of egg mortality caused by these species can be very high, and in the 1977–78 dry season, for example, 58% ($n = 1340$) of egg pods sampled had been destroyed by natural enemies (Popov 1980). Surveys in northern Mali also revealed that in areas of egg pod densities of 20–40 egg pods m^{-2}, mortality due to *X. oophaga* alone reached 90–100% (Colvin, unpublished data). As pods can contain up to 36 eggs (Colvin and Cooter 1995), natural enemies obviously play an important role in determining *O. senegalensis* numbers and in preventing serious outbreaks.

An important difference between the life-history strategy of *O. senegalensis* and its major egg predator in northern Mali is that *X. oophaga* adults emerge in the laboratory irrespective of whether they experience wet conditions as pupae. As previously mentioned, quiescent *O. senegalensis* eggs will only resume embryonic development if they receive sufficient moisture. In the northern Sahel, therefore, the *X. oophaga* population would be expected to emerge each year irrespective of rainfall, whereas grasshopper emergence would be closely linked to both the quantity and distribution of rainfall.

Population model

A mathematical model was developed to examine the interactions between the *O. senegalensis* grasshopper population, the number of egg pods in the soil or "egg pod bank", the bombyliid predator population and rainfall. As a simplification, the model assumes the whole of the *O. senegalensis* population to occupy a single habitat, obviating the need to consider migration.

The model predicts that when periods of drought alternate with periods of good rains, grasshopper numbers oscillate with rainfall, whereas the predator population slowly dies out (Colvin and Holt, 1996). Under continuously good conditions, the predators play a significant role in determining the size of the grasshopper population, and the egg pod bank effectively disappears. The model also shows that the size of the egg pod bank does not affect the general principle that drought severity reduces predator efficacy. Large egg pod banks, however, improve predator survival during droughts, allowing the predators to reduce the size of the grasshopper outbreak when the good conditions return. After dry periods, the predator population always takes time to catch up with the grasshoppers, and therefore outbreaks inevitably occur after significant periods of drought (Colvin and Holt, 1996).

Discussion

This study suggests a possible mechanism underlying the development of major *O. senegalensis* outbreaks. It also provides an important contribution to future attempts at outbreak forecasting which egg pod surveys on their own cannot provide. For example, it would probably be concluded from the low numbers of viable egg pods in the soil after a period of drought that, when the good conditions return, there is no immediate danger of an outbreak occurring. The model, however, suggests that exactly the opposite may be true.

Rigorous validation of the model is difficult, mainly because *O. senegalensis* outbreaks prior to the late 1960s were rare (G.B. Popov, personal communication). Since then, however, the Sahel has experienced a period of below-average rainfall which has coincided with a significant increase in the frequency of outbreaks (Popov 1988; Cheke 1990; Maiga 1992). Arguably, the most serious and widespread of these occurred in 1974, when good rains fell over most of the Sahel, ending an extended period of pan-Sahelian drought (Popov 1988).

Acknowledgements
I am very grateful to Dr M. Sanghata, Dr B. Maiga and Moussa Sissoko of the Service de la Protection des Végétaux, Mali, for permission to work at Mourdiah and for their help with the experiments presented in this article. I also thank Dr Cooter for constructive criticism of the manuscript.

References

Burt PJA, Colvin J, Smith SM (1995) Forecasting the early-season eclosion of *Oedaleus senegalensis* in the Sahel: the role of remotely sensed rainfall data. Proceedings of the International Conference on new strategies in locust control. This volume

Cheke RA (1990) A migrant pest of the Sahel: the Senegalese grasshopper, *Oedaleus senegalensis*. Phil Trans R Soc Lond B 328: 539–553

Colvin J, Cooter RJ (1995) Diapause induction and colouration in the Senegalese grasshopper, *Oedaleus senegalensis*. Phys Ent 20: 13–17

Colvin J, Holt J (1996) Modèle d'étude des effets de la pluviométrie, de la prédation et de la quiescence des œufs sur la dynamique des populations du Criquet sénégalais, *Oedaleus senegalensis* . Sécheresse 7: 145–150

Diop T (1993) Observations préliminaires sur le role de la photopériode sur la diapause embryonnaire du criquet sénégalais, *Oedaleus senegalensis* (Krauss, 1877). Insect Sci Appl 14: 471–475

Fishpool LDC, Cheke RA (1983) Protracted eclosion and viability of *Oedaleus senegalensis* (Krauss) eggs (Orthoptera: Acrididae). Entomologist's Monthly Magazine 119: 215–219

Launois M (1978) Modélisation écologique et simulation opérationnelle en acridologie. Application à *Oedaleus senegalensis* (Krauss, 1877). Ministère de la Coopération, Paris, 212 pp

Maiga B (1992) Mali: notes on the acridid problem in Mali. Pages 82–85 in Lomer CJ, Prior, C (eds) Biological control of locusts and grasshoppers. Wallingford, UK, CAB International

Popov GB (1980) Studies on oviposition, egg development and mortality in *Oedaleus senegalensis* (Krauss) (Orthoptera: Acrididae) in the Sahel. Centre for Overseas Pest Research, Miscellaneous Report 53, 48 pp, London

Popov GB (1988) Sahelian Grasshoppers. Overseas Development Natural Resources Institute Bulletin, no 5, vi + 87 pp, London

Riley JR, Reynolds DR (1983) A long-range migration of grasshoppers observed in the Sahelian zone of Mali by two radars. J Anim Ecol 52: 167–183

Saraiva AC (1962) Plague locusts – *Oedaleus senegalensis* (Krauss) and *Schistocerca gregaria* (Forsk.) – in the Cape Verde Islands. Estudos Agronomicos 3: 61–89

New Strategies in Locust Control
S. Krall, R. Peveling and D. Ba Diallo (eds)
© 1997 Birkhäuser Verlag Basel/Switzerland

Modelling brown locust outbreaks in relation to rainfall and temperature

S.A. Hanrahan and D. Horne

University of the Witwatersrand, Department of Zoology, Johannesburg, Wits 2050, South Africa

Summary. A simulation model of its population dynamics was constructed to aid understanding brown locust outbreaks. Known details of the life history of the brown locust have been synthesised into a rule-based model which generates changes in population size in response to rainfall and temperature. Simulated outbreaks for particular areas have been compared to numbers of brown locust swarms reported destroyed during control operations in the same period.

Résumé. Le biomodèle sur la dynamique des populations du Criquet brun a été mis au point pour mieux connaître le mécanisme des invasions de ce locuste. Les détails sur le cycle de vie du Criquet brun ont été synthétisés dans un modèle basé sur des règles de décision et générant des modifications de la taille des populations en fonction des précipitations et des températures. Des invasions simulées pour des zones particulières ont été comparées au nombre d'essaims de Criquets bruns qui selon les rapports obtenus ont été décimés lors d'opérations de lutte conduites durant la même période.

Introduction

The brown locust, *Locustana pardalina* (Walker), has outbreak areas in the semi-arid Karoo region of South Africa (Lounsbury 1915; Du Plessis 1938; Lea 1958). Under suitable plague conditions swarms have spread into the northern grain-producing areas of South Africa and neighbouring countries of Namibia and Botswana. Chemical control has been used to attempt to contain the swarms within the outbreak areas. Locust control by farmers is enforced by law, but is the financial responsibility of the government. Although the government bears the cost, the actual implementation of control procedures is carried out by farmers who are supplied with insecticide and reimbursed for all expenses, a system that encourages spending.

Details of brown locust life cycle have recently been reviewed (Price 1988; Nailand and Hanrahan 1993). The brown locust is remarkably well adapted to its semi-arid environment, particularly in the development of the egg stage (Matthee 1951). Eggs can remain viable for long periods in dry soil, where they become quiescent and suspend development. They are able to absorb moisture from the soil if light rains fall, returning to the quiescent state a number of times should conditions become dry. Diapause eggs exposed to wet conditions enter a deeper level of diapause broken by as yet unquantified factors. Once diapause has ended, at least 5% of the diapause eggs do not hatch under favourable conditions but remain viable for at least 12 months (Botha 1967). Rainfall is thus a key factor in egg viability and egg development. Outbreaks were first associated with rainfall in 1915 (Loundsbury) and have been noted to follow periods of drought (Smit 1939; Lea 1958). Price (1988) suggested that swarms arise after a build-up of solitary forms which lay proportionately more diapause eggs (Mathee 1951). Egg numbers increase prior to winter because hatching is limited, or after prolonged dry periods, so that when adequate rains fall there is large-scale hatching.

Few studies have systematically recorded locust numbers in the field (Smit 1939; Lea 1969). Numbers of swarms eradicated have been recorded by magisterial district, areas of many hundreds of square kilometres. Du Plessis (1937, 1938) and Lea (1968) used number of magisterial districts recording swarms and expenditure on control as a measure of the outbreak size. This is a very crude record of swarm activity, and the pattern is not sufficiently regular for accurate prediction of outbreaks. Considerable success has been achieved in modelling locust populations and life cycle (Wright 1987; Symmons et al. 1981; Reus and Symmons 1992). Given the wealth of biological information about the brown locust and the limited surveillance and field information about swarming activity, this seemed to be an ideal area in which to develop a simulation model.

Our aim was to develop a model to simulate the brown locust life cycle and establish changes in population number based on climate data, and to use the model to test sensitivity of key factors in swarm development and decline.

Methods

Model formulation

A simulation model of a brown locust population based on its life cycle was constructed (Nailand and Hanrahan 1993) using a rule-based decision system (Starfield and Bleloch 1991). This first version of the model used Turbo Pascal language but was found to be inadequate because of memory requirements. The model presented here is a modification of the Nailand-Hanrahan version and is run on Mathsworks Matlab with Simulink under Windows. Program development under Matlab is significantly faster than with Pascal. Matlab has the advantage of using memory only as it is needed and can be run on a 486 PC. The Simulink simulation software allows one to visualise the model operation through the layout graphics and adjust the parameters during a simulation, without having to recompile code. It is possible to optimise the model parameters without knowing how to write source code.

The model was based on the locust life cycle, which was divided into discrete egg, hopper and adult classes. Known biological data were formulated into 'rules' to govern development of locusts in each class and define the conditions that have to be met for an individual to progress to the next stage of its life cycle. This information was gathered from literature and from observations by Dr D. Brown and his staff, Locust Research Unit, Institute for Plant Protection, Pretoria. Each stage also has simulation parameters, i.e., fixed values based on the biological information. The rule-base or decision-making code has been written as a set of Matlab functions. The model takes the environmental inputs on each day and tests the individuals with the rules to decide if they are ready to graduate to the next class.

Model 'inputs' are rainfall, which is regarded as the driving variable for transitions between egg stages and sustained egg viabilty and hatching, and temperature, which determines the rate of hopper and adult maturation. Raw climate data is processed in 'starting' files and manipulated before the model is run. The number of days that the soil could be expected to be wet after different amounts of rainfall is an example of one of the factors calculated. The starting file also uses the temperature data to calculate the degree day contribution of each day. A linear triangulation assumption is used, and the degree days are calculated from maximum and minimum air and soil temperature values (Zalom et al. 1983). Smit (1939) estimated mortality over the life cycle to be as high as 96%, with highest levels occurring in the early instars.

Actual simulations

To test the model, actual rainfall and temperature data sets from four widely spread stations, namely Middelburg, Pofadder, Graaff Reinet and Douglas, were used as model input. These results were compared with the numbers of hopper bands reported destroyed by the Directorate of Resource Conservation. Rainfall provides a very clear stimulus for egg hatching. At Middelburg and Graaff Reinet its pattern is complex, and falls are rare at Pofadder and Douglas.

The model was tested by running the climate data at the four different stations with different model parameters and comparing the results with known field data. It was possible to follow all stages of the life cycle, but for graphing purposes numbers of hoppers were totalled for each month of the outbreak season and adults were ignored.

Results

Some of the results obtained are presented in Figure 1. No single set of model parameters gave
equally good simulation results at all stations. It was found that in the dry Douglas and
Pofadder areas a mortality rate of 95% was far too high and hopper numbers increased only if
mortality dropped to 70%, whereas in Middelburg 95% mortality allowed for dramatic population increases. Use of soil temperatures to calculate egg development improved the match to real

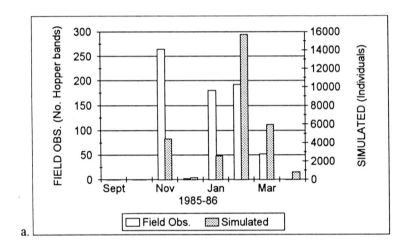

a.

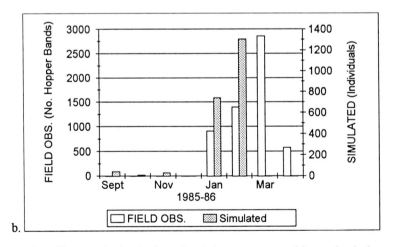

b.

Figure 1. Number of hoppers simulated using soil and air temperatures and hopper bands destroyed during
1985–1986 season. a = Middelburg; b = Pofadder.

data in Middelburg, but far better simulation was achieved in Douglas when all calculations were made on air temperatures only. Previous work indicated that 14 °C (Smit 1941) was the temperature at which development of eggs ceased. Trial and error showed that 14 °C was too low as the lower threshold and best results were obtained by using 20 °C. This figure had also been suggested by Price from personal observations.

Conclusions

Even in this very simplistic form the model was able to predict a pattern of increase and decrease in locust numbers in all four areas to a greater or lesser degree. More assessment is required to sort out the significance of different factors on locusts living under different environmental conditions and poor quality data used as input. For example, with no organised system of locust monitoring in place, locust swarms may not have been recorded in these vast unpopulated areas even though they may have been present. Recorded rainfall events may have been very localised and may not have occurred in areas where the egg beds were present. More accurate data will be available, as map co-ordinates are now being used in the recording of locust swarms and we have access to data from additional weather stations.

Areas that could benefit from further research and therefore provide more reliable input are the following. The survival rate under different rainfall and therefore different vegetation cover requires further study. The water-holding capacity of the soil after rain has important implications for egg development and could vary greatly from station to station with differing soil types. The details of egg diapause and sensitivities of the embryo in catatrepsis need to be determined accurately.

The model succeeds as a compilation of biological and climate data used to drive change in population size but has serious shortcomings if it is to be considered as a tool for prediction of swarming events. No attempt has been made to deal with generation of real swarming numbers. An indication of increase and decrease in number does not automatically imply that swarm formation will occur. Major events other than changes in rainfall and temperature still need to be included, for example emigration and immigration factors.

Acknowledgements
The authors would like to acknowledge the following: Dr H.D. Brown, Mr R.E. Price of the Locust Research Unit, Institute for Plant Protection, for data and advice; the South African Weather Bureau for rainfall and temperature data; the Climatology Research Group of the University of the Witwatersrand for processed rainfall data; Mr I. G. Venter of the Directorate of Resource Conservation for information on locust swarms destroyed; Mr P. Hanrahan for assisting with the Matlab conversion; Dr J. Magor for discussion, encouragement and funding; the University of the Witwatersrand for research funding.

References

Botha DH (1967) The viability of brown locust eggs *Locustana pardalina* (Walk.) S Afr J Agric Sci 10: 445–460

Du Plessis C (1937) Economic importance of the locust problem in the Union of South Africa and South West Africa. 4th Int. Loc. Conf., Cairo, approx. 46 pp

Du Plessis C (1938) The influence of weather conditions on the incipient swarming of the brown locust, *Locustana pardalina* (Walker). Sci Bull Dep Agric Un S Afr 186: 1–60

Lea A (1958) Recent outbreaks of the brown locust, *Locustana pardalina* (Walk.),with special reference to the influence of rainfall. J Ent Soc Sth Afr 21: 162–213

Lea A (1968) Natural regulation and artificial control of brown locust numbers. J Ent Soc Sth Afr 31: 97–112

Lea A (1969) The distribution and abundance of brown locusts, *Locustana pardalina* (Walker), between 1954 and 1965. J Ent Soc Sth Afr 32: 367–398

Lounsbury CP (1915) Some phases of the locust problem. S Afr J Sci 11: 33–45

Matthee JJ (1951) The structure and physiology of the egg of *Locustana pardalina* (Walk.) Sci Bull Dept Agric, S Afr 316: 1–83

Nailand P, Hanrahan SA (1993) Modelling brown locust, *Locustana pardalina*, outbreaks in the Karoo. S A J Science 89: 420–424

Price RE (1988) The life cycle of the brown locust, with reference to egg viability. Pages 27–40 in McKenzie B, Longridge M (eds) Proceedings of the Locust Symposium, Kimberley, 1987. South African Institute of Ecologists Bulletin Special Issue

Reus J, Symmons PM (1992) A model to predict the incubation and nymphal development periods of the desert locust, *Schistocerca gregaria* (Orthoptera: Acrididae). Bull Ent Res 82: 517–520

Smit CJB (1939) Field observations on the brown locust in an outbreak area. Sci Bull Dep Agric of Un S Afr 6: 1–48

Smit CJB (1941) Forecasts of incipient outbreaks of the brown locust. J Ent Soc Sth Afr 4: 206–221

Starfield AM, Bleloch AL (1991) Building models for conservation and wildlife management. 2nd ed, Minnesota, Burgess International

Symmons PM, McCulloch L, Balogh C (1981) A model to estimate incubation and nymphal development from daily temperatures and rainfall. Pages 6–8 in Plague Locust Commission Annual Report Research Supplement *1979–1980*. Canberra: Australian Plague Locust Commission

Wright DE (1987) Analysis of the development of major plagues of the Australian plague locust *Chortoicetes terminifera* (Walker) using a simulation model. Aust J Ecol 12: 423–437

Zalom FG, Goodell PB, Wilson LT, Barnett NW, Bentley WJ (1983) Degree days: the calculation and use of heat units in pest management. Div Ag and Nat Res, University of California Leaflet 21373, 10 pp

New Strategies in Locust Control
S. Krall, R. Peveling and D. Ba Diallo (eds)
© 1997 Birkhäuser Verlag Basel/Switzerland

Metapopulations of locusts and grasshoppers: spatial structures, their dynamics and early warning systems

M.G. Sergeev

Department of General Biology, Novosibirsk State University, 2 Pirogova Street, Novosibirsk 630090 Russia, and Institute for Systematic and Ecology of Animals, Siberian Branch of Russian Academy of Sciences, 11 Frunze Street, Novosibirsk 630091 Russia

Summary. A metapopulation analysis allows us to distinguish acridid groups with similar relations to ecological factors, including landscape heterogeneity, to determine the possible paths and barriers for dispersion and to describe landscape differences in dynamic patterns. The boundaries between the different parts of a metapopulation seem to be very distinct. Often movements of grasshoppers (including good flyers) are limited by the frontiers of the local landscape.

Résumé. L'analyse des metapopulations permet à distinguer les groupes des acridiens avec ressemblant relations à facteurs écologiques, dont notamment hétérogénéité des paysages, déterminer les voies possible et barrières de diffusion et décrire les différences de paysage en régularités dynamiques. Il se suppose que les frontières entre différents parts des metapopulations sont très distincts. Souvent déplacements des acridiens, dont notamment bien volants, limitent par les frontières des paysages local.

Introduction

Many problems of modern biogeography and ecology may be solved by studying population distributions over species ranges. A number of classic papers (Richards and Waloff 1954; Uvarov 1977) considered not only the internal structures of some local populations but also their dynamics and inner organisation. As a rule, local populations (dems) are distributed over a range in accordance with natural conditions, especially landscape structures. Exchange usually occurs via migrant individuals, but a level of gene flow is often determined by different barriers (mountains, rivers, boundaries between terraces etc.). This kind of population distribution is called a *metapopulation* (Levins 1970) or a *spatial population structure* (Shilov 1977) and thus describes a system of local populations of a species within the limits of its range (area). This approach is expected to be very useful both for general ecology and biogeography of locusts and grasshoppers and for developing early warning systems. Uvarov (1977: 445) emphasized "both the environmental factors and the biological properties of a species are variable in time and space, so that their mutual relations can be understood only by systematic studies of populations of a species in all its stages throughout its total distribution area, usually comprising a range of habitats, and extending over a period of years. Such an approach is difficult in practice, but this should not be a reason for abandoning it as an ideal goal." To date, the principal spatial organisation, especially the dynamics, of species metapopulations remains unknown, because to solve this problem we have to establish where population structures, including inter- and intrapopulation boundaries of different ranks and migration paths, are located and how and why they change in space and time.

Material and methods

The samples were collected from 1976 to 1992 in southern Siberia, Kazakhstan, Kirgizstan, Uzbekistan, Turkmenistan, Tajikistan and the North Caucasus. Two methods were mainly adapted for abundance estimation: capturing individual insects for a fixed time with a net (Gause 1930; Kashkarov 1933; Sergeev 1986), and estimating densities in small sample plots during a survey (Kashkarov 1933; Riegert 1968). A sample area and time could vary in different landscape units and were limited by landscape unit area. Usually insects were caught for 10–40 min with a standard net within 200–500 m^2 and densities were estimated over an area of 25 m^2. About 200,000 specimens belonging to 338 species of Orthoptera were analysed. These were collected during 3000 quantitative surveys using nets. We exclude data for outbreaks.

Calliptamus italicus (L.) (the Italian Locust) and *Chorthippus parallelus* (Zett.) have been chosen as the main model species. Both are the common and abundant species of the Palaearctic. The former is mainly connected with the semi-desert biotopes of the Mediterranean and Central Asia; the latter is distributed over the meadows and meadow steppes of Europe, and North and Central Asia.

Spatial structures and metapopulations of model species

We have peviously described the four principal parts of a distribution area (range) of a species (Stebaev and Sergeev 1982; Sergeev 1986; Stebaev et al. 1989; Kazakova and Sergeev 1992): (1) the *main part*, within the limits of which a species is distributed in abundance over all available habitats (the optimum of a range) (Fig. 1, H); (2) the *transitional part* (K) associated with the beginning of population dismemberment (bifurcation) into the watershed and valley colonies; (3) the *basic part* (C), where the species populations are found over watershed plains and flood plains or/and low terraces, sometimes over watersheds only, species abundance may be

i   ii

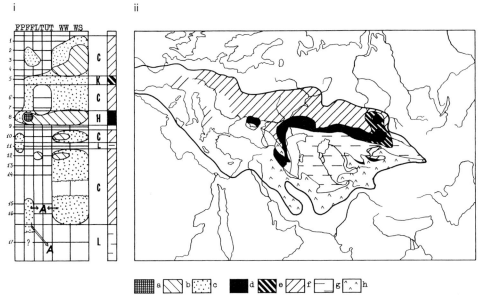

Figure 1. Colony distribution of *C. italicus* (i, landscape scheme for the eastern part of the range along the profile from Omsk to South Tajikistan; ii, map of general metapopulation structure).

a–c   levels of abundance (a, more than 0.5; b, 0.1–0.5; c, less than 0.1 per square metre);
d–h   parts of range (d, main; e, transitional; f, basic; g, marginal; h, montane)
A   spreading through anthropogenic ecosystems;
H, K, C, L   parts of range (see text);
FP   low flood-plains; FF, upper flood-plains; LT, low and UT, upper terraces; WW and WS, watershed plains (WW, upland; WS, non-drained plains);
1–17   investigated transects (1, northern steppe; 2–4, typical steppes; 5, southern steppe; 6–8, semi-deserts; 9–14, northern deserts; 15–17, southern deserts).

high locally; (4) the *marginal part* (L) characterized by connection of colonies with flood plains and low terraces, and insular or linear populations. Although not always the case, both model species (*C. italicus* and *C. parallelus*) have a well-described population structure with a full set of distribution area parts (cf. Stebaev and Sergeev 1982; Stebaev et al. 1989; Kazakova and Sergeev 1992).

C. *italicus* is a common species in the Mediterranean and the semi-deserts and the deserts of Central and East Asia (Fig. 1). Many outbreaks have occurred in these areas and in the neighbouring steppes and mountains. Comparison of a set of transects including a number of sample plots from the local watershed plain to the flood plain allows us to describe the distribution pattern of *C. italicus* colonies along the profile from Omsk in South Siberia to Dusti in South Tajikistan (Fig. 1.i).

The main part (H) of the species range is in the limits of the semi-desert zone (Fig. 1.i, 8). There is its optimum where many outbreaks have been observed intermittently. As a rule, species abundance is great. The transitional part (K) is situated in the southern steppe (Fig. 1.i, 5) and the basic ones – in the northern and typical steppes (1–4), the semi-deserts (partly) (6, 7) and the deserts (partly) (10, 12–16). Here the populations of *C. italicus* are associated with watersheds, the slopes of low mountains, and sometimes with dry parts of low terraces (e.g. natural levees or scroll dunes). Species abundance may be high locally. Sometimes the outbreaks may be observed. The marginal part (L) of the range is observed in some deserts of Central Asia where the species colonies are distributed over flood plains (including meadows) and low terraces (Fig. 1.i, 11, 17). In agricultural landscapes, *C. italicus* usually spreads through irrigated fields (especially alfalfa) (Fig. 1.i, A). Outbreaks may develop.

Comparison of this profile with additional profiles and some published data (see Sergeev 1986) permits us to create a map of the general metapopulation structure of *C. italicus* (Fig. 1.ii). The local optima of *C. italicus* are in the sandy steppes of western Siberia and the Irtysh River basin and in the piedmont plains of the Tien Shan Mountains. The basic parts of its metapopulation are chiefly confined to the steppes, to the European forest-steppes and forests (partly), and also to the Mediterranean region. In the Turanian Plain, *C. italicus* mainly inhabits river valleys. In mountain regions, *C. italicus* often inhabits the local southern slopes. These population groups are isolated from the populations of the plain. An especially significant difference is observed in the southern part of Central Asia where two subspecies of *C. italicus* coexist: short-winged *C. i. reductus* (in the mountains) and normal *C. i. italicus*.

The metapopulation structure of *C. parallelus* was described by Kazakova and Sergeev (1992). This species has a comparatively correct pattern of colony distribution with an optimum in the northern steppes, and thus is suitable for spatial extrapolations. On the other hand, *C. italicus* has some additional local optima (Fig. 1), and its metapopulation should be studied more closely.

Spatial features of dynamics

Dynamic patterns are variable in the different parts of species ranges. This is true both for locusts and for grasshoppers. For example, in the northern Siberian steppes, maximum grasshopper abundance usually occurs in the middle of summer. But in the southern steppes, semi-deserts and deserts, it may be at the beginning of summer. Both in central Yakutia and in the steppe, forest-steppe and semi-desert regions, outbreaks of non-swarming grasshoppers and *C. italicus* (in the steppes and the semi-deserts) begin after droughts. In the deserts, the outbreaks are chiefly connected with above-average annual precipitation, especially with spring rains. Our unpublished data allow us to propose that the beginning of each outbreak is usually confined to a definite type of microhabitat. For example, *C. italicus* is clearly associated with sagebrush plots in the steppes and semi-deserts and with highly localised meadow flood plains in the deserts.

Our data also allow us to propose that the dynamics of *C. italicus* and grasshoppers may be very different in neighbouring habitats (Sergeev et al. 1988; Sergeev, unpublished data; see also Kopaneva and Dorokhova 1987). It is unlikely to result from species migrations, because the majority of species do not significantly change their local habitat distribution during seasons and years (Sobolev and Sergeev 1985). In central Kazakhstan, in non-outbreak years, the local movements of *C. italicus* are mainly connected with male wanderings. Often, observing individuals in unusual habitats is simply the result of their moving from one favourable site to another (Sobolev and Sergeev 1985).

Conclusions

Distribution of biotopes available for grasshoppers and locusts allows them to inhabit regions and landscape units (including anthropogenic) more or less widely but mainly not at random. On the other hand, important eco-geographical barriers are essential not only for limiting the spreading of whole species but also for metapopulation differentiation. In addition, observed patterns may change essentially at various scales of study. The general results of insecticide application by an aerosol fogger are evidently and strongly associated with spatial heterogeneity of species colonies (Sobolev and Sergeev 1985; Sergeev et al. 1988). So creating a system of early warning thus requires studying the spatial and temporal variations of the landscape and the geographical units inhabited by the metapopulation of each species. Investigations should be long-term and should also examine the organisation of acridid communities. The current emphasis on outbreaks needs to be supplemented with study of conditions between outbreaks, especially in connection with the organisation of populations and communities in space and time.

Acknowledgements
I am most grateful for fruitful discussion of these ideas with A. Emeljanov, K. Gorodkov, A. Joern, O. Kryzhanovskij, J. Lockwood, M. Samways, and I. Stebaev. I thank the State Committee for High Education (Russian Federation) (Programme "Universities of Russia" and grant B-42-4) and the State Programme for "Biological Diversity" (grant 1.19) for vital financial support. I appreciate an anonymous referee's careful reading of the manuscript, which greatly improved its readability and content.

References

Gause GF (1930) Studies on the ecology of the Orthoptera. Ecology 11: 307–325
Kashkarov DN (1933) Environment and community. Moscow: Gosmedgiz, 244 pp (in Russian)
Kazakova IG, Sergeev MG (1992) Spatial organisation of species populations system of short-horned grasshopper *Chorthippus parallelus*. Zhournal Obstshej Biologii 53: 373–383 (in Russian)
Kopaneva LM, Dorokhova GY (1987) Population dynamics of non-gregarious locusts and *Calliptamus* L. in the mountains of Kirgizia. Pages 51–57 in Shumakov EM (ed) Saranchovye - ecologia i mery borjby. Leningrad: VIZR
Levins R (1970) Extinction. Pages 77–107 in Gustenhaver (ed) Some mathematical questions in biology. Vol 2. Providence, Rhode Island
Richards OW, Waloff N (1954) Studies on the ecology and population dynamics of British grasshoppers. Anti-Locust Bulletin 17: 1–182
Riegert PM (1968) A history of grasshoper abundance surveys and forecast of outbreaks in Saskatchewan. Memoir of Entomological Society of Canada 52: 3–99
Sergeev MG (1986) Patterns of Orthoptera distribution in North Asia. Novosibirsk: Nauka, 237 pp (in Russian)
Sergeev MG, Bugrov AG, Kazakova IG, Sobolev NN (1988) Regulation of population dynamics of grasshoppers in agrocoenoses with aid of the aerosol fogger. Pages 63–69 in Zolotarenko GS (ed) Landshaftnaja ecologia nasekomyh. Novosibirsk: Nauka (in Russian)
Shilov IA (1977) Ecologo-physiological base of population relations of animals. Moscow: University Press, 262 pp (in Russian)
Sobolev NN, Sergeev MG (1985) Population dynamics of grasshoppers in the agrocoenoses of North Kazakhstan. Pages 96–104 in Zolotarenko GS (ed) Antropogennye vozdejstvija na soobstshestva nasekomyh. Novosibirsk: Nauka (in Russian)
Stebaev IV, Murav'eva VM, Sergeev MG (1989) Ecological standards of Orthoptera in herbaceous biotopes in the Far East. Entomological Review 68 (2): 1–10 (English translation)
Stebaev IV, Sergeev MG (1982) The internal landscape-population structure of area, as exemplified by Acrididae. Zhurnal Obstshej Biologii 43 (2): 399–410 (in Russian)
Uvarov BP (1977) Grasshoppers and locusts: a handbook of general acridology. Vol 2. London: Centre for Overseas Pest Research, 613 pp

New Strategies in Locust Control
S. Krall, R. Peveling and D. Ba Diallo (eds)
© 1997 Birkhäuser Verlag Basel/Switzerland

Forecasting seasonal dynamics of the Asiatic migratory locust using the *Locusta migratoria migratoria* – *Phragmites australis* forecasting system

A.G. Antonov and V.E. Kambulin

Kazakh Scientific Research Institute of Plant Protection, P.O. Box 483117, Almaty, Republic of Kazakhstan

Summary. Many species of grasshoppers and locusts cause economic damage in Kazakhstan. In 1992 the authors formulated a seasonal dynamics model, describing behaviour of the Asiatic migratory locust, *Locusta migratoria migratoria,* and the *Phragmites australis* system in the Balkhash-Alacol basin. This paper presents the computer model used in forecasting locust development stages, density, population trends, estimate of potential forage losses and production for *L. m. migratoria.* Such forecasting allows to decide when to spray and to optimise the date of application and size of target area and to minimise the environmental impact.

Résumé. De nombreuses espèces de sauteriaux et de criquets causent des dommages économiques au Kazakhstan. En 1992, les auteurs ont élaboré un modèle de dynamique saisonnière, décrivant le comportement du criquet migrateur asiatique, *Locusta migratoria migratoria,* et le système écologique *Phragmites australis,* dans le Bassin Balkhash-Alacol. Cette publication présente le modèle de simulation informatique utilisé pour la pré-vision des phases de développement des criquets, de la densité et de l'évolution des populations, de l'estimation des pertes de fourrage et de production agricole pour *L. m. migratoria.* De telles prévisions nous permettent de décider quand pulvériser et d'optimiser les dates d'application et la superficie traitée et de minimiser l'impact sur l'environnement.

Introduction

The Republic of Kazakhstan occupies an area of about 2.8 million km^2, situated in the following geographical zones: forest-steppe and steppe (27% of the area), semi-desert (22%), desert (40%) and mountainous regions (11%). More than 180 million ha of natural rangeland is utilised for fodder for livestock breeding. The greater part of this area is situated in the arid zone, where desertification has resulted from intensive land use.

Active reclamation of land for agricultural use has considerably reduced the natural vegetation, and in common with other factors, has impacted negatively on species diversity and abundance of insects, including locusts, whose natural habitat has become reduced. However, these changes have not reduced the economic importance of locusts, their main centres of breeding remaining unaffected. In recent years the importance of the phytobiont economic grasshoppers, such as *Dociostaurus, Chorthippus* and *Stenobolthrus,* and the phytogeobiont species, *Oedaleus deco-rus* and *Calliptamus italicus,* have actually increased. The natural cycle typical for *C. italicus, D. maroccanus* and *Locusta migratoria migratoria,* which produces periodic widespread outbreaks, suggests that the locust and grasshopper problem in Kazakhstan has not lost its economic significance.

In 1988–1994, 87% of locust and grasshopper control in the Commenwealth of Independent States (CIS, former USSR) occurred in Kazakhstan. Large-scale pest control measures have mainly been carried out by aerial treatments using different chemicals. This has resulted in increased pesticide contamination of treated areas, sometimes beyond acceptable limits. In recent years, because of escalating costs of aircraft hire, fuel and costs of chemicals (the last purchased in US dollars), the costs of control have risen sharply, and it is therefore necessary to re-examine the problem.

At the same time, analysis has shown that locust control operations were inefficient. In fact, the area infested expanded despite control, and existing control methods only provided a temporary reduction in locust populations. Large-scale chemical treatments adversely affected the natural enemy complex, thus creating good conditions for pest resurgence in the future. It was therefore concluded:

- The existing level of forecasting locust outbreaks and the methods of control have serious shortcomings.
- The absence of a scientific database and proper monitoring network of locust breeding sites is the main reason for the current situation.

Simulation models of the dynamics of natural systems form an integral part of monitoring and include complex mutually influencing factors factors such as natural climatic conditions, food plants, locust populations and anthropogenic factors. The successful realisation of such computer models is dependent on the corresponding input of information for forecasting the state of natural systems at any given date to plan future management strategies for pest control.

In recent years, simulation models have proven effective instruments for operational evaluation of the phenology and seasonal dynamics of locusts (Capinera et al. 1982; Dennis and Kemp 1988; Berry et al. 1991). The negative significance of locusts in Kazakhstan for non-gregarious grasshopper species has been repeatedly discussed and experimentally demonstrated (Serkova 1961; Kambulin and Bugayev 1982; Dormidontova 1987; Starostyn and Shumakov 1987). Concerning the gregarious locust species, damage has obviously expanded (Popov 1987). Nevertheless, during the course of several years a model describing the seasonal dynamics of the *L. m. migratoria – Phragmites australis* system both under natural conditions and under the influence of anthropogenic factors has been developed by the authors (Kambulin 1989; Antonov and Kambulin 1992).

Material and methods

The Asiatic migratory locust in Kazakhstan occurs on the coastal delta parts of large basins, such as the Caspian and Arals Seas and Lakes Balkhash, Alakol and Sasykhol, where it inhabits reed (*P. australis*) thickets. The main reason for creating a model was for short-term forecasting of the number of locusts and probable loss of reeds as well as recommending control measures, and correlating this with locust ecology and economics.

To some extent the task of simulating the dynamics of the system has been made easier for following reasons:

- In simulating the districts, the reed thickets usually grow as pure communities and are preferred by all stages of development of the Asiatic migratory locust.
- No other species of locust is as abundant in these reed communities. There is thus no competition for food.
- Because of the relatively few districts utilised by people, simulating the anthropogenic influence on the system is restricted to the impact of insecticides on the pest population and their impact on the environment.

The model consists of several sections: the main section simulates the seasonal dynamics of *L. m. migratoria* population from the start of egg development, after diapause, up to death of the adults in autumn. A second section determines the yield of biomass of the food plant *P. australis*, while a third simulates chemical control measures. A fourth section simulates ecological and economic after-effects (evaluation of the simulated processes can be distinguished).

In the beginning of the model's run, fine-tuning of the parameters was required for setting the fixed lots. Such characteristics as soil type on a lot, depth of groundwater and degree of mineralisation, size of the reed community and calorific value of the unit of dry plant biomass, average value sets of daily air temperature over many years, and analogous sets for the heat quantity of the air and other sets are given.

For determining the expected reed productivity on the lot, the following formula is used (Plisak 1981): $h = a_0 + a_1 x_1 + a_2 x_2 + a_3 x_3 + a_4 x_4 + a_5 x_5$, where x_1 = layering depth of groundwater on the lot, x_2 = mineralisation of the groundwater, x_3 = stock of moisture in soil layer $0-100$ cm, x_4 = salt store in the same layer, x_5 = average weighed summary effect of toxic ions in the $0-100$ cm layer, and the value of a_0, a_1, a_2, a_3, a_4 and a_5 coefficients depends on the type of soil on the lot. The total yield of reeds on the lot is determined by the formula $H = h\, S_{rd}$, where S_{rd} is area of the reed community. In the simulation of the seasonal dynamics of migratory locust populations, that fact is taken as a baseline, which in the process passes through a number of developmental stages, such as hatching of $1-5$ nymphal instars, wing formation, mating, ovipositing etc. Each stage is characterised by the beginning date, d_i, and duration, l_i. Mutual disposition of dates on the temporary axis d relative to each other can be introduced by the next step:

$$\underrightarrow{d_0 \quad d_1 \quad d_2 \quad d_3 \quad d_4 \quad d_5 \quad d_6 \quad d_7 \quad d_8 \quad d_9 \quad d_{10} \quad d_{11} \quad d_{12} \quad d_{13} \quad d_{14} \quad d_{15}} \ d \quad (1)$$

where d_0 = date of the spring passing of average daily temperatures through 0 °C, d_j = date of the beginning of jth instar nymph hatching ($1 \leq j \leq 5$), d_6 = date of the beginning of wing formation, d_7 = date of the beginning of imago mating, d_{k+7} = date of the beginning of kth oviposition ($1 \leq k \leq 7$), d_{15} = date of the autumn death of adults (depending on the fixed natural-climatic conditions, where such situations occur when d_{15} comes before one of the preceding dates).

The dates d_1-d_{14} are given by the formula:

$$d_j = d_{j-1} + D_j \ (1 \leq j \leq 14) \quad (2)$$

where D_j = number of the days between d_{j-1} and d_j. The value of D_j can be calculated by one of three methods, based on the accuracy, complexity and required amount of initial data. In the first method for deriving D_j the mean duration of the corresponding interstage period for this district is computed.

The second method is based on the sum of average daily temperatures. For the period from the date d_j to the date d_{j-1}, the sum of average daily air temperatures, or the "degree days" passed, is T_j. In this case

$$D_j = k_{T_j} T_j = k_{T_j} \sum_i t_i \quad (3)$$

where t_i = mean daily temperatures, and k_{T_j} = coefficient of transferring degree-days into days.

The third method is based on the quantity of heat in the air. As in the second method, the sum of average daily heat, Q_j, is computed for the period from d_{j-1} to d_j (Kambulin 1989). Thus

$$D_j = k_{Q_j} Q_j = k_{Q_j} \sum_i q_i \quad (4)$$

where q_i = mean daily heat content, and k_{Q_j} = coefficient of transferring kilogram-calories/kilogram into days. Because it is based on experimental data, the third method is the most exact, but it is also the most labourious and requires more data than the others (Dinasilov 1995).

Duration of periods l_j, beginning at a date d_j ($1 \le j \le 14$), is calculated analogously. Along with weather conditions, it depends both upon the fixed physico-geographical peculiarities of the simulated lot (latitude and longitude, relief, altitude) and on insect physiology. Different methods of calculation may be used both on the alternative base and jointly.

In simulating the Asiatic migratory locust population dynamics during the period from the beginning of 1st instar nymph hatching up to the end of wing formation, its state on date d ($d_1 \le d \le d_6 + l_6$) is characterised by the number, age structure and by the area occupied.

As noted before, the existing period of ith instar locusts ($1 \le i \le 6$) in the simulated population depends on a series of factors, and duration is $d_i - d_{i-1} + l_i$ days. Hatching of this instar occurs in the first l_i days and passage into the ($i + 1$)th instar in the last l_{i+1} days. The model is based on the assumption that an even proportion (l / l_i) of ith instar hatches every day. Thus, up to the simulated date in the population model, several instars may be present simultaneously, with the following parameters: number, survival and quantity of reeds eaten. The number of ith instar on a day d is

$$N_i(d) = b_i [N_i(d-1) + n_{i-1}(d-1) - n_i(d-1)] \qquad (5)$$

where $n_i(d-1)$ = number of ($i-1$)th instars hatched during the course of the previous day, and the coefficient b_i is calculated on the base of corresponding survival coefficients for ith instar. Having summed up the obtained values for all instars in the population to date d, we obtain the total population by determining its instar structure and weighted mean instar.

The daily food requirement f_i of the ith instar individual with a mass m_i is determined by the next formula (Stoljarov 1975; Antonov and Kambulin 1992):

$$f_i = 16.5 \, m_i^{3/4} k_e k_c k_a / K_{rd} \qquad (6)$$

where k_e = the coefficient of energy exchange of the active individual, k_c = the coefficient of food consumption, k_a = the coefficient of food assimilation and K_{rd} = the caloricity of unit dry mass of reeds on the simulated lot. The total loss of reeds from the population $F(d)$ on a day d will thus be

$$F(d) = \sum_i f_i N_i(d) = 16.5 \, k_e k_c k_a / K_{rd} \sum_i m_i^{3/4} N_i(d) \qquad (7)$$

Having summed up the everyday yield losses from date d_1 up to date d, we can forecast both the absolute and the relative damage caused by locusts to this day. The economic loss can be calculated both by value and its effect on live stock production (meat in this case).

The average daily area $S(d)$ occupied to date d is

$$S(d) = S(d-1) + R(d-1) \qquad (8)$$

where the adherence of area $R(d-1)$ for the previous day is calculated on the basis of the coefficient of expanding area. For such a case, when the locust populations exceed density and area thresholds (Tsyplenkov 1970), the possibility of migration is foreseen.

The period from the beginning of mating to death in autumn $(d_7 \leq d < \leq d_{15})$ simulates the development of the locust population, when during the period from d_{k+7} until $d_{k+7} + l_{k+7}$ surviving female locusts oviposit kth egg pods ($1 \leq k \leq 7$).

Assuming that sex ratio in the population is 1 and the process of oviposition takes place evenly, redoubling the number of females $N_{k+7}(d)$, oviposited kth and non-oviposited $(k+1)$th egg pods on day d, are defined analogous to (5):

$$N_{k+7}(d) = b_{k+7}[N_{k+7}(d-1) + n_{k+7}(d-1) - n_{k+8}(d-1)] \qquad (9)$$

where $n_{k+7}(d-1)$ = redoubling the number of females that oviposited kth pods for a day $d-1$. The number of locust ovipositions for this day, $P_k(d)$, is

$$P_k(d) = P_k(d-1) + n_{k+7}(d-1)/2 \qquad (10)$$

and the number of eggs in these pods, $E_k(d)$, is:

$$E_k(d) = E_k(d-1) + A_k n_{k+7}(d-1)/2 \qquad (11)$$

where A_k = average number of eggs in kth pod. The formulas (9–11) are easily modified for another sex ratio.

Summing up all the eggs laid in one day from date d_8 to date d_{15}, we obtain the total number laid by the locust population for a simulated season. It allows us to "close the model" and to forecast the population dynamics for the next season, assuming the coefficient of egg survival is known and the environmental conditions remain stable, i.e., no flooding of oviposition sites occurs and food is available.

For the date in autumn when the locusts die (d_{15}), we take the autumn date passing of average daily temperature through 0 °C on the simulated lot. Though the possibility of simulation for seven ovipositions is foreseen, in most cases d_{15} comes earlier than d_{14} or d_{13}. In addition, as the data of natural control show, at the end of seasonal development, the number of Asiatic migratory locust populations is abruptly reduced but does not influence the main forecast, which is dependent on the quantity of exterminated reed biomass and on the number of eggs laid. It is thus possible to finish seasonal forecasting at an earlier date (for example on the date $d_{10} + l_{10} =$ the end of 3rd oviposition).

Thus, the model allows us to determine the assumed reed losses from locust feeding on the lot, both in terms of total yield and in terms of costs. On this basis an informed decision about treating the lot with insecticides can be made. Treatments can be simulated and optimised by date of treatment, treated areas and volume of chemicals required. At the economic level we can evaluate and minimise expenditures and measure environmental impacts.

The date $d_1 + l_1$ at the end of hatching of the 1st instar nymphs is usually selected for treatment, when the highest density of locusts is concentrated in the smallest possible area. However, other dates can also be selected. The recommended insecticides may differ in price, rate of application, biological efficiency and impact on the environment. As a standard measure, the integrated ecotoxicological index I_{et} (Vasiljev et al. 1982) calculated from this formula is used: $I_{et} = I_{av} D_s S_p / (I_p S_l)$, where I_{av} = average evaluation index of insecticidal toxicity, D_s = specific dosage of chemical, I_p = intensity of natural soil purification, S_p = area treated with chemicals and S_l = area of lot. When calculating expenditures for treated lots, the price of chemicals and costs of application will depend on the costs of transport, application method (air or ground treatment) and the volume rate applied to the site.

Results and discussion

A practical working model is being developed based on the collection of field observations and databases which function in the FoxPro environment. Stored database information describing the fixed lots of the Balkhash-Ily-Alakol breeding areas of the Asiatic migratory locust, based on autumn inspections of oviposition sites and the use of meteorological data, make it possible to forecast locust development and apply control measures with the aid of the *L.m.m. – P.a.* model.

A feature of the computer model is that vector $x(d)$, describing the state of the system for a day d $(d_0 \leq d \leq d_{15})$, is a function of vector $x(d-1)$, which describes the state of the system on the previous day:

$$x(d) = F[x(d-1)] \tag{12}.$$

It allows for accurate forecasts in the case of detailed information coming in for any date within the indicated time interval. Variation of initial data and parameters within given bounds allows us to anticipate different scenarios, including the best, worst and most probable.

The following shortcomings of the model should be mentioned:

- The full collection of all the parameters and the initial data necessary for successful function of the model are difficult to obtain owing to special features of the locusts, the simulation of their behaviour and the insufficient development of a suitable material and technical base for control.
- The absence in the model of key evaluation factors subject to long-term variation (e.g. sun activity, climate, lake levels etc.), which require periodic correction of parameters used for determining required natural control, does not permit accurate long-term forecasting at this stage.

Despite these deficits, it appears that plant protection specialists planning locust control operations as well as conservationists analysing the environmental impact of these operations will benefit from this model. If the monitoring network of locust breeding sites is improved in Kazakhstan, the model could be highly effective in predicting information.

We note in conclusion that the same thesis based on the above model could be used when simulating other natural systems involving other locust and grasshopper species, e.g. *C. italicus* and *D. maroccanus.*

In the first case, the main changes describing these insect populations must concern the section simulating the growth of preferred food plants (or sets of such plants). Determination of the total harvest from the simulated site may not be sufficient, and all the different stages of plant development will be required depending on the time and the degree of damage produced.

When forecasting yield losses from a grasshopper complex, it is necessary to define the number and pest status of each of M species entering this complex. In this case the task of simulation is complicated, because each of the different species has a typical set of dates. Different populations compete for the same food resources, and to keep account of each of them formulas analogous to (2–11) can be used. Summing up the data on a given day d, it will be possible to find both the absolute and relative damage caused by each species on a simulated lot. Such information will allow us to determine if control measures are justified. In that event, the most harmful species can be identified, based on the relative increase in damage caused by the complex of m species ($m \leq M$), and optimal volume rates and application requirements can be calculated for an effective and environmentally sound control of these species.

References

Antonov AG, Kambulin VE (1992) The season dynamics of the "reed – Asiatic locust" system simulated model. Doklady VASHNYL 6: 44–47

Berry JS, Kemp WP, Onsager JA (1991) Integration of simulation models and an expert system for management of rangeland grasshoppers. Applications in Natural Resource Management 5: 1–74

Capinera JL, Palton WJ, Delting JK (1983) Application of a grassland simulation model to grasshopper pest management on the North American shortgrass prairie. Pages 335–344 in: WK Lauenroth, GV Skogerboe and M Flug (eds) Works of the Third International Conference on State-of-the-Art in Ecological Modelling, Colorado State University, 24–28 May , 1982

Dennis B, Kemp WP (1988) Further statistical methods for a stochastic model of insect phenology. Environmental Entomology 17: 887–893

Dinasilov AS (1995) Substation of the common reed protection from pest insects in the Balkhash-Alakol depression. Thesis. Almaty

Dormidontova GN (1987) Harmfulness of non-gregarious locusts in Kazakhstan. Pages 84–91 in: EM Shumakov (ed.) Locusts – ecology and control measures. Leningrad: Kolos

Kambulin VE (1989) Forecasting of Asiatic locust harmfulness on the base of simulation model of possible losses. Pages 56–70 in: EM Shumakov (ed.) Principles and methods of simulation modelling in plant protection. Alma-Ata:

Kambulin VE, Bugaev GS (1982) Methods of evaluating population and harmfulness of locusts on haymowings and pastures. Pages 90–96 in: EM Shumakov (ed.) Cereal crops protection in the North of Kazakhstan from pests, diseases and weeds. Alma-Ata:

Plisak RP (1981) Delta vegetation change of the river Ily by regulating water runoff. Alma-Ata: Nauka

Popov GA (1987) Dynamics of locust's population and harmfulness. Pages 12–25 in: EM Shumakov (ed.) Locusts – ecology and control measures. Kolos. Leningrad:

Serkova LT (1961) To biology and harmfulness of locusts in summer steppes of Sary-Arka. Scientific works of Kazakh Scientific Research Institute of Plant Protection, vol 6. Alma-Ata

Starostyn SP, Shumakov EM (1987) Modern problems of plant protection from pest locusts. Pages 5–11 in: EM Shumakov (ed.) Locusts – ecology and control measures. Kolos. Leningrad:

Stoljarov MV (1975) Experiment of using energetic principles for determining the size of being consumed vegetation by orthoptera on the high-mountain pastures of the East Georgia. Ecology 1: 5–9

Tsyplenkov EA (1970) Noxious grasshopper insects of the USSR. Leningrad: Kolos

Vasiljev VP, Bublic LI, Gorokhovsky NA (1982) Methodical recommendations on evaluating the degree of potential contamination of the environment during pesticide treatment of agricultural crops. Kiev: Urozjai

Forecasting and modelling

Poster contributions

New Strategies in Locust Control
S. Krall, R. Peveling and D. Ba Diallo (eds)
© 1997 Birkhäuser Verlag Basel/Switzerland

The SGR biomodel: a synoptic model for surveillance and early warning specific to the desert locust over the whole of its distribution habitat

M. Launois

CIRAD-GERDAT-PRIFAS, B.P. 5035, 34032 Montpellier Cedex 1, France

In order to attempt to build a model of the bio-ecology of the desert locust *Schistocerca gregaria* (Forskål 1775), it was necessary to start with the available information, recognising that it was not all of a scientific nature nor was it all published. Priority had to be given to local information and the assistance of locust specialists of many years' standing.

The SGR biomodel makes use of all the bio-ecological data relating to the types of environment to which this locust is sensitive in its habitat, which covers 20% of the land area of the world. Inputs consist of transformed meteorological data from the European Centre for Medium Term Weather Forecasting (transmitted by METEO-FRANCE), the eco-geographical characteristics of different habitats and the possible biological responses for each biological and development phase of the desert locust. The biomodel can also manage supplementary data in the form of any information from the locality, once it has been checked. The biomodel covers the years 1985 to 1994. It is descriptive, quantitative, demographic and synoptic.

The aim of building the model is to be able to determine, at the synoptic level of a country or continent, for each degree and each tenth of a degree, those zones that are most favourable to its survival, breeding and gregarisation, as well as the demographic development of natural populations (taking into account birth rate, mortality and dispersal). By locating the zones of high risk, it is possible to select ground areas for inspection and to implement appropriate control measures in advance.

New Strategies in Locust Control
S. Krall, R. Peveling and D. Ba Diallo (eds)
© 1997 Birkhäuser Verlag Basel/Switzerland

Anti-locust early warning systems: recent experiences from eastern Africa

P.O. Odiyo

Desert Locust Control Organisation for Eastern Africa (DLCO-EA), P.O. Box 4255, Addis Ababa, Ethiopia

The Desert Locust Control Organisation for Eastern Africa (DLCO-EA) operates a data collecting, forecasting and early warning system for the area covered by the member countries. This note gives an example of the operation of the service by describing events in the Horn of Africa and around the Red Sea during 1993–94.

Widespread rain led to widespread breeding between July and October (Fig.1). All the breeding areas, with the exception of Wad Medani, were listed in the DLCO-EA sitrep/forecast

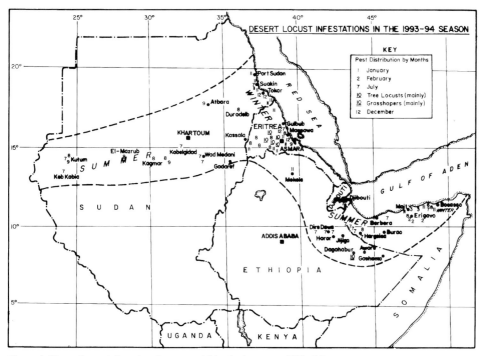

Figure 1. Desert locust infestations in eastern Africa in the season 1993–94.

for July. This helped to ensure timely control action. The areas within which infestations were reported in Sudan declined from a maximum of 420,000 ha in August to 40,000 ha in September and nil in October. In Eritrea the areas decreased from 9000 ha in July to 3600 ha in August and nil in September. No control was possible in northern Somalia, but action was taken in Djibouti and in eastern Ethiopia where locusts are believed to have moved.

What appeared likely to be a significant upsurge did not materialise, and it is tempting to suppose that early warning and prompt control were at least contributory causes.

Forecasting and modelling

Working group

New Strategies in Locust Control
S. Krall, R. Peveling and D. Ba Diallo (eds)
© 1997 Birkhäuser Verlag Basel/Switzerland

Results and recommendations of the working group *Forecasting and modelling*

K. Cressman (Chairman and Secretary)

The group noted that forecasting is most difficult during recession periods when, in fact, it plays the most important part of an early warning system. Nevertheless, early warning is essential to the management of the desert locust. A main component of early warning is locust forecasts, which depend on the quality and timeliness of information. There is little chance for early warning to be of use if ground surveys do not occur on a regular basis and forecasts are not acted upon.

Status of present systems

It was the opinion of the group that the forecasts provided by the FAO are extremely useful to the various target audiences, since they themselves do not have access to such information nor can they produce it themselves. Countries depend on short-term FAO forecasts to organise survey and control operations and on longer-term forecasts for campaign planning. However, recipients, especially those in locust-affected countries, should provide the FAO with feedback on possible improvements. This could be done under the auspices of an informal workshop with plant protection directors within a region on an annual basis that would encourage a frank and technical review of the forecasts and what follow-up action was taken. Efforts are required to ensure that the most appropriate technical person in locust-affected countries, usually the plant protection director, receives forecasts in a timely manner.

The group discussed the various tools that are available in forecasting and noted that these tools cannot be used in isolation but could supplement existing data and perhaps fill in some of the gaps.

Remote sensing products

It was noted that plant protection departments in locust-affected countries probably do not have the resources or capabilities to collect and process satellite data for producing maps that indicate vegetation and rainfall and can be used on an operational basis. In fact, these products, as well as other existing satellite-derived biotope maps, still require ground truthing and refinement in order to clarify their usefulness. The latter should also reflect minimum and maximum fluctuations in vegetation distribution. Geographical information system (GIS) technology may offer some assistance in validation. If such products are found to be useful, it is probably better for regional and international organisations to provide products that have already been processed.

GIS

Although a proven technology in other fields, GIS has yet to be used in work with locusts. The introduction of SWARMS offers new possibilities in data management, manipulation and analysis as well as in useful outputs for affected countries. The group felt that GIS should eventually be introduced into national and regional organisations after experience has been gained in using SWARMS. However, such systems should be simple yet be compatible with SWARMS and meet the differing needs of the countries. Even in this form, GIS will require experienced users.

Models

For the most part, models remain an academic exercise and are not yet applicable to forecasting except for simple models that synthesise information. Using models for predictive purposes is not considered feasible at present.

Improvements and further developments

Improvements are required in two primary areas: information and communications. These are inter-related.

Information

Data collection needs to be strengthened by encouraging regular surveys and involving other potential sources that already exist, namely nomads and security forces. For example, the latter group could be trained by National locust units in basic observation and reporting. The use of GPS should continue and each survey team should have one. Computers should be used for data management (entry, display and storage) and communication (see below). The group noted that efforts have been made by FAO to improve data collection by standardised survey forms and encouraged locust-affected countries to use these forms. Training programmes should be implemented on how to use such forms.

Communications

National communication systems need to be strengthened. Although this is generally outside the scope of locust projects and assistance, affected countries should encourage their Governments to improve such systems. In the meantime, efforts must continue to establish fax and email facilities at the Plant Protection Departments and at present radios still offer the best possibilities of data transfer from the field to the PPDs.

Nevertheless, forecasters are still hampered by the lack of direct communications in some countries. Hence, the group believed that the single most useful development for early warning would be a robust self-powered hand-held device that would enable the locust field officer to enter locust and environmental data, obtain the location of the site and transmit all of this by satellite from the field directly to the PPD headquarters copied to FAO and the appropriate regional organisation. This would overcome the current difficulties in communications and the resulting delays in reporting, and reduce the undesirable necessity of assessing assessments and trying to forecast from highly summarised and sometimes exaggerated information. Lastly, new technology is rapidly developing and efforts should continue to review such technology in terms of its usefulness in early warning.

Control agents and methods

Overview and challenges of new control agents

W.F. Meinzingen

Consultant, P.O. Box 30470, Nairobi, Kenya

Summary. Since the banning of persistent pesticides, the search has begun for new and environmentally safer control agents. These potential new control agents are insect growth regulators (IGRs), botanicals and pathogens. Due to the remanence and safety aspects of IGRs, there is hope that barrier spraying will resume importance for the control of hoppers. Botanicals or pathogens such as *Metarhizium flavoviride* could be used for spraying locusts. Ultra low volume (ULV) drift spraying will remain the most common control technique, as most new control agents will be formulated in oil, but some of them might be formulated in dust or used as bait or repellents. Conventional chemicals are still going to be widely used in the near future. Their effectiveness can be further improved through better application techniques and formulations. As most of these new control agents are used best for the control of hoppers, the early detection of locust hoppers is essential and governs the success of control results. New control strategies are needed, and the concept of controlling locusts in recession areas has to be reviewed.

Résumé. Depuis l'interdiction de l'usage des pesticides rémanents, les chercheurs s'emploient à trouver des substances moins dangereuses pour l'environnement. Ces nouveaux agents potentiels de la lutte antiacridienne sont les dérégulateurs de croissance, les biocides végétaux et les agents pathogènes. En raison des avantages qu'ils présentent sur le plan de la rémanence et de la sécurité, les IGR devraient bénéficier d'un regain d'intérêt pour les applications en barrière contre les bandes larvaires. Les biocides végétaux ou les agents pathogènes tels que *Metarhizium flavoviride* pourraient être utilisés en pulvérisation contre les locustes adultes. La pulvérisation UBV en dérive continuera à être la technique la plus employée étant donné que la plupart des nouveaux agents sont disponibles dans des formulations huileuses. Certains pourront cependant être appliqués par poudrage ou utilisés pour appâter ou repousser les criquets. Les substances chimiques conventionnelles continueront à être largement utilisées dans un avenir proche. Leur efficacité pourra être améliorée par de meilleures formulations et techniques d'application. L'efficacité et la réussite des actions de lutte utilisant ces nouveaux agents antiacridiens dépendent de la rapidité de détection des locustes. De nouvelles stratégies de lutte sont nécessaires et le concept de lutte dans des zones de récession devra être révisé.

Introduction

The prevention of locust plagues, particularly in regions where desert locusts (*Schistocerca gregaria*) occur, is an important objective not only for countries where an upsurge can occur but also for international organisations which have been given the mandate to forecast, monitor and control these migrant pests. Furthermore, the donor community helping to fund research and emergency control operations has a deep interest in a long-lasting solution to the problem.

Preventive control programmes have been repeatedly developed and rewritten by international locust control organisations. They involve constant monitoring of the locust population in recession areas and control of gregarious populations, at times over vast and remote regions.

Upsurges often remain undetected. Some take place far away from crop land or the control poses a major logistical problem and is therefore not carried out.

According to Food and Agriculture Organisation of the United Nations (FAO) sources, in 1986–1989 26 million ha of locust infestation areas were treated, during which 16 million l of liquid and 14 million kg of dust pesticides were used, putting a severe environmental pressure on the desert locust habitat. Although during this period US$ 315 million was spent, it is widely believed that the effect of chemical control on the overall decline of the desert locust population was insignificant.

Due to the lack of funds and implementation of proper forecasting and monitoring concepts and strategies, the control of desert locusts in recession areas has never worked satisfactorily. It has to be reviewed: New control strategies, which share responsibilities in a more cost-effective way are needed, as well as mechanisms using control agents and methods with better-structured locust control organisations, both at regional and national levels. Control efforts aiming to prevent locust upsurges only in specific outbreak areas are to be further developed.

Present control methods

Pesticides

Since the banning of dieldrin and BHC, replacement acridicides such as organophosphates or synthetic pyrethroids or combinations of these have been used for the control of hoppers and adult locusts. Organophosphates generally have a high mammalian toxicity, while synthetic pyrethroids often adversely affect aquatic organisms or beneficial insects. Most of these conventional chemicals are applied as concentrated ultra low volume (ULV) formulations. Others such as propoxur and bendiocarb are also produced in dust formulation and are used for the control of hoppers.

To minimise the risk of insecticides to the environment intensive research has been conducted in order to:
- reduce the amount of pesticide used;
- determine the optimum droplet size for different application techniques;
- develop specific ground and air spray equipment such as rotary atomisers;
- use better formulations for a target-specific control operation and
- combine the physiology and behaviour of insects with the correct application technique.

Baiting, which involves the mixing of insecticides and a suitable carrier such as bran or groundnut husks, has been almost forgotten, and dusting techniques, which require less logistical support and were used extensively by farmers for the control of hoppers in the past, are rarely practised nowadays. For the next five years, or even longer, the use of insecticides will still remain the first option for locust control.

In the search for more environmentally friendly and safer product alternatives, new chemicals and formulations which produce good knock-down effects and show persistence in the field are presently being developed. Their toxicity and environmental side-effects have yet to be checked and intensive environmental studies have to be conducted before they are recommended by FAO.

Formulation

Besides the active ingredient, the carrier in which the chemical is formulated is essential for achieving the desired results; the ULV formulations are generally recommended for migrant pest control. ULV formulations are already pre-mixed ex-factory and can be applied directly by ULV spray equipment. Good formulations enhance the mode of entry, produce a better droplet spectrum, better distribution and a longer remanence of the chemical in the field.

ULV formulations consist of:

- suitable oils used as carrier;
- a stabiliser to avoid deterioration of the pesticide due to temperature or prolonged storage;
- active ingredients which can be either in solid or liquid state;
- solvents to dissolve the active ingredients and sometimes the UV stabiliser.

The use of ULV application implies that the maximum application rate does not exceed 5 l/ha with a droplet spectrum ranging between 30–150 μm. Due to the ready-mixed oil base, ULV spray has a longer persistence in the field and does not evaporate as rapidly as water-based formulations.

Spray equipment

For locust control, ULV and conventional spray equipment are used. The latter applies the spray through hydraulic nozzles which atomise the liquid by means of pressure. This method produces a wide droplet spectrum and is gradually being replaced by rotary atomisers which utilise centrifugal force to produce a relatively narrow droplet spectrum, evenly distributing the spray over a large target area. Rotary atomisers, normally fitted to aircraft, have also been developed for ground spraying and are mounted on a vehicle or used as hand-held sprayers.

Pesticide distribution depends on the following factors:

- size of spray droplets;
- number and type of nozzles and the way they are arranged on the spray boom;
- emission height and track spacing;
- forward speed and spray platform;
- meteorological conditions.

The number and size of spray droplets which are produced by the individual spray equipment onto the target, be it hopper bands or adult swarms, determine the biological efficiency. For effective control of locust hoppers, a droplet spectrum with a volume median diameter (VMD) size of 100–120 μm for hoppers and a VMD of 70–90 μm for adult swarms is recommended (Meinzingen 1993). In order to reduce the dosage rate of pesticides, more research in application techniques and further development of application equipment has to be carried out. In addition, more training is needed for spray operators and field officers.

Overview of potential new control agents

Over the past years intensive research has been carried out on alternative products to control locust and grasshopper species. Available products and their effectiveness, including their present stage of development, are briefly described as follows.

Insect growth regulators (IGRs)

Products such as teflubenzuron, triflumuron and diflubenzuron have been tested with good results for the control of hopper bands (Scherer and Rakotonandrasana 1993).

These products are derivatives of benzoyl urea, which inhibits chitin synthesis and in return effects the formation of the insect cuticle. IGRs act slowly but have a relatively long persistence in the field, which varies from 10 days to several weeks depending on the amount of active ingredient applied per hectare. Their mode of entry is through ingestion and contact. IGRs are produced in formulations which allow application by hand-held sprayer, vehicle- mounted sprayer or aircraft fitted with rotary atomiser at application rates between 10 and 100 g a.i./ha, depending on the application technique used which can either be barrier spraying or total-cover spraying. Ecotoxicology tests are still incomplete and further environmental studies are required.

Insect growth regulators have greater persistence and are suitable for barrier spraying and should be applied against early hopper instar. IGRs are suitable products for the prevention of locust outbreaks. However, they are not suitable for direct crop protection because of their slow action.

Juvenile hormone analogues (JHAs)

The effects of JHAs (e.g. fenoxycarb) on hopper bands have not fully been evaluated for practical use in the field. Their mode of entry is both through contact and the stomach. Action is by suppression of the gregarisation process, scattering of hopper bands and malformation of parts of the insect body. JHAs are slow acting. Careful assessment is required to clarify if further research and development should be continued.

*Botanicals (*Azadirachta indica *and* Melia volkensii)

A. indica, or neem, has been tested in the field to control nymphs of *S. gregaria* (Schmutterer and Freres 1990). The results are promising. Neem extracts produce a repellent effect and also act as an anti-feeding agent when applied on crops at all growth levels (Nasseh et al. 1993a). Depending on the dosage and concentration of neem formulations, a good mortality rate of hoppers and, in special cases, adults can be achieved if directly treated (Wilps et al. 1993a). Small amounts of neem extracts minimise overall activities (Meinzingen unpublished reports) and lead to a considerable reduction of flight abilities (Wilps et al. 1993b). In parts of East Africa simple neem extracts prepared from fruits or tree bark are widely used against malaria and yellow fever. It is recommended that neem formulations be further tested against adult locusts. ULV-formulated neem extract can be produced and is applied with ULV spray equipment.

However, mass production of neem extract and registration of the product is still a problem which has to be resolved. In the United States, neem extract is already commercially available but has yet to be screened for locust control. Neem extract can be safely handled and has no negative effect on human or domestic animals.

Melia volkensii has similar characteristics to those of neem. It can be used for controlling hoppers and adult locusts (Nasseh et al. 1993b). *M. volkensii* is in an advanced experimental stage but is not yet commercially available. From *M. volkensii* extract a ULV formulation can be produced and applied with appropriate spray equipment. More training in production technology is necessary in order to develop botanicals into alternatives to present control methods in the coming years.

Pathogens

The use of pathogens for the control of agro-forest insect pests has long been recognized but their operational use against locusts has yet to be implemented. They are still in the experimental stage of development.

Bacterial pathogens like *Bacillus thuringiensis* have already replaced pesticides in agriculture, forestry and vector control. Furthermore, products based on insect pathogenic viruses, fungi, nematodes and protozoa are increasingly being used in the control of pests. All these pesticides are considered safe and most of them are environmentally acceptable.

Although not yet used in large-scale operations, mycopesticides have proven effective against locusts and many grasshopper species (Delgado unpublished results) and research efforts by national and international institutions must continue. The advantages of some of these pathogens are that they can be established and formulated locally. However, commercial production and stability for field operations is still a problem. For locust and grasshopper control, fungal pathogens such as *Metarhizium flavoviride* and *Beauveria bassiana* are showing promising results.

Metarhizium flavoviride

This pathogen offers an alternative for controlling hopper bands and shows potential for upsurge prevention. Applied to settled swarms it changes their behaviour, causing no or late departure from their roosts and exposure to sun radiation. They are slow acting with good mortality rates after 6 days. Oil-based or water-based formulations have been tested for application; they can be applied by ULV or conventional sprayers (Zimmermann et al. 1994).

M. flavoviride is directly applied to hopper bands at a rate of approximately 100 g a.i./ha. The technology to produce and formulate *M. flavoviride* still needs to be optimised before it can be used operationally. *M. flavoviride* can be produced and formulated locally in locust countries, involving different processing procedures depending on whether conidia or blastospores are used. However, their short shelf-life is a disadvantage. *M. flavoviride* is not suitable for crop protection. More fieldwork on the adult desert locust is required and environmental impact studies on non-target organisms need to continue.

Beauveria bassiana

B. bassiana has similar characteristics to *M. flavoviride* but has a wider host range and is less tolerant of high temperatures. More field tests need to be carried out. Other bioagents, namely protozoa, Sarcomastigophora (*Malamoeba locustae*) and the Microsporidian *Nosema locustae* have not achieved satisfactory results (Krall 1992). Combinations of botanicals with pathogens are in the process of being tested.

Semiochemicals

These products are still in the experimental stage. They could be used as a means to monitor gregarization of locusts and the early detection of outbreaks. Semiochemicals could be used for integrated pest management programmes. However, their potential still requires further investigation and probably more than 10 years will be needed to understand the complexity of these chemicals.

Locust control techniques

Current locust control techniques involve the use of insecticides and have almost completely replaced traditional control methods. Most locust insecticides act by contact and are applied by the impingement of spray droplets onto the target, or indirectly by the ingestion of sprayed vegetation. When the use of dieldrin was discontinued one of the best application methods for large-scale control operations, namely barrier spraying, was abandoned. With the development of new remanent compounds, it is hoped that barrier spraying will be reinstated.

Application techniques and new control agents

Drift-spraying

The most common locust control technique is drift spraying. It uses wind of not more than 3 m/sec to disperse spray droplets over the target area. The technique requires the use of specialised equipment and the use of ULV formulations that can be applied either by aircraft or by ground spray equipment (Meinzingen 1993). The advantage of drift spraying is that large areas can be treated using small amounts of pesticides. Provided ULV formulations are used, all control agents can be applied.

Barrier spraying

This method is essentially a drift-spraying technique which does not aim to give blanket coverage but treats strips or barriers within the target area. Barrier spraying is a technique that was developed for dieldrin application and is probably the most successful method developed for hopper control.

Depending on density and the stage of the hoppers, dieldrin was applied directly to the vegetation at intervals of 300 to 2000 m through which the hoppers marched and fed. The advantage of barrier spraying is that large infestation areas can be controlled quickly, treating only a relatively small fraction of the total area. In addition, operational expenditure is low because constant monitoring of a given area is not required. It is hoped that with the development of IGRs barrier spraying will be reintroduced. IGRs are remanent, and depending on the dosage rate remain active in the field for a period of time. Hoppers are affected by consuming treated vegetation and promising results have been obtained in the field. However, more large-scale field trials are still to be carried out. For successful control, IGRs should be applied in the early hopper stage.

New chemicals such as phenylpyrazoles also have long persistence in the field, and tests carried out in laboratories have shown good control results on the desert locust (DLCO-EA, personal communication). However, more ecotoxicological studies have to be carried out.

Hopper band spraying

This technique involves directly spraying hopper bands or the concentrated spraying of hoppers. Control is best carried out when nymphs are roosting. Conventional chemicals will still be used for the foreseeable future. Pathogens and botanicals should be tested in outbreak areas. The availability of proper ULV formulations of these products will be the key element for success.

Locust swarm spraying

Flying swarms are controlled by aircraft using air-to-air spraying. To control settled swarms, ULV ground spray equipment can be used. In the years to come, pesticides will still be the most common means to control locust swarms. Botanicals, or even pathogens, might be considered for controlling flying locust swarms. However, they are slow acting, hence immediate control results are not expected, but through stress or behavioural changes good indirect control results might be achieved. To increase the number of impingeing droplets to flying locusts, electrostatic application techniques might be applied.

Dusting and baiting

The use of alternative compounds for dusting and baiting should be studied. Its use will largely depend on the availability of storage facilities, shelf-life of the ready-formulated compound, application equipment and additional manpower. Apart from conventional chemicals, IGRs and pathogens could be considered for this application.

Repellents

M. volkensii and *A. indica* have a repellent effect, and ULV or emulsifiable concentrate (EC) formulations applied directly to crops could limit damage caused by some locusts and grasshoppers.

Control through stress or behavioural changes

Some of the new control agents, specifically botanicals but also *M. flavoviride*, cause stress or changes in locust behaviour which expose them to natural enemies or premature death through hyperactivity or exposure to solar radiation.

Challenges of future strategies

Over many years the role of regional locust control organisations has been emphasised. Yet very few organisations have successfully fulfilled this task and in most cases operational control activities have reverted to individual plant protection services at the national level. Regional organisations should concentrate their efforts in co-ordinating these national plant protection services.

Taking into account the expense and the complex task of locust control in recession areas, it might be better in the future to carry out locust control in upsurge areas only. Thus more efforts need to be made to monitor and forecast locusts in upsurge areas. Research activities by institutions from different donor communities and the locust emergency programme must be better co-ordinated and be implemented faster and more effectively.

With regard to new locust control strategies, drastic changes are unlikely to occur. The use of conventional insecticides remains the only reliable option to control locusts in the foreseeable future. Most pathogens, bioagents and insect growth regulators are only effective when applied during the larval stage. The early detection of hoppers is essential and governs the success of control results. If, in addition to IGRs, pathogens and botanicals can be produced in the required quantity and quality, the following control strategies could be suggested:

- Control of hoppers away from crops using IGRs, pathogens and botanicals. Methods: baiting, dusting, barrier and direct ULV spraying.
- Control of roosting or swarming locusts away from crops using contact insecticides, botanicals, possibly pathogens. Method: ULV drift-spraying technique.
- Control of hoppers or swarms near crops using fast-acting pesticides. Methods: ULV drift spraying (ground and aerial application), low-volume application using knapsack sprayer etc.

IGRs are already available and manufacturers are trying to register their products in countries where locusts and grasshoppers occur. It is hoped that botanicals and pathogens can be produced in sufficient quantities, equal qualities and hopefully, will also be registered in the near future. IGRs, botanicals and pathogens, together with the use of different application methods and equipment, could form the basis for new and environmentally safer control strategies.

However, the incorporation of new locust compounds with existing application techniques has yet to prove its effectiveness. New control agents and methods have to be tested against all locust and grasshopper species. For environmental reasons it is also important to continue tests on their impact on non-target organisms. New control strategies and better locust control techniques require considerable research.

Acknowledgements
I would like to express my thanks to the Deutsche Gesellschaft für Technische Zusammenarbeit (GTZ) for inviting me to the International Conference on New Strategies in Locust Control in Bamako/Mali, from 3–7 April, 1995. Special thanks goes to Stephan Krall and Dr Hans Wilps for their advice and useful discussions held in Eschborn and Bamako.

References

Krall S (ed) (1992) Efficacy and environmental impact for biological control of *Nosema locustae* on grasshoppers in Cape Verde: a synthesis report. GTZ, Germany, 16 pp

Meinzingen WF (ed) (1993) A guide to migrant pest management in Africa. FAO: Rome, 184 pp

Nasseh O, Freres T, Krall S (1993a) Fraßabschreckender Effekt von *Azadirachta indica* A. Juss auf adulte *Schistocerca gregaria* Forskål. Mitt Dtsch Ges Allg Angew Ent. 8: 835–838

Nasseh O, Wilps H, Rembold H, Krall S (1993b) Biologically active compounds in *Melia volkensii*. J. Appl Ent 116: 1–11

Scherer R, Rakotonandrasana MA (1993) Barrier treatment with a benzoyl urea insect growth regulator against *Locusta migratoria capito* (Sauss) hopper bands in Madagascar. Int J of Pest Manag 39: 411–417

Rembold H (1989) The azadirachtins – their potential for insect control. Econ Med Pl Res 3: 57–72

Schmutterer H, Freres T (1990) Beeinflussung von Metamorphose, Färbung und Verhalten der Wüstenheuschrecke *Schistocerca gregaria* (Forskål) und der Afrikanischen Wanderheuschrecke *Locusta migratoria migratorioides* (R. & F.) durch Niemsamenöl. Z PflKrankh PflSchutz 97: 431–438

Wilps H, Nasseh O, Krall S (1993a) Neemprodukte – Natürliche Insektizide gegen *Schistocerca gregaria*. Mitt. Dtsch. Ges. Allg Angew Ent 8: 827–833

Wilps H, Nasseh O, Krall S (1993b) Application to flying locusts a powerful method for combatting *S. gregaria* (Forskål) adults. Trends in Comp Biochem Physiol 1: 1073–1082

Zimmermann G, Zelasny B, Kleespies R, Welling M (1994) Biological control of African locusts by entomopathogenic microorganisms. Pages 127–138 in Krall S, Wilps H (eds) New Trends in Locust Control . TZ-Verlags-Gesellschaft, Rossdorf, Germany

New Strategies in Locust Control
S. Krall, R. Peveling and D. Ba Diallo (eds)
© 1997 Birkhäuser Verlag Basel/Switzerland

Field investigations on *Schistocerca gregaria* (Forskål) adults, hoppers and hopper bands

H. Wilps and B. Diop[1]

GTZ Eschborn, P.O. Box 5180, D-65726 Eschborn, Germany
[1]Division of Plant Protection, PB 180-Nouakchott, Mauritania

Summary. In the course of five years of investigations in the natural habitats of *Schistocerca gregaria* in West Africa, botanicals, mycocides and insect growth regulators (IGRs) were tested. Several of the botanicals were effective, as were all the mycocides and IGRs. The latter were also well suited for barrier application because of their remanence for 12 days and longer. None of the products showed any notable knock-down effect, and moreover, their slow action makes them unsuitable to protect crops at risk. But because of their environmental tolerability, they are definitely useful for preventive control. The mortality rates achieved with the IGRs reached 40% after 6 days and maximum values of 100% after 10 days. Similar results were also obtained after treatment with mycocides and botanicals. In these cases, however, the differences observed were due to the dosages applied, the incubation time and the type and origin of the various products. Investigations on feeding preferences and food consumption reveal that *S. gregaria* consumes less than had been generally assumed namely 30±8% of its own body weight only.

Résumé. Diverses substances appartenant à la classe des biocides végétaux, des mycocides et des dérégulateurs de croissance (insect growth regulators – IGR) ont été testées au cours d'une campagne d'essais de cinq années conduite dans les habitats naturels de *Schistocerca gregaria* (Forskål) en Afrique de l'Ouest. Une partie des biocides végétaux s'est montrée efficace, de même que l'ensemble des mycocides et des IGR. Ces derniers convenaient aussi parfaitement aux applications en barrière grâce à leur persistance durant 12 jours et plus, mais aucun des agents employés n'a eu un effet de choc notable et la lenteur de leur mode d'action les rend peu aptes à une protection de cultures directement exposées. Toutefois, puisque ces substances ne sont pas déprédatrices de l'environnement, leur utilité dans la lutte préventive est certaine. Les taux de mortalité obtenus avec les IGR étaient de 40% après 6 jours pour atteindre le maximum de 100% après 10 jours. Des résultats semblables ont été obtenus après traitement avec les mycocides et les biocides végétaux. Mais dans ces derniers cas, l'efficacité a été extrêmement variable selon les dosages employés, le temps d'incubation, ainsi que selon la nature et l'origine des différents produits. Des études sur les préférences alimentaires et les habitudes de nutrition de *S. gregaria* ont montré que ce criquet consommait moins que ce qui était généralement admis, soit seulement 30±8% de son propre poids corporel.

Introduction

The GTZ project Integrated Biological Control of Grasshoppers and Locusts started its field trials in 1990 in In Abangharit, followed in 1991 by investigations in Anoue Mekkerene. Because of security problems, it was necessary to leave the Niger and to relocate in Mauritania. A new station was set up in Akjoujt in 1992. From here the operations were conducted in northern Mauritania, in Inchiri, as well as in the southern part of the country in the region around Boumdeid. In this area there are substantial, interesting differences in habitat conditions compared with those in Inchiri, so in 1993 another field station was opened in Kiffa. Since the locusts appear first in the southern and south-eastern parts of Mauritania, and then some four to eight weeks later in Inchiri, the working season was extended. In this field research, the following main goals were set. The basic goal was to test new products against nymphs and adults of *S. gregaria*. These products included botanicals, entopathogenic fungi and chitin synthesis inhibitors, generally known as insect growth regulators (IGRs) and belonging to the product class of benzoyl phenyl ureas (BPUs).The effectiveness of the products was initially tested under semi-field conditions, i.e., in field-cage trials, and then examined using other methods, for example, against flying adults and then in the field, against roosting hopper bands or by barrier spraying migrating hopper bands. During additional trials conducted as mentioned above, seed extracts of another Melicaeae, *Melia volkensii*, were tested on *S. gregaria* nymphs. The results obtained indicated high mortality rates, malformations, retarded development and an effect on the phase transformation (Nasseh et al. 1993). Besides the trials conducted with nymphs, mycocides, some botanicals and IGRs were also applied on resting and flying adults with satisfactory success (Wilps and Nasseh 1992a, b; Wilps et al. 1992a, 1993a). Furthermore, intensive investigations were made to calculate hopper band sizes, food preferences and food consumed by nymphs and hopper bands.

Materials and methods

Test insects and rearing conditions, products tested, and food trials

The locusts used in the tests, the breeding and rearing conditions, as well as the application methods, are described elsewhere (Wilps et al. 1992a, b; Wilps et al. 1993c; Nasseh et al. 1992a, b).The origin of the products used and their content of active ingredients, as well as the amounts applied, correspond to the descriptions given previously (Nasseh et al. 1992b, 1993; Wilps and Nasseh 1994b).

The food choice and food consumption experiments were carried out in cages $(40 \times 40 \times 60$ cm) which were placed, as opposed to laboratory trials, under natural conditions in the field. The tests were designed as food-choice and no-choice tests in which the hoppers were offered either one or three different plant species. Twenty hoppers of the same instar and comparable weight were introduced to each cage. Their weight and the weight of the plants were determined daily before and after feeding. Thirty grams of vegetation was distributed per cage. Daily food consumption was calculated by subtracting the weight loss values from the evaporation controls.

Determination of hopper band sizes

Observations on migrating hopper bands

Small plots of 100–200 cm^2 were marked off in the sand in the areas covered with migrating hoppers, and their number was counted repeatedly. The size of the plots was chosen to be small enough that all the hoppers present could be counted before they left or new ones entered. The number of insects per square metre was then calculated (number of observations 3 to 10, depending on the hopper band size and the different hopper densities). The total area covered was determined by pacing off or driving alongside the whole band while estimating its width at regular intervals. Based on these data the size of the total area infested as well as the total number of hoppers per band were calculated.

Estimation of the numbers of hoppers in bushes

It is very difficult to estimate the number of hoppers roosting in bushes. This was not regularly quantified, as two or three observers were required at a time. To improve reliability of estimates, observers were trained as follows: First the number of live hoppers was estimated, and then they were treated with a pesticide with a high knock-down effect. Dead hoppers were counted, and the results were compared with the initial estimates.

Calculation of the number of hoppers during resting periods on the ground

In the morning, before the hopper bands start to migrate, they concentrate on fairly large areas which are usually sandy, vegetation-free spots for basking. In such situations, the number of hoppers can be estimated fairly accurately. First, the observer estimates the size of the covered area, then notes hopper density, that is how large the distance is between individuals, as measured in body widths. Finally, individual insects are caught and their development stage is determined. The length and width of the hoppers were measured using a calliper rule in order to calculate the surface covered by one hopper.

Results

Treatments and mortality rates

The foremost tests carried out with *S. gregaria* hoppers and adults were essentially all field-cage trials because of the sparse occurrence of locusts between 1990 and 1993. Here adults were

Table 1. Mortality rates in percent of *S. gregaria* adults

Class	Products	Dosage	1991/1992 after		1992/1993 after	
			6 days	12 days	6 days	12 days
Botanicals	Neem oil	1 g a.i./ha	88	92	38	95
	Azal-F	1 g a.i./ha	62	80	-	-
	M. volkensii	10 g a.i./ha	-	-	32	88
Mycocides	*M. flavivoride*	10^{13} spores/ha	0	88	-	95
	B. bassiana	10^{13} spores/ha	20	50	-	-
		2.5×10^{13} spores/ha	-	-	33	88
Benzoyl	Triflumuron	25 g a.i./ha	-	-	25	70
phenyl ureas	(Alsystin)	50 g a.i./ha	48 (1990)	69 (1990)	30	65
(BPUs)	Teflubenzuron					
	(Nomolt)					

The heading spanning the mortality columns reads: "Highest mortality achieved in % during the seasons:".

The data presented summarise trials conducted with adult *S. gregaria*, part of which were published elsewhere (Wilps et al. 1992a; Wilps et al. 1993a).

treated both during flight activity and on the ground during resting periods. The mortality rates obtained using the latter method, as a rule, lay substantially below 50%. In contrast, the rates for locusts treated in flight were up to 98% (Tab. 1).

The different products were tested against hoppers (instar 2 to 5) also. These tests were initially performed as field-cage trials (due to a shortage of locusts, but also in order to determine dose-effect relationships), then in 1993/94 against hopper bands. Botanicals and mycocides acted only as a contact poison, while BPUs, in contrast, were effective both as a feeding poison and a contact poison (Tab. 2).

In current control practice, contact pesticides such as pyrethroids, organophosphates and carbamates are used for blanket treatments of infested areas. Apart from adverse effects on the non-target organisms, blanket treatments require a tremendous amount of pesticides. This can be substantially reduced by targeted treatment of hopper bands in their roosting places, and by barrier treatment with adequately remanent insecticides. With both methods, it seems that up to 80% of insecticide may be saved, but this must be further verified (Tab. 3).

Table 2. Mortality rate in percent of *S. gregaria* hoppers

Class	Product	Dosage (g a.i./ha or conidia/ha)	Highest mortality rate (%) 6 and 12 days after treatment in seasons 1991–1995							
			1991/92		1992/93		1993/94		1994/95	
Botanical	Neem oil	0.8–2.4	38	90	33	60	80	85	38	56
	Neem Azal	1	50	94	-	-	45	78	-	-
	M. volkensii	10	-	-	10	50[a]	42	66	46	91
Micro-sporidia	*N. locustae*	baits	0 (1990)	0 (1990)	-	-	-	-	-	-
Fungi	*B. bassiana*	2.5×10^{13}	-	-	42	66	-	-	-	-
	M. flavivoride	1.3×10^{13}	-	-	-	-	50	92	47	98
Benzoyl phenyl ureas	TFM	12.5	-	-	48	72	-	-	-	-
		25	70	100	43[b]	70[b]	40[c]	60–70[c]	75[e]	100[e]
		50	-	-	60	100	20–30[d]	80[d]	40[f]	93[f]
	TFB	25	40	81	-	-	-	-	-	-
		50	-	-	72	82	-	-	-	-
	DFB	60	-	-	-	-	-	-	44	73

In all tests, mortality was <10% in untreated controls and <22% in vehicle controls. Sources of products: Neem oils (Prof. Schmutterer, Univ. Giessen; Trifolio Co., Lahnau; SROM Corp., India); *Melia* extracts (Prof. Rembold, MPI Munich; Prof. Mwangi, Univ. Nairobi); benzoyl phenyl ureas (TFM = Triflumuron/Alsystin: Bayer Corp.; TFB = Teflubenzuron/Nomolt: Shell-Agro; DFB = Diflubenzuron/Dimilin: Rhône-Poulenc Co.); microsporidia and fungi (Dr Prior, IIBC; Dr Crawford, Myco Tech Co.; Dr Welling, BBA).
[a] *Melia*-treated hoppers did not undergo adult moulting
[b] Topical application in field-cage trials
[c] Topical application on a hopper band
[d] Barrier application (1993)
[e] Topical application on roosting places
[f] Barrier treatment
The amounts applied for barrier treatments varied between 0.12 and 0.16 l/ha.
These data are also summarised values of representative trials conducted from 1990 to 1994. Some of them were published in detail previously (survival curves, dose-response relationships) (Nasseh et al. 1992c, 1993; Wilps and Nasseh 1994a).

Table 3. Mortality rates after roosting-place treatment and barrier applications and pesticide saved in comparison to blanket treatments

Trial	No. of roosting places (A) or hopper density (B/C)	area treated (ha)	mortality rate (%)	mortality rate after day	total size of protected area (3)	insecti-cides used (1)	insecticides needed by blanket treatment (2)	insec-ticides saved (%)
A	10	<0.1	100	7	10 ha	1.6 l	10 l	84
B	6–9/m²	3.85	90	20	42 ha	4.5 l	42 l	86
C	8–17/m²	4.6	95	15	46 ha	6.9 l	46 l	85

A: Treatment of hoppers at their roosting places using a motorised sprayer with equipped for ultra light volume applications. The treatments took place between 8 and 9 a.m. B: Barrier treatment with Micro Ulva. C: Barrier treatment with the same motorised backsprayer. The percentage of pesticides saved is calculated as follows: The pesticides actually used (1) are compared with the amounts of pesticides needed (2) for blanket spraying. These amounts are based on the assumption that the areas protected (3) are normally treated at 1 l/ha.

Hopper band sizes, food preferences, weight gain and food consumption of hoppers

Determination of hopper band sizes

A sound knowledge of hopper band sizes is a prerequisite for evaluating control efficiency, estimating the loss of vegetation and investigating other parameters, like the impact of predators on hopper band decimation. Besides the methods described above (see Materials and Methods), in some cases the number of hoppers can be fairly accurately calculated provided that the surface covered by one hopper can be quantified. Corresponding data are given in Table 4.

Food preferences

Regarding the amount of food consumed daily by *S. gregaria*, Davey's (1952) results are commonly cited, mostly in an extremely oversimplified form and often without even mentioning his name. According to Davey, *S. gregaria* is supposed to consume an amount equal to its own body weight every day. This value is taken as a general basis without taking into consideration that this is the maximal value between two moults. However, the value was determined in laboratory experiments with grasses provided as a sole food and under particular maintenance conditions. To verify these data under natural conditions, the food preference of *S. gregaria* hoppers was first investigated in choice and no-choice experiments (Fig. 1).

Increase in weight and food consumption

According to the results obtained in the feeding experiments in the following trials, *S. thebaica* and maize were offered as no-choice food and a choice between *S. thebaica, V. unguiculata* and *Heliotropium* offered. The daily food uptake and increase in body weight did not differ signifi-

Table 4. Surface covered by hoppers of instar 1 to 5

Instar	Surface ± SD in cm^2	Number of hoppers/m2, based on the distance between the single insects		
		hoppers close together, no distance in between	distance: width of 1/3 hopper	distance: width of 1/2 hopper
L_1	0.146±0.03	68,500	45,500	32,250
L_2	0.439±0.06	22,700	15,100	11,350
L_3	0.684±0.10	14,600	9,700	7,300
L_4	0.684±0.10	8,000	5,300	4,000
L_5	2.886±0.40	3,600	2,400	1,800

$n = 20$ for each instar

cantly according to the various food supplied. Figure 2 represents the data achieved with the mixed food supply.

Calculated food consumption of hopper bands

Based on the daily food uptake of a single nymph, the food consumption of a hopper band can be calculated approximately.

As depicted in Figure 2, the hoppers double their weight through a nymph instar. Because this doubling follows an approximate linearity, hopper weight halfway through an instar amounts to

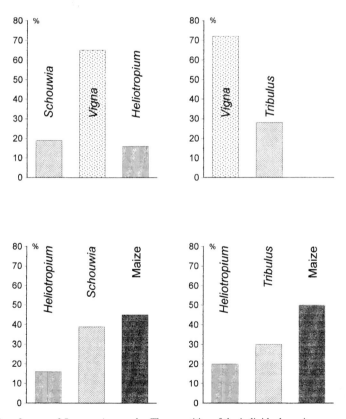

Figure 1. Food preference of *S. gregaria* nymphs. The quantities of the individual species consumed are expressed as % of the total food amounts consumed. Of all species offered, the cow pea was clearly the most preferred. On the other hand, *Schouwia* thebaica was consumed to about the same extent as maize. *Vigna unguiculata* and maize were unequivocally preferred over *Tribulus terrestris*. *Heliotropium* sp. was taken up in all trials to a comparable extent.

half the sum obtained by adding the initial and end weights of each instar. The values achieved for each instar amount to (compare also Fig. 2):

$$L_1 = 0.022 \text{ g}; L_2 = 0.055 \text{ g}; L_3 = 0.176 \text{ g}; L_4 = 0.414 \text{ g and } L_5 = 0.849 \text{ g}$$

On the basis of this approximate linearity of the two parameters weight and food uptake within the short time of one stage, and given the observation that the average quantity of vegetation consumed amounts to one-third of body weight, a simplified vegetation loss quota can be calculated. From these relations it follows that the daily food intake of a hopper or a hopper band can be calculated as follows:

average weight (g) × 0.3 = g/day (average weight = weight of hoppers halfway through a stage)

Calculated as the daily food consumption of a band in kilograms, one obtains the following expression:

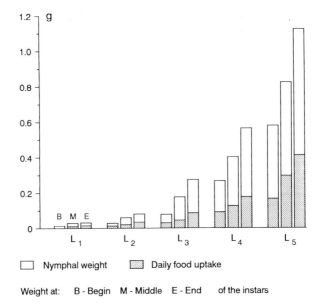

Figure 2. Weight increase and food uptake of S. gregaria hoppers. The daily food uptake was 30±8% of the body weight. This is a rounded-off average value. In these experiments the drastically reduced uptake just before and after each moult was also measured, as well as the maxima lying between two moults. The body weight data are the average of 60 weightings for each instar. The food uptake was determined three times in separate experiments for each instar and each food plant. These experiments were repeated in the 1994/95 season and gave comparable if somewhat higher results of about 35%. Within a stage, food uptake and gain of body weight both increase more or less linearly. But viewed over the entire nymphal development, it becomes clear that these increases follow a quadratic ($x^2 + a$) function.

$$\frac{\text{number of hoppers} \times \text{average weight} \times 0.3}{1000} = \text{kg vegetation/day}$$

Using these values, food consumption can be calculated for each individual stage; for example, for an L_1 band:

$$\text{number of hoppers} \times \frac{0.022 \times 0.3}{1000} = \text{kg vegetation/day}$$

Since

$$\frac{0.022 \times 0.3}{1000} \quad \text{equals nearly} \quad \frac{1}{150,000}$$

it follows in this case that the amount of vegetation consumed daily is:

$$\frac{\text{number of 1st instar nymphs}}{150,000} = \text{kg/day}$$

The denominators for the other stages are as follows:

$$L_2 = 60,000; \; L_3 = 20,000, \; L_4 = 8000, \; L_5 = 4000$$

These calculated values yield inaccurate estimates when applied to a single day. For example, in a uniform band of equal instar they are too high at the beginning and too low at the end. In addition, the time period spent in a certain area is important. But if a band stays for several days or during an entire instar in defined areas and the expressions derived above are multiplied by the number of days, reliable estimates of potential loss can be made.

Table 5. Biomass of wild and cultivated plants

	Sorghum sp. leaves and panicles	young maize* leaves	*V. ungiuculata* whole plant	*S. thebaica* leaves	*F. olivieri* leaves	*T. terrestris* leaves	*H. muticus* leaves
Coverage	10 plants per 10 m²	12 plants per 10 m²	12.5 plants per m²	90%	70%	30%	90%
Biomass (kg/ha)	2500	1600	4500	9300	5600	3500	9900

*The maize plants had an average height of 0.7±0.1 m and did not yet have panicles

In order to estimate potential losses, however, rough estimates of the size of the areas affected and the biomass available to *S. gregaria* must be provided. Some of these estimates are shown in Table 5.

The values given in the tables are the mean of 10 individual plants (*S. thebaica, Sorghum* sp. and maize) or the weight of the plants removed from six sample plots with a vegetation coverage of 100%. All calculations included only those parts of the plants consumed by *S. gregaria*, namely leaves and fruits. The calculation on a hectare basis for *Sorghum*, maize, and *V. unguiculata* is based on the way these plants are generally cultivated in Mauritania. That means a plant density of 10, 12 and 12.5 per 10 m^2 was assumed respectively, and for wild plants, different degrees of coverage varying between 30% to 90% were taken which represent the biomass of wild plants found in the field during the locust season. As regards the cultivated plants, wide variations are possible, because they are planted at quite variable times after the rainy season.

The extent of possible plant losses is demonstrated in the following worst-case scenario: A hopper band which has concentrated on one hectare and with an initial size of (L_1) 2 million hoppers (density 200/m^2) and a final size (L_5) of 0.5 million (= 50/m^2), remains in the same area for its entire development until adult moult. This contains a natural mortality rate of 75%, significantly less than the value of 92% measured by Roffey and Popov (1968). Assuming a developmental time of 36 days, the natural mortality already mentioned and the food consumption rates already indicated, the total food uptake of this hopper band amounts to 2450 kg. That means maize and sorghum suffer 100% damage, that is, all the available biomass would be consumed. Normally, it can be assumed that infested areas will be deserted after a few days. In this case the damage will be much less, especially since the plants have the ability to regenerate. This is also true of grazing land. Furthermore, it should be added here that the biomass estimates taken for wild plants in Table 5, based on a single species, are too low. Normally, one finds a mixed vegetation of plants covering the ground completely (e.g. *T. terrestris* and *F. olivieri*), with other species emerging above this cover *(S. thebaica)*. The higher damage inflicted on cultivated plants, especially in the case of maize and sorghum, is primarily due to their lower proportion of plant parts which can be used by *S. gregaria* (leaves, panicles and cobs) in relation to those that may not be used (stalks).

Discussion

No effects were essentially obtained in the tests with the microsporidian *Nosema locustae*, nor with several cold-pressed neem oils, which had less than 200 ppm of active ingredients (Wilps and Nasseh 1994a). Some other neem oils yielded high mortality rates, but were not tested further, because the content of active ingredients varied too much between different batches (Wilps et al. 1993b; Wilps and Nasseh 1994b). Commercially produced neem products were, as a rule, very effective, but were omitted from the tests because so far they have been too expensive for large-scale application (Nasseh et al. 1992a, b; Wilps and Nasseh 1994b). In contrast, the IGRs, several species of fungal spores (*B. bassiana and M. flavivoride*) and various botanicals caused sufficient mortality rates. In addition, all these products were shown to be ecologically tolerable and harmless to the environment (Peveling et al. 1994). The results obtained under field conditions with the various botanicals support findings made in the laboratory (Schmutterer and Freres 1990; Nicol and Schmutterer 1991; Mwangi 1982; Mwangi and Rembold 1986, 1988). The IGRs tested were not only effective but are also suitable for barrier treatments because of their persistence for 14 days or longer. This method, also used successfully by Scherer and Rakotanandrasna (1993) against *Locusta migratoria*, also permits a large amount of insecticides to be saved. Similar savings are also possible by treating roosting places and resting areas. For this purpose, botanicals are excellent as well, and they cause an additional significant reduction in fitness (loss of hoppers' mobility), so that they become an easy prey for predators (Wilps, unpublished data). Another important advantage of botanicals is that they are formulated with pure plant oil, and thus present no problems of contamination after application and are easily biodegradable.

The investigations on food preference and consumption show that the average daily food consumption is substantially lower than had been previously assumed (Davey 1952). Regarding the total food uptake of 2450 kg by a hopper band with an initial size of 2 million, its daily migrating behaviour on the one hand and the biomass of wild plants after favourable rainy seasons (see Tab. 5 and text) on the other, it becomes clear that *S. gregaria* is not a competitor of grazing livestock. The preference for cultivated plants, especially for cow pea, might be due to a lower content of alkaloids and terpenoids in food plants in comparison to wild plants. In general, damage to plants may reach high levels but the extent to which this damage can be overcome by the plants' regeneration ability must be investigated. Nevertheless, the data obtained so far demonstrate that losses may be assessed, although more data regarding the biomass of different plants, locusts' feeding habits and migrating behaviour are still needed.

Acknowledgements
We would especially like to thank our co-workers at the station in Akjoujt, especially Ba Ousmane, Issa Sy and Ahmed ould Hadj, as well as the team members of the Force Maghrebine, who gave us timely information about the location of numerous hopper bands. Thanks are also due to the National Plant Protection Service in Mauritania, which gave us constant support in all our activities during our investigations. Last but not least, our sincere thanks to Volkhard Leffler, who gave his untiring assistance and provided logistical support.

References

Davey PM (1952) Quantities of food eaten by the desert locust, Schistocerca gregaria (Forsk.) in relation to growth. Anti Locust Research Centre: 539–551

Mwangi RW (1982) Locust antifeedant activity in fruits of Melia volkensii. Ent Exp Appl 31: 277–280

Mwangi RW, Rembold H (1986) Growth-regulating activity of Melia volkensii extracts against the larvae of Aedes aegypti. Proc 3rd Int Neem Conf, Nairobi: 669–681

Mwangi RW, Rembold H (1988) Growth-inhibiting and larvicidal effects of Melia volkensii extracts on Aedes aegypti larvae. Ent Exp Appl 46: 103–108

Nasseh O, Wilps H, Krall S (1992a) Neem Products – effective biocides for combatting the desert locust Schistocerca gregaria (Forsk.). Report on investigations carried out on field and laboratory-reared locusts under natural conditions in the Tamesna Desert (Republic of Niger). Zschr Pflkr Pflsch 100: 611–621

Nasseh O, Wilps H, Krall S (1992b) Efficacy of neem, Azadirachta indica A. Juss, in controlling the laboratory-reared and field-captured larvae of Schistocerca gregaria (Forsk.) in field cage trials in the Republic of Niger. Pages 79–90 in Kleeberg H (ed) Practice-oriented results on use and production of neem ingredients

Nasseh O, Wilps H, Krall S, Salisossou, MGM (1992c) Les effectes d'inhibiteurs de croissance et de biocides végétaux sur les larves de Schistocerca gregaria (Forscål). SAHEL PV INFO 45: 5–19

Nasseh O, Wilps H, Rembold H, Krall S (1993) Biologically active compounds in Melia volkensii – larval growth inhibitor and phase modulator against the desert locust Schistocerca gregaria (Forsk.). J Appl Ent 116: 1–11

Nicol CMJ, Schmutterer H (1991) Kontaktwirkungen des Samenöls des Niembaumes Azadirachta indica (A. Juss) bei gregären Larven der Wüstenheuschrecke Schistocerca gregaria (Forsk.) J Appl Ent 111: 197–205

Peveling R, Weyrich J, Müller P (1994) Side-effects of botanicals, insect growth regulators and entomopathogenic fungi on epigeal non-target arthropods in locust control. Pages 147–176 in Krall S, Wilps H (eds) New trends in locust control. Rossdorf: TZ-Verlags-Gesellschaft

Roffey J, Popov GB (1968) Environmental and behavioural processes in a desert locust outbreak. Nature 219: 446–450

Scherer R, Rakotanandrasna MA (1993) Barrier treatment with benzoyl urea insect growth regulator against Locusta migratoria capito (SAUSS) hopper bands in Madagascar. Int J Pest Management 39: 411–417

Schmutterer H, Freres T (1990) Beeinflussung von Metamorphose, Färbung und Verhalten der Wüstenheuschrecke Schistocerca gregaria (Forsk.) und der afrikanischen Wanderheuschrecke Locusta migratoria migratorioides (R. &.F) durch Niemsamenöl. Zschr Pflkr Pflsch 97: 431–438

Wilps H, Kirkilionis E, Muschenich K (1992a) The effects of neem oil and azadirachtin on mortality, flight activity and energy metabolism of Schistocerca gregaria Forskål – a comparison between laboratory and field locusts. Comp Biochem Physiol 102C: 67–71

Wilps H, Nasseh O (1992a) The effects of insect growth regulators, plant compounds and pathogens on larvae and adult of the desert locust Schistocerca gregaria: results of laboratory and field investigations in Agadez and Anou Mekkerene (North-Niger), 1991. GTZ Report, 68 pp

Wilps H, Nasseh O (1992b) The effect of various neem products on the fitness of adult Schistocerca gregaria. Pages 337–346 in Lomer CJ, Prior C (eds) Biological control of locusts and grasshoppers. Proceedings of a workshop held at the International Institute of Tropical Agriculture, Cotonou, Republic of Benin, 29 April–1 May 1991

Wilps H, Nasseh O (1994a) Field tests with botanicals, mycocides and chitin synthesis inhibitors. Pages 51–79 in Krall S, Wilps H (eds) New trends in locust control. Rossdorf: TZ-Verlags-Gesellschaft

Wilps H, Nasseh O (1994b) Current status and future prospects of natural products for locust control. Pages 24–33 in Rembold H, Benson JA, Franzen H, Weickel B, Schulz FA (eds) New strategies for locust control in natural-product and receptor research. Proceedings of the CEC workshop held in Hamburg, Germany, 10–11 June 1993. Bonn: ATSAF

Wilps H, Nasseh O, Krall S (1993a) The effects of various neem formulations on mortality rate and morphogenetic defects upon Schistocerca gregaria (Forskål) larvae. – Report on investigations carried out on field and laboratory-reared locusts under natural conditions in the southern Sahara Desert (Republic of Niger). Pages 221–236 in RP Singh, MS Chari, AK Raheja, W Kraus (eds) Neem and Environment; vol. 2., Bangalore, Lebanon, New Hampshire

Wilps H, Nasseh O, Krall S (1993b) Application to flying locusts – a powerful method for combatting S. gregaria (Forsk.) adults. Trends in Biochem and Physiol India: 1073–1082

Wilps H, Nasseh O, Rembold H, Krall S (1993c) The effect of Melia volkensii extracts on mortality and fitness of adult Schistocerca gregaria (Forsk.) J Appl Entomol 116: 12–19

New Strategies in Locust Control
S. Krall, R. Peveling and D. Ba Diallo (eds)
© 1997 Birkhäuser Verlag Basel/Switzerland

Persistence of benzoylphenylureas in the control of the migratory locust *Locusta migratoria capito* (Sauss.) in Madagascar

R. Scherer and H. Célestin

Deutsche Gesellschaft für Technische Zusammenarbeit (GTZ), Projet Protection des Végétaux, Bureau GTZ, B.P. 869, Antananarivo, Madagascar

Summary. The benzoylphenylureas (BPUs), insecticides classified as insect growth regulators (IGRs), are potential products to replace dieldrin in barrier locust control because of their relatively long persistence. A short literature review of their use in pest control is documented in this paper. To study the persistence of diflubenzuron and triflumuron (two derivatives of BPU) on nymphs of *Locusta migratoria*, tests in cages were carried out in the field in south-west Madagascar. Plots were treated with each product at doses of 50 and 100 g/ha. Cages containing 200 hoppers each were installed on plots 0, 14 and 28 days after treatment. After 2 days the cages with hoppers were moved to untreated plots. The mortality was 100, 70 to 80 and 30 to 70% for animals placed on vegetation 0, 14 and 28 days after treatment respectively. The results of these experimental treatments indicate that the persistence of BPUs is sufficient for use in barrier treatment against hopper bands of *L. migratoria*.

Résumé. A la recherche de produits pouvant remplacer la dieldrine pour le traitement par barrières en lutte contre les locustes l'attention fut attirée sur les benzoylphenylurées (BPU), insecticides classés parmi les dérégulateurs de croissance (IGR). Ces produits ont montré une rémanence assez importante dans la lutte contre divers ravageurs. Des exemples documentés sont présentés. Pour étudier l'effet rémanent du diflubenzuron et du triflumuron (deux dérivés des BPU) sur les larves de *Locusta migratoria*, des tests sous cages ont été effectués en plein air dans le Sud-Ouest de Madagascar. Des parcelles ont été traitées avec chacun des produits aux doses de 50 et 100 g/ha. Les cages avec 200 larves chacune furent installées sur les parcelles 0, 14 et 28 jours après le traitement. Après 2 jours elles ont été déplacées sur terrain non-traité. L'efficacité du traitement fut calculée à 100, 70 à 80 et 30 à 70% respectivement pour les tests à 0, 14 et 28 jours après le traitement. Selon ces résultats et des traitements expérimentaux les BPU ont un effet rémanent suffisamment long pour être utilisés en traitement par barrières contre des bandes larvaires de *L. migratoria*.

Introduction

Since the ban of dieldrin no product has been found with sufficient persistence to be useful in the control of locusts by barrier treatment. To date, pesticides replacing dieldrin have to be sprayed repeatedly to cope with reinvasions. Industry is interested in developing persistent products for food crops not because of residue problems, but for locust control and non-food crops.

Eventually, research on new products with limited persistence led to the development of the benzoylphenylureas (BPUs). Several studies with different pests have shown that, depending on conditions, these products remain active for one to twelve months after application.

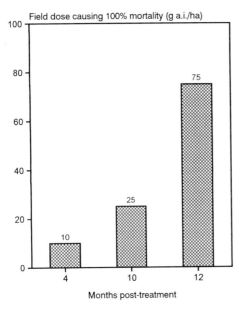

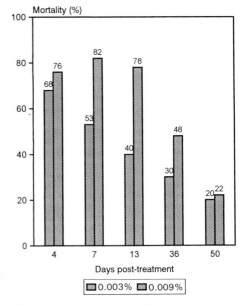

Figure 1. Minimum field dose of diflubenzuron required to achieve 100% mortality in *Lymantria monacha*. Treated pine needles were fed to caterpillars at various periods after treatment (after Skatulla 1989).

Figure 2. Mortality in caterpillars of *Spodoptera littoralis* fed on cotton treated with diflubenzuron at different times after treatment (after Ascher and Nemmy 1984).

Experiments conducted in Germany using different doses indicate that BPUs degraded much more slowly than other insecticides on the surface of pine leaves (Skatulla 1989). Lepidopteran larvae raised in cages were fed on treated vegetation at different intervals after treatment. The dose required to achieve 100% mortality was 10, 25 and 75 g a.i./ha at 4, 10 and 12 months post-treatment respectively (Fig. 1). Teflubenzuron and triflumuron had a shorter persistence. In another assay leaves were treated with diflubenzuron at the recommended dose and at one-tenth of this dose. Treated leaves were fed to larvae once a week for a period of 10 weeks. One hundred percent mortality was achieved up to 10 weeks post-treatment at the recommended dose and up to 4 weeks at the lower dose.

Ascher and Nemmy (1984) treated cotton fields with teflubenzuron and diflubenzuron and fed the leaves to lepidopteran larvae at different times after treatment. With diflubenzuron applied at doses of 0.003 and 0.009%, the mortality never reached 100% (Fig. 2). However at a dose of 0.009%, the product had retained its initial effect even 13 days after treatment. The other IGR tested, teflubenzuron, remained very effective up to 28 days post-treatment at a dose of 0.009%

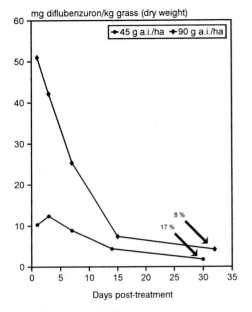

Figure 3. Residues of diflubenzuron on grasses, Senegal, 1990.

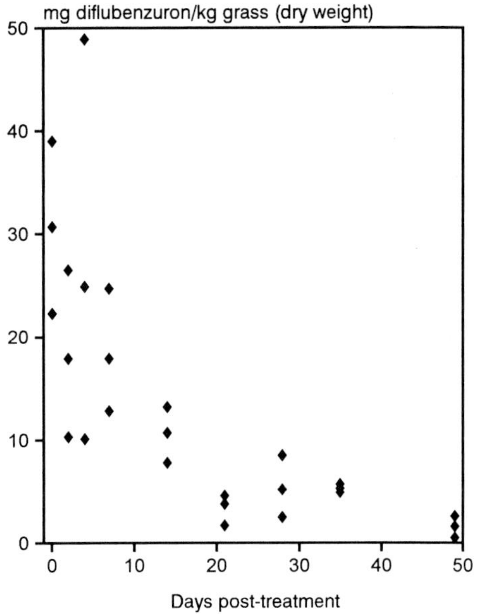

Figure 4. Residues of diflubenzuron on grasses, Mali, 1990.

and 50 days post-treatment at doses of 0.003 and 0.009%. Herbert and Harper (1985) also conducted tests with teflubenzuron on cotton and found a high efficacy for up to 55 days after treatment.

Pouwelse and Allan (1991, 1992) studied the persistence of diflubenzuron on grassy vegetation by taking samples for chemical analysis at different times after treatment. In Senegal, the doses applied were 45 and 90 g/ha. Seventeen percent and 8% (1.8 and 4.2 mg/kg of dry vegetation) of the quantity found one day after application was recovered after 30 days (Fig. 3). In Mali, treatments at 62 (originally meant to be 60), 62 and 64 g/ha were conducted. In all three cases an average of 17% of the amount found in samples taken two hours after the treatment was recovered one month later (Fig. 4). The residual was more than 5 mg of diflubenzuron per kilogram of dried vegetation.

These biological tests and chemical residue analyses confirm that the BPUs remain active for weeks or even months after treatment.

Materials and methods

The study area selected was near the village of Besatra and 9 km to the south of Betioky. The vegetation consisted of grasses dominated by *Heteropogon contortus*. In this area four plots for treatment and one as control (40 × 40 m each) were selected. Treatments were with diflubenzuron and triflumuron each at 50 and 100 g/ha. In each plot, 36 subplots measuring 5 × 5 m were marked for placing cages.

The assays were performed in field cages. Each cage (3 × 3 × 1.5 m) could be entered for evaluating the organisms. Immediately after the application three cages were at 3 of the 36 subplots randomly in each of the four treatments and control. After installation of the cages, 200 4th and 5th instar hoppers of the migratory locust were placed in each cage. The hoppers tested were in the transient and gregarious phases and captured from hopper bands in the vicinity, but sometimes as far away as 250 km from Betioky. Hoppers were allowed to acclimatise for a period of two or three days in a cage near the experimental site. The cages with hoppers remained on the treated plots for two days and subsequently were taken to untreated vegetation.

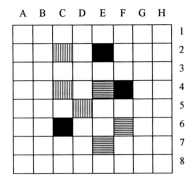

Plot (40 x 40 m) treated with diflubenzuron
at 100 g/ha. Date of treatment: 14.02.1994

Hatch fill	Stocking of field cages (date)	Days post-treatment	Code of site
■	14.02.1994	0	E2,F4,C6
▥	28.02.1994	14	C2,C4,D5
▤	14.03.1994	28	E4,F6,E7

Figure 5. Arrangement of cages on the plot treated with diflubenzuron at 100 g/ha.

This treatment simulates a barrier treatment situation, in which hoppers would not permanently ingest the products, but remain for most of the time between the treated barriers.

Two weeks after the treatment, the first test was terminated. Thereafter the empty cages were shifted to subplots not used previously and restocked with 200 nymphs each, following the same procedure as described for the first test. Again, 4th and 5th instar nymphs were placed in the cages. In this way they were exposed to vegetation which had been treated two weeks previously. For this test we proceeded in exactly the same way as in the preceding test. In the fourth week a third test was carried out in the same manner. Figure 5 shows the arrangement of the cages for the plot treated at 100 g of diflubenzuron per hectare.

Observations were made every two days for a period of two weeks. Survival, developmental stage and malformations were recorded. The efficacy was determined for each day according to the formula of Henderson and Tilton (1955):

$$E = 100 \times \left(1 - \frac{Tb \times Na}{Ta \times Nb} \right)$$

E = Efficacy in % on the day of evaluation
Ta = Treated plot: number of hoppers tested
Tb = Treated plot: number alive on the day of evaluation
Na = Untreated plot: number of hoppers tested
Nb = Untreated plot: number alive on the day of evaluation

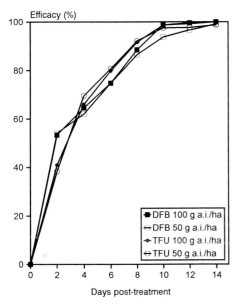

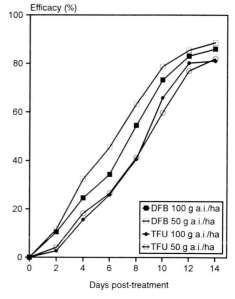

Figure 6. Mean efficacy of diflubenzuron (DFB) and triflumuron (TFU) on nymphs of *L. migratoria* 0 weeks post-treatment.

Figure 7. Mean efficacy of diflubenzuron (DFB) and triflumuron (TFU) on nymphs of *L. migratoria* 2 weeks post-treatment.

Results and discussion

Efficacy of the benzoylureas diflubenzuron and triflumuron decreased from about 100% for both products at all doses immediately after application (Fig. 6) to 81 and 89% two weeks later (Fig. 7) and 34 and 70% after four weeks (Fig. 8), depending on product and dose. The summary in Figure 9 shows a satisfactory efficacy at 14 days after treatment with slightly better results for diflubenzuron at the two doses used. After 28 days an effect could still be noted, but was reduced depending on the product and dose. The best results were found for diflubenzuron, with an efficacy of 50 and 70% at 50 and 100 g/ha.

In the controls an average mortality of 63, 42 and 77% were found in the first, second and third tests respectively. Physiological stress during transport (up to two days) may have contributed to the low survival (Fig. 10). More important in our opinion may have been the high level of parasitoid infestation and fungal disease in nymphs of the migratory locust observed during the 1994 campaign. Despite this high non-treatment mortality Figure 10 shows a considerable rate of mortality due to treatment in tests 1 and 2 and for the diflubenzuron groups in test 3.

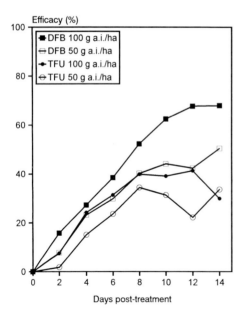

Figure 8. Mean efficacy of diflubenzuron (DFB) and triflumuron (TFU) on nymphs of *L. migratoria* 4 weeks post-treatment.

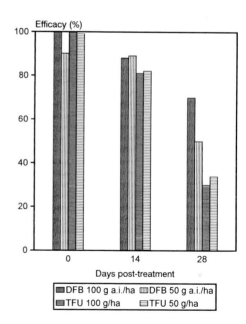

Figure 9. *Summary* of the efficacy of diflubenzuron (DFB) and triflumuron (TFU) 0, 14 and 28 days post-treatment.

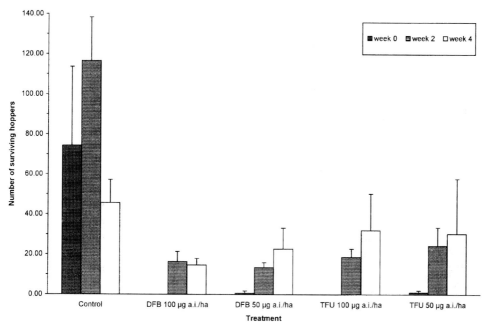

Figure 10. Survival in nymphs exposed for two days to vegetation treated with diflubenzuron (DFB) and triflumuron (TFU) on the same day and two or four weeks previously. Initial number of nymphs: 200. Values are the mean of three replicates ± Standard deviation (SD).

The results of this study show that BPUs are sufficiently persistent, up to two weeks, under the climatic conditions of Madagascar for lasting effects on the migratory locust similar to those found for other pests. Therefore, it may be recommended that the practice of barrier treatment against the pests can be resumed if barrier spacing is 300 to 600 m and the vegetation is low, conditions under which hopper bands enter a barrier within a few days after treatment (Scherer and Rakotonandrasana 1993; Cooper et al. 1995).

References

Ascher KRS, Nemmy NE (1984) The effect of CME 134 on *Spodoptera littoralis* eggs and larvae. Phytoparasitica 12: 13–27

Cooper J, Dobson HM, Scherer R, Rakotonandrasana A (1995) Sprayed barriers of diflubenzuron (ULV) as a control technique against marching hopper bands of migratory locust *Locusta migratoria capito* (Sauss) (Orthoptera: Acrididae) in Southern Madagascar. Crop Protection 14: 137–143

Henderson CF, Tilton EW (1955) Tests with acaricides against the brown wheat mite. Journal of Economic Entomology 48: 157–161

Herbert DA, Harper DJ (1985) Field trials and laboratory bioassays of CME 134, a new insect growth regulator against *Heliothis zea* and other lepidopterous pests of soybeans. Journal of Economic Entomology 78: 333–338

Pouwelse AV, Allan E (1991) Diflubenzuron residues in grass (Senegal, 1989) Report Duphar B. V. The Netherlands NO. 56630/118/1990 DI - 8175

Pouwelse AV, Allan E (1992) Diflubenzuron residues in grass (Mali, 1990) Report Solvay Duphar B. V. The Netherlands NO. 56637/44/1989 DI - 8554

Scherer R, Rakotonandrasana A (1993) Barrier treatment with a benzoyl urea insect growth regulator against *Locusta migratoria capito* (Sauss) hopper bands in Madagascar. International Journal of Pest Management 39: 411–417

Skatulla U, Kellner M (1989) Zur Persistenz einiger Häutungshemmer auf Kiefernnadeln. Anzeiger für Schädlingskunde Pflanzenschutz Umweltschutz 62: 121–123

New Strategies in Locust Control
S. Krall, R. Peveling and D. Ba Diallo (eds)
© 1997 Birkhäuser Verlag Basel/Switzerland

Evaluation of insect growth regulators for the control of the African migratory locust, *Locusta migratoria migratorioides* (R. & F.), in Central Africa

A.C.Z. Musuna and F.N. Mugisha[1]

International Red Locust Control Organisation for Central and Southern Africa (IRLCO-CSA), Ndola, Zambia

Summary. The insect growth regulators (IGRs) flumuron, hexaflumuron and teflubenzuron were field-tested against *Locusta migratoria migratorioides* (R. & F.) hoppers in Malawi and Zambia in 1993. They were sprayed at three different dose rates: 25 (teflubenzuron only), 50 and 100 g a.i./ha (all IGRs). All IGRs tested adversely affected moulting of 3rd and 4th instar hoppers at any of the applied dose rates. Mortality was low in Zambia (5 to 38% 5 days post-treatment) at dose rates of 50 and 100 g a.i./ha, but high in Malawi (50 to 87% on day 5 and 73 to 100% on day 7 post-treatment) at dose rates of 25, 50 and 100 g a.i./ha. However, no clear-cut dose-response relationship was observed, and conclusions as to which of the IGRs tested was the most promising control agent could not be drawn. Despite these shortcomings, the results obtained suggest that, in general, IGRs may play an important role in preventive locust control.

Résumé. Les insecticides dérégulateurs de croissance (insect growth regulators – IGR) flumuron, hexaflumuron et téflubenzuron ont fait l'objet en 1993 d'essais sur le terrain contre *Locusta migratoria migratorioides* (R. & F.) au Malawi et en Zambie. Les épandages ont été effectués à différentes doses: 25 m.a./ha (téflubenzuron seulement) 50 et 100 g m.a./ha (pour chacun des IGR). En Zambie, le taux de mortalité n'a été que faible (5 à 38% 5 jours après traitement) aux doses 50 et 100 g m.a./ha, mais il a par contre été élevé au Malawi (50 à 87% le 5ème jour après traitement et 73 à 100% le 7ème jour après traitement) aux doses 25, 50 et 100 g m.a./ha. Toutefois, l'existence d'un rapport précis entre dose et effet n'a pu être constatée et il n'a pu être tiré de conclusions quant à la supériorité de l'un ou l'autre des IGR testés. Néanmoins, les résultats obtenus semblent indiquer que d'une manière générale les IGR pourront jouer un rôle important dans la lutte antiacridienne préventive.

Introduction

The African migratory locust, *Locusta migratoria migratorioides* (R. & F.), is prevalent in many countries in Africa south of the Sahara desert (Anonymous 1992a, b). Upsurges of this locust species occur, from time to time, in Central and Southern Africa. Synthetic, non-specific organic insecticides are widely used to control migratory locusts in outbreak situations.

The widespread use of these insecticides is of global concern with respect to environmental hazards in general and side-effects on non-target organisms in particular. It is in this regard, therefore, that the International Red Locust Control Organisation for Central and Southern

---

[1]F.N. Mugisha died on 24 October 1995.

Africa (IRLCO-CSA) embarked on evaluating alternative locust control agents including insect growth regulators (IGRs) (Anonymous 1992a, b, 1993). Due to their persistence of several weeks, IGRs have potential as barrier treatments in preventive locust control. Thus, in 1993, IRLCO-CSA evaluated the effects of IGRs on hoppers of *L. m. migratorioides*.

Materials and methods

Three IGRs, flumuron (Cascade 5 ULV), hexaflumuron (Consult 250 ULV) and teflubenzuron (Nomolt 5 ULV) were field-tested as blanket sprays on 3rd and 4th instar hoppers of *L. m. migratorioides* in the Lake Chiuta plains (14°9.2'S/35°8.3'E) in southeastern Malawi and at Kasaya (17°5.5'S/24°9.7'E) in southern Zambia in November and December 1993, respectively. Dose rates were 25 (teflubenzuron only), 50 and 100 g a.i./ha (all IGRs), following the supplier's recommendations. The IGRs were suitably diluted with Shellsol AB and diesel in order to attain the appropriate rate of application. A control comprising a mixture of Shellsol AB and diesel was included in each trial. Each treatment was replicated three times. Separate, relatively stationary hopper bands, each covering at least 0.5 ha, were taken as treatment plots. The vegetation mainly consisted of *Hyparrhenia* spp.

Treatments were carried out between 9.00 and 10.00 h using hand-held battery-powered Micro-ULVA sprayers. The air temperature at this time ranged from 20 °C to 30 °C. Three samples, each of 20 hoppers, were randomly collected from each plot 30 minutes after spraying. Hoppers were maintained indoors at ambient temperature in cages (18 cm × 18 cm × 6 cm) for subsequent observation. In a first series (I; Malawi and Zambia), grasses were harvested from teflubenzuron- and hexaflumuron-treated plots and fed ad libitum to caged hoppers. Thus, the route of pesticide uptake was twofold in this series, via direct contact during spraying and via ingestion of treated food thereafter. In a second series (II; Zambia), which also included flumuron, unsprayed hoppers were collected and starved for 36 h before being fed on grasses sprayed with the respective IGRs. In this series, pesticide uptake was predominantly via ingestion. Mortality and moulting success of caged hoppers was assessed daily from 7.00 to 8.00 h until five days (Zambia) or seven days (Malawi) post-treatment. Data shown in tables and figures are means of three replicates. No statistical data analysis is presented in this paper.

Results

Series I

In Malawi, 65% of the hoppers in the control moulted successfully from 3rd to 4th instar within seven days post-treatment, but none of those sprayed with hexaflumuron or teflubenzuron did. Hexaflumuron (100 g a.i./ha) and teflubenzuron (50 g a.i./ha) were very effective, since they caused 100 and 97% mortality, respectively, six days after spraying (Tab. 1). At lower dose rates the two IGRs were less effective. Seven days after spraying only 10% hopper mortality occurred in the control.

In Zambia, all hoppers in the control moulted successfully from the 4th to 5th instar four days after spraying, while at least 48% of the hoppers treated with an IGR failed to moult (Fig. 1). Less than 40% hopper mortality was caused by IGRs treatment five days after spraying (Tab. 2).

Table 1. Mean mortality (%) of hoppers of *L. m. migratorioides* sprayed with teflubenzuron and hexaflumuron at various dose rates within seven days post-treatment in Malawi

Treatment	Dosage g a.i./ha	Days after treatment						
		1	2	3	4	5	6	7
Teflubenzuron	25	0	23	23	43	50	53	73
Teflubenzuron	50	0	13	17	53	55	97	99
Hexaflumuron	50	0	10	53	53	53	83	83
Hexaflumuron	100	0	37	73	83	87	100	100
Control	-	0	0	0	0	3	7	10

Table 2. Mean mortality (%) of hoppers of *L. m. migratorioides* sprayed with teflubenzuron and hexaflumuron at various dose rates within five days post-treatment in Zambia

Treatment	Dosage g a.i./ha	Days after treatment				
		1	2	3	4	5
Teflubenzuron	100	0	8	10	28	38
Teflubenzuron	50	0	0	3	18	20
Hexaflumuron	100	0	0	0	0	18
Hexaflumuron	50	0	0	0	0	5
Control	–	0	0	0	0	0

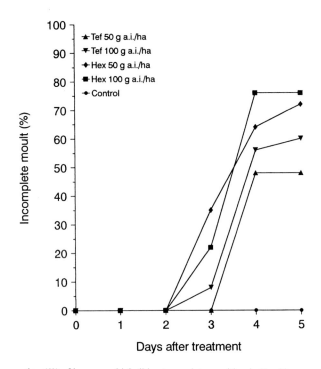

Figure 1. Mean proportion (%) of hoppers which did not complete moulting in Zambia.

Series II

Four days post-treatment the moulting success of hoppers having fed on treated grasses was 57% (flumuron, 100 g), 73% (flumuron, 50 g), 67% (hexaflumuron, 100 g), 85% (hexaflumuron, 50 g), 45% (teflubenzuron, 100 g) and 65% (teflubenzuron, 50 g), respectively, while 80% of the hoppers in the control groups moulted successfully. On the same day, mortality was still relatively low (<40%) in all treatments (Fig. 2).

Discussion

L. m. migratorioides hoppers normally undergo five moults (Steedman 1993). At the time the studies were conducted, the hoppers had already moulted two or three times, hence the population was a mixture of the 3rd and 4th instars (3:1 proportion). IGRs are known to be more effective on early instars (Krall and Nasseh 1992). Even though the hoppers used in these trials were in their advanced stages of development, the IGRs caused hopper mortality and moult disruptions especially in Malawi (Tab. 1). The results obtained in Zambia were not as good as expected: the observed responses, both mortality and moult disruptions, were not dose dependent. For example, teflubenzuron evoked higher mortality at a dose rate of 50 g a.i./ha than at 100 g (Fig. 2). However, statistical significance could not be proved. Moreover, delayed responses that may have shown up later than five days (Zambia) or seven days post-treatment have been missed due to an unavoidable early termination of the observations. Also, comparison of the efficacy of the three IGRs tested is not possible on the basis of the current data.

In series II (ingestion only) the effects on both moulting and mortality were not as pronounced as in series I (combined contact plus ingestion). These findings support the view that IGRs, though originally designed as stomach poisons, are more effective when used as contact insecticides. However, because no pure contact spray treatments (without subsequent feeding on trea-

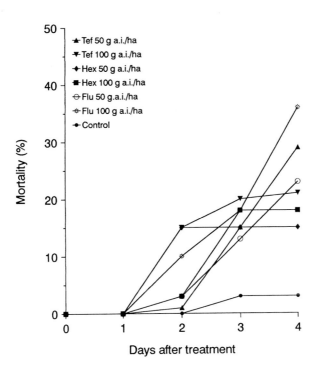

Figure 2. Mean mortality (%) in hoppers fed on treated grasses in Zambia.

ted grasses) were included as a variant, no conclusions can be drawn regarding the comparative efficacy of residual or contact spraying.

Despite these shortcomings, the results obtained suggest that, in general, IGRs may play an important role in preventive locust control.

Acknowledgements
This paper is presented with the permission of the director of the International Red Locust Control Organisation for Central and Southern Africa. The authors wish to thank the National Resources Institute (NRI), UK, for supplying the IGRs tested.

References

Anonymous (1992a) The locust and grasshopper agricultural manual. Centre for Overseas Pest Research. London
Anonymous (1992b) Report of the director for the year 1992. IRLCO-CSA, Ndola, Zambia
Anonymous (1993) Report of the director for the year 1993. IRLCO-CSA, Ndola, Zambia
Krall S and Nasseh O M (1992) GTZ – the integrated biological control of locusts and grasshoppers – a GTZ research project. Pages 44–49 in Lomer CJ and Prior C (eds) Biological control of locusts and grasshoppers. IIBC\IITA, CAB, UK
Steedman A (ed) (1993) Locust handbook. NRI, Chatham, UK 204 pp

New Strategies in Locust Control
S. Krall, R. Peveling and D. Ba Diallo (eds)
© 1997 Birkhäuser Verlag Basel/Switzerland

Field application of the juvenile hormone analogue fenoxycarb against hopper bands of *Locusta migratoria capito* in Madagascar

A. Dorn[1], M. Schneider[1], F.F.W. Botens[1,2], M. Holtmann[1] and I. Petzak[1]

[1]*Institute of Zoology, University of Mainz, D-55099 Mainz, Germany*
[2]*Bureau GTZ B.P. 869, Antananarivo (101), Madagascar*

Summary. Field trials have been carried out to examine the suitability of the JHA fenoxycarb in locust control. Laboratory tests have shown that a variety of JHAs, including fenoxycarb, applied to last instar larvae increased mortality, induced morphogenetic defects during metamorphosis, reduced fertility and provoked solitarisation of gregarious hoppers. The phase shift was indicated by green coloration and the acquisition of morphological and behavioural characteristics typical for solitary locusts. The present field experiments should clarify whether or not the effects observed in the laboratory are also observed with hopper bands in their natural habitat and if swarm formation and emigration from the recession areas can be prevented. The results from the topical application (ultra light volume [ULV] method) of six hopper bands of different sizes and composition (in respect to developmental stage of hoppers and their phase expression) with a broad range of fenoxycarb doses were quite comparable to those obtained in the laboratory. Colour transition started at day 2 after treatment. It was obvious that coherence and marching behaviour were strongly disturbed. Even the lowest dose applied, 50 g a.i./ha, caused a whole array of morphogenetic defects impairing jumping and flight. Fitness in general was greatly reduced, making the treated animals more vulnerable to many predators. Although a quantitative evaluation of the field trials, especially concerning mortality, was not possible, it was shown unequivocally that fenoxycarb exhibited the same activity profile as in the laboratory tests at a reasonably low dose. Thus, further field trials with even lower doses and quantitative calculations are of interest.

Résumé. Des essais sur le terrain ont été conduits pour étudier l'utilisation possible du fenoxycarbe, un analogue de l'hormone juvénile (AHJ) des insectes dans la lutte antiacridienne. Des essais de laboratoire avaient montré qu'une variété de AHJ, dont le fenoxycarbe, appliquée sur des larves de dernier stade, provoquait des perturbations d'ordre morphogénique durant la métamorphose, réduisait la fertilité et entraînait la solitarisation des insectes grégaires. Le changement de l'état phasaire se signalait par la coloration en vert des criquets et l'acquisition de caractéristiques morphologiques et comportementales typiques des locustes solitaires. Les expérimentations menées actuellement sur le terrain devraient permettre de savoir si oui ou non les effets observés en laboratoire sont également observables sur des bandes de criquets dans leur habitat naturel et s'il est ainsi possible d'éviter la formation d'essaims et leur départ des aires de récession. Les résultats de l'application topique (méthode ULV) sur six bandes de criquets de taille et de composition différentes (en ce qui concerne le stade de développement des insectes et leur expression phasaire) de fenoxycarbe à des doses très variées ont été très proches de ceux obtenus en laboratoire. Le changement de couleur a commencé le jour 2 suivant l'application. Il est apparu clairement que la cohérence et le comportement sur le plan du déplacement avaient été fortement perturbés. Même la dose la plus réduite, 50 g m.a./ha, a provoqué un grand nombre d'altérations morphogéniques gênant le saut et le vol. Les insectes traités étaient d'une manière générale dans une très mauvaise forme physique et étaient devenus une proie facile pour de nombreux prédateurs. Bien qu'une évaluation quantitative des essais sur le terrain, en particulier ceux concernant la mortalité, n'ait pas été possible, il a pu être démontré de façon univoque que le fenoxycarbe présentait sur le terrain le même profil d'action que dans les tests de laboratoire à une dose raisonnablement réduite. D'autres essais sur le terrain avec des doses encore plus réduites et des évaluations quantitatives seront donc d'un grand intérêt.

Introduction

It is of general interest that the conventional neurotoxic insecticides, which are potentially harmful to all animals and humans, will be replaced by selective, target-specific agents or biological control devices. Juvenile hormone analogues (JHAs) are a group of highly selective substances which disturb morphogenetic processes and are confined to insects. They occur naturally in certain plants (Bowers et al. 1966; Toong et al. 1988), probably serving as defence chemicals against herbivorous insects, but are also accessible to chemical synthesis. One of the latter, fenoxycarb (Dorn et al. 1981), has already gained commercial importance, and several others are at the stage of laboratory as well as field trials. Whether or not they are suited for locust control is the subject of our current study.

The most common mode of JHA action is the inhibition of metamorphosis. In hemimetabolous insects, including the migratory locusts, the transition from the last instar larva to adulthood is dependent on the cessation of juvenile hormone (JH) synthesis during the moult. If JH or JHAs are applied to last instar larvae, metamorphosis is suppressed, and supernumerary larval instars are induced which fail to develop to the reproducing stage. Even very low doses produce crippled, larval-adult intermediates, unable to reproduce or to fly (Dorn et al. 1994).

JH may also serve another function in migratory locusts – it might be involved in phase expression (Pener 1991). The devastating damages to farming caused by these insects is due to the swarm formation that takes place when environmental conditions are favourable. *Schistocerca gregaria* and *Locusta migratoria* normally live as solitary insects in semi-arid and arid recession areas. But if rainfall is exceptionally high and vegetation richer than normal, the locust populations grow. When their density has reached a certain level, the solitarious hoppers change colour, morphological expression and behaviour. Passing through transient stages, they switch from the solitarious into the gregarious phase (Uvarov 1966, 1977). Hoppers form large bands, which synchronize their development, form huge adult swarms and undertake long-distance flights. Those migratory flights are fuelled by stored lipids mobilised from the fat body shortly after take-off (Beenakker et al. 1984). This adipokinetic reaction is initiated by the adipokinetic hormone. Lipid storage and strength of adipokinetic reaction are additional phase characteristics (Schneider and Dorn 1994; Schneider et al. 1995). The internal regulatory processes directing and stabilising phase expression are largely unknown. JH has been discussed repeatedly as one of the factors closely involved in phase polymorphism, since in several independent studies on *S. gregaria* and *L. migratoria* as well a higher JH content has been found in solitary than in gregarious locusts (reviewed in Botens et al., in press). If it is true that there is a causal relationship between JH titre and phase behaviour, and that the solitary expression is based upon a higher hormone level, it should be possible by JHA treatment of gregarious locusts to reverse their phase expression into a solitary one. This would mean that the marching of hopper bands and migratory flights could be suppressed. A preventive JHA treatment of hopper bands or still immature adult swarms in recession areas could stop an infestation of farmland. In this case, it is not necessary to kill the locusts, because they would eventually die from starvation. The present investigations on the suitability of JHAs in the control of migratory locusts follow this strategy. Here, we report the results of the first field trials using the JHA fenoxycarb against hopper bands of *Locusta migratoria capito* in Madagascar.

Materials and methods

The field trials were carried out from March 1 to April 22 1993, in south-west Madagascar near Anakao at the Indian Ocean. After the rainy season, which ended in March, the climate was dry with maximum temperatures of 35 °C and minimum temperatures of 18 °C at night. Winds of moderate speed (1 – 5 m/sec) usually came from the east in the morning and from the west in the afternoon. The area is rather flat except where the sandy soil forms dunes. Figure 1 gives an impression of the vegetation, which consists of thorny bushes that sometimes form woodlike thickets, and patches of grass.

Six hopper bands of different sizes, developmental stages and somewhat varying phase characteristics were topically treated with a broad range of fenoxycarb concentrations (Tab. 1). Most hopper bands were observed two weeks prior to application in order to recognise a possible shift

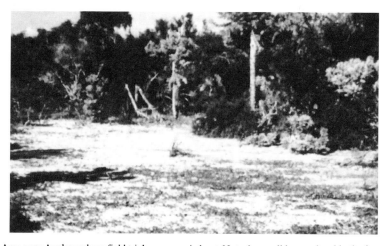

Figure 1. Area near Anakao where field trials were carried out. Note the small hopper band in the foreground.

Table 1. Habitat and characteristics of treated hopper bands at application

No.	Dose applied	Size of band marching speed/day	Age phase of hoppers	Area treated
A	600 g/ha	200 × 100 m 200–600 m/day	70% L5, 25% L4, few adults totally gregarious	2.6 ha dense wood with some grass
B	600 g/ha	35 × 100 m 20–50 m/day	mostly L5 close to adult moult, few adults totally gregarious	0.7 ha dense wood
C1*	200 g/ha	100 × 30 m 100–300 m/day	mostly L5, few L4, few adults	3.4 ha sparse grassland with a few bushes at the periphery
C2*	200 g/ha	50 × 20 m 100–300 m/day	mostly gregarious few solitary and transient	
C3*	200 g/ha	40 × 20 m 100–300 m/day	hoppers	
D	50 g/ha	band not compact, very low marching activity	mostly L4 and L5, few L3 mostly gregarious but with notable amounts of solitary and transient hoppers	3.5 ha mostly grass with scattered bushes

*The three hopper bands were close together, showed the same characteristics and were treated together

in behaviour provoked by the treatment. It was known from long-term observations that the experimental animals represented the third generation of gregarious locusts of the 1992/93 season. During the time of observation there was a surge of gregarisation and formation of huge bands (up to several square kilometres) in the vicinity. The hopper bands selected for treatment were constantly monitored from 7 a.m. when they were still at their sleeping places, until 5 p.m., when they had settled for the night. Marching direction and speed, eating habits, pausing and fitness were registered twice a day.

Fenoxycarb was provided by Ciba-Geigy (Basel) in a formulation (200 g a.i./l) that allowed dilution in diesel oil for hand-spraying with the ultra low volume (ULV) method. Doses were topically applied at the rate of 50, 200 and 600 g a.i./ha either in the evening (preferentially) or morning when the locusts were resting. In order to mark the treated animals, the fluorescent dyes Brilliant Yellow (6 g/l) or Helios (8.3 g/l) (both granted from Ciba-Geigy) were added to the solution. ULV Micron Sprayers and other parameters were adjusted so that in each test 3 l of a solution was applied per hectare.

Results and discussion

The hopper bands observed during our field studies varied in some characteristics (Tab. 1) which, apparently, depended primarily on band size: larger bands (> 50 × 100 m) showed highly synchronised development, uniform gregarious phase expression, were compact with a distinct head and marched with relatively high speed (several hundred metres per day), mostly without much change of direction. Smaller bands often included larvae of several instars, transient or even solitary coloured animals (which, however, always displayed gregarious behaviour); they were not as coherent as large bands and often changed direction without progressing very much. In such cases it was necessary to withhold the treatment until the majority of the hoppers within a band had reached the fifth larval instar, except for band D (Tab. 1).

In spite of the considerable differences between the treated hopper bands and the doses applied, the results were quite comparable and revealed a strong correlation to our laboratory tests (Dorn et al. 1994). A few days after treatment, starting at day 2, hoppers and adult locusts developed an intense green colour, often greener than in solitary animals. Moulting was not a prerequisite for colour change. Many adults that subsequently hatched showed morphogenetic defects: coiled and crippled wings, deformed hindlegs, intermediate larval-adult characteristics or even represented supernumerary larval instars (Fig. 2). Figure 3 depicts a qualitative evaluation of the effects produced after the fenoxycarb treatment. Adults with deformed wings were unable to fly; but also many animals with no obvious wing defects were unwilling to take off in response to charging (in contrast to normal young gregarious adults). The lowest dose of 50 g/ha

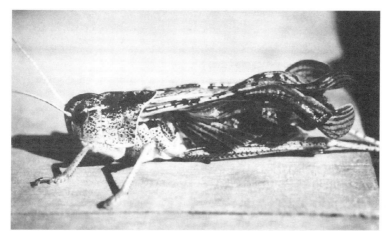

Figure 2. Wing malformations of a locust treated as L5 with 200 g a.i./ha.

still produced the full scale of morphogenetic defects, except for the induction of supernumerary larval instars. Thus, in future even lower concentrations may be considered for testing.

For several reasons it was not possible to determine mortality in treated hopper bands and fertility of surviving adults quantitatively (see below). We found in laboratory tests that a dose of 10 µg/hopper, topically applied to last instar larvae, killed 50% of the animals prior to or during moulting (Dorn et al. 1994). Much lower doses caused morphogenetic defects as observed in the field trials. Defective adults did not reproduce in laboratory tests. In cases where mating and egg deposition were observed, the eggs were not viable.

As pointed out above, an important goal of the studies was to demonstrate a possible change

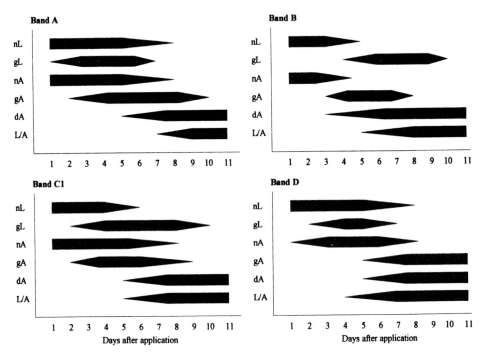

Figure 3. Evaluation of the fenoxycarb treatment of four hopper bands, Band A, Band B, Band C1 and Band D, which are characterized in Table 1. The treated hopper bands were observed at least until day 11 after fenoxycarb application. At the time of treatment the bands consisted predominantly or exclusively of gregarious locusts (nL = larvae of gregarious coloration (as in non-treated larvae); nA = adults of gregarious coloration). Green larvae (gL) and green adults (gA) appeared soon after fenoxycarb treatment. At day 10 after treatment all larvae had attempted or completed adult moult. In numerous cases the adults exhibited morphogenetic defects (dA) (crippled wings, deformed hindlegs and/or genital appendages) or represented larval-adult intermediates (L/A). Many animals died during metamorphic moult. Whereas the deformed adults and larval-adult intermediates remained close to the site of treatment, normal adults (nA, as non-treated adults) and green adults (gA) dispersed and/or died. At day 10 they were no longer observed (except in Band D).

of phase behaviour by the JHA fenoxycarb from a gregarious to solitary phase in field populations as was shown to occur in laboratory tests (Wiesel et al. 1995). Whereas a phase shift in colour and morphological parameters can be clearly demonstrated in the field, a solitarisation effect on behaviour was sometimes difficult to monitor due to several difficulties. For example, treated bands were overrun by non-treated bands, hoppers underwent a moult soon after treatment and one band was sprayed with a neurotoxic insecticide by the Madagascan plant protection service. Most advantageous for behavioural studies proved the largest hopper band (A in Tab. 1). This hopper band continued its strong unidirectional march for two days after application. At day 3, the head of the band broke up, and the hoppers gave an impression of disorientation. Even 23 days after treatment, animals were still found in the vicinity where application had taken place. They all were in the adult stage and exhibited different degrees of malformations.

Beginning two to three days after application of fenoxycarb, the locusts revealed signs of a strongly reduced fitness, i.e., erratic behaviour, abortive attempts to moult and morphogenetic defects impairing walking, jumping and flight. Such animals were easy prey to birds and other predators as well as to other locusts as could frequently be observed.

Earlier tests with fenoxycarb on different locust and grasshopper species produced ambiguous results. These inconsistencies could rest on differential species-specific responses and/or the mode of application. It has been observed repeatedly that topical application is much superior to oral treatment (Fuzeau-Braesch 1989; Capinera et al. 1991; Dorn et al. 1994). Thus, the poor performance of fenoxycarb in field trials in Mali may be due to the oral treatment (Ramseier 1991) and the presence of mixed grasshopper populations (including for instance *Oedaleus*) (Duffield and Clayton 1991; Langewald 1991). On the other hand, Fuzeau-Braesch (1989) and Capinera et al. (1991) found a high efficacy when topically applied in *L. migratoria migratorioides* and *Melanoplus sanguinipes*, respectively. The results in the latter species are quite comparable with ours in *L. migratoria capito* reported here: reduction of nymphal survival, reduction in egg production by grasshoppers treated as nymphs, induction of morphological deformities, especially wings, which would greatly inhibit or prevent normal behaviour of adults, induction of green coloration which may be indicative (together with an altered behaviour) of transformation from the more damaging gregarious phase to the less damaging solitary phase (Capinera et al. 1991; Dorn et al. 1994). Additional field trials with doses of 50 g a.i./ha and lower appear desirable for a full evaluation of the efficacy of this JHA, in particular in respect to its novel mode of action on the phase polymorphism in migratory locusts.

Acknowledgements
The studies are part of the project Integrated Biological Control of Grasshoppers and Locusts organised and sponsored by the Deutsche Gesellschaft für Technische Zusammenarbeit (GTZ); we acknowledge their financial

and logistic support. We greatly appreciate the help of the members of the Cooperation Germano-Malgache: W. Zehrer, M. Rakotobe, R. Scherer, M. Lie. Local helpers – Edimont, Ernest, Gabriel, Gilles and Tsyamauiri – gave valuable technical assistance. We thank Ciba-Geigy (Basle) for materials (fenoxycarb, fluorescent markers and detection lamps) as well as financial support.

References

Beenakker AMT, van der Horst DJ, van Marrewijk WJA (1984) Insect flight muscle metabolism. Insect Biochem 14: 243–260

Botens FFW, Rembold H, Dorn A (in press) Phase-related JH determinations in field catches and laboratory strains of different *Locusta migratoria* subspecies. J Insect Physiol

Bowers WS, Fales HM, Thompson MJ, Uebel EC (1966) Juvenile hormone: identification of an active compound from balsam fir. Science 154: 1020–1021

Capinera JL, Epsky ND, Turick LL (1991) Responses of the grasshopper *Melanoplus sanguinipes* and *M. differentialis* to fenoxycarb. Results communicated by Ciba-Geigy (Basel)

Dorn A, Wiesel G, Schneider M (1994) Juvenile hormone analogues in locust control. Pages 91–106 in Krall S, Wilps H (eds) New trends in locust control. Schriftenreihe der GTZ, no 245. GTZ, Eschborn, Germany

Dorn S, Frischknecht ML, Martinez V, Zurflüh R, Fischer U (1981) A novel non-neurotoxic insecticide with a broad activity spectrum. Z Pfl Krankh Pfl Schutz 88: 268–275

Duffield S, Clayton JS (1991) Investigation into the efficacy of fenoxycarb and polytrin C on mixed grasshopper populations in Mali. Results communicated by Ciba-Geigy (Basel)

Fuzeau-Braesch S (1989) Action du fenoxycarb sur les larves L5 du criquet *Locusta migratoria migratorioides* en phase gregaire. Results communicated by Ciba-Geigy (Basel)

Langewald J (1991) Effects of treatment with oil from the neem tree (*Azadirachta indica* Juss) compared to the insect growth regulator fenoxycarb on two grasshopper species in northern Mali (preliminary report). Results communicated by Ciba-Geigy (Basel)

Pener MP (1991) Locust phase polymorphism and its endocrine relations. Adv Insect Physiol 83: 1–79

Ramseier U (1991) Trial report: fenoxycarb and CGA229188 against *Locusta migratoria*. Results communicated by Ciba-Geigy (Basel)

Schneider M, Dorn A (1994) Lipid storage and mobilisation by flight in relation to phase and age of *Schistocerca gregaria* females. Insect Biochem Molec Biol 24: 883–889

Schneider M, Wiesel G, Dorn A (1995) Effects of JH III and JH analogues on phase-related growth, egg maturation and lipid metabolism in *Schistocerca gregaria* females. J Insect Physiol 41: 23–31

Toong XC, Schooley DA, Baker FC (1988) Isolation of insect juvenile hormone III from a plant. Nature 333: 170–171

Uvarov BP (1966) Grasshoppers and Locusts. Vol 1. Cambridge: Cambridge University Press

Uvarov BP (1977) Grasshoppers and Locusts. Vol 2. London:Centre of Overseas Pest Research

Wiesel G (1993) Der Einfluß von Juvenilhormon-Analoga auf Entwicklung, Reproduktion und Phasenpolymorphismus von Wanderheuschrecken. Doctoral Thesis. University of Mainz

Wiesel G, Tappermann S, Dorn A (1996) Effects of juvenile hormone and juvenile hormone analogues on the phase behaviour of *Schistocerca gregaria* and *Locusta migratoria*. J Insect Physiol 42(2): 385–395

New Strategies in Locust Control
S. Krall, R. Peveling and D. Ba Diallo (eds)
© 1997 Birkhäuser Verlag Basel/Switzerland

Locust control with *Metarhizium flavoviride*: New approaches in the development of a biopreparation based on blastospores

D. Stephan, M. Welling and G. Zimmermann

Federal Biological Research Centre for Agriculture and Forestry, Institute for Biological Control, Heinrichstraße 243, D-64287 Darmstadt, Germany

Summary. In order to develop a dry and stable biopreparation of blastospores of *Metarhizium flavoviride*, a special spray-drying technique was used which did not reduce the viability of blastospores (germination rate 91%). In bioassays against *Locusta migratoria* (L$_3$), the efficacy of spray-dried blastospores was comparable to freshly produced blastospores (mortality > 90%), although the time to kill 50% of the nymphs was slightly extended. For long-term storage, spray-dried blastospores were incubated at different constant temperatures between 5 and 50 °C under dry and oxygen-reduced conditions. After 52 weeks of storage at 5, 20 and 30 °C, the germination rate was 73.1, 68.0 and 38.3%, respectively. Storage at 40 and 50 °C for about eight and two weeks, respectively, resulted in a loss of viability of 50%. In Mauritania, different formulations of spray-dried blasto-spores were tested in semi-field trials against larvae of *Schistocerca gregaria* using an ultra low volume (ULV) application technique. Spray-dried blastospores were highly infective in a water-based formulation, an oil/water emulsion and an oil formulation. The highest mortality of nearly 100% after 15 days was observed with the water-based formulation (20% molasses, 80% water). The investigations were carried out within the framework of the Deutsche Gesellschaft für Technische Zusammenarbeit (GTZ) project "Integrated Biological Control of Grasshoppers and Locusts".

Résumé. Les travaux de recherche menés pour mettre au point une bio-préparation sèche et stable de blastospores de *Metarhizium flavoviride* ont conduit à l'élaboration d'une technique spéciale de séchage par pulvérisation qui offre l'avantage de ne pas réduire la viabilité des blastospores (taux de germination de 91%). Des bio-essais contre *Locusta migratoria* (L$_3$) ont montré que l'efficacité des blastospores séchées par pulvérisation était comparable à celles de blastospores fraîchement produites (mortalité > 90%), bien que le temps écoulé pour tuer 50% des larves ait été légèrement plus long. Pour étudier leur comportement pendant un entreposage prolongé, des blastospores séchées par pulvérisation ont été incubées à différentes températures constantes entre 5 °C et 50 °C, à sec et sous oxygène réduit. Après 52 semaines de stockage à 5 °C, 20 °C et 30 °C, le taux de germination était respectivement de 73,1%, 68,0% et 38,3%. L'entreposage à 40 °C et 50 °C pendant respectivement environ huit et deux semaines s'est traduit par une perte de la viabilité de 50%. Différentes formulations à base de blastospores séchées par pulvérisation ont été testées en Mauritanie dans des conditions semi-naturelles contre des larves de *Schistocerca gregaria* en utilisant la technique d'application en ULV. Les blastospores séchées par pulvérisation ont été hautement infectantes dans une formulation aqueuse, une émulsion huile/eau et une formulation huileuse. La plus forte mortalité de près de 100% après 15 jours a été constatée avec la formulation aqueuse (20% de mélasse, 80% d'eau). Ces travaux ont été conduits dans le cadre du projet GTZ «Lutte biologique intégrée contre les sauteriaux et les locustes».

Introduction

At present, the entomopathogenic fungus *Metarhizium flavoviride* is the most promising patho-gen for biocontrol of African locusts. Special attributes such as cheap mass production, storage of preparations for long periods under tropical conditions and the efficacy of formulations

which allow a controlled droplet application at ultra low volume (ULV) rates evoked great interest (Kleespies and Zimmermann 1994; Lomer et al. 1993; Stathers et al. 1993).

In liquid media, *M. flavoviride* produces hydrophilic blastospores. However, blastospores
stored in different water-based formulations at room temperature have only a relatively short
shelf-life (Kleespies and Zimmermann 1994). Drying of blastospores could be a more suitable
way to reduce their metabolic activity. So far, little work has been done on the development of
drying techniques for blastospores of entomopathogenic fungi (Fargues et al. 1979; Fargues et
al. 1983).

Stathers et al. (1993) demonstrated that the water content of conidia of *M. flavoviride* influence the storage quality. In oil-based formulations dried conidia can be stored for a long time.
One aspect of our research is to study the viability and pathogenicity of spray-dried blastospores of *M. flavoviride* during long-term storage.

With regard to conidia, formulation and application in vegetable oils increase their efficacy
against locusts compared with water-based formulations (Prior et al. 1988). In order to find a
suitable formulation for spray-dried blastospores, we compared a water-based, an oil-based formulation and an oil-water emulsion in semi-field trials in Mauritania.

Material and methods

Fungal culture

The following fungal strains of *M. anisopliae* (Ma) and *M. flavoviride* (Mfl) were tested (isolate
no., origin, host insect): Ma 97, Philippines, unknown lepidoptera; Ma 106, Australia, *Austracris
guttulosa* (Acrididae); Ma 131, Madagascar, soil sample; Mfl 5, Madagascar, *Locusta migratoria* (Acrididae); Mfl 6, Niger, *Ornitacris turbida cavroisi* (Acrididae).

Production of blastospores

Blastospores were produced in a liquid medium containing 2% glucose, 2% yeast extract, 1.5%
corn steep and 0.2% Tween 80.

Viability tests of blastospores

Spray-dried and freshly harvested blastospores were distributed on phyton-yeast agar (containing antibiotics) and incubated at 25 °C for 8 hours (Experiment: Comparison of fresh and spray-dried blastospores) or for 24 hours (Experiment: Storage of spray-dried blastospores at different temperatures). The germination rate of 300 blastospores (germinated: germ tube longer than the width of the blastospore) was assessed. Three replicates were carried out.

Bioassays

The efficacy of spray-dried and fresh blastospores of Mfl 5 was tested in laboratory bioassays. Dried and fresh blastospores were suspended in deionised water with a final blastospore concentration of 1×10^7 blastospores per millilitre. Five microlitres of the suspension was applied topically under the pronotum of 20 *L. migratoria* (L_3/L_4). Treated locusts were incubated at a day/night temperature of 35 °C (8 h) and 25 °C (16 h). The bioassays were monitored daily over a period of 14 days. Three replications were carried out.

Storage

For long-term storage, spray-dried blastospores were incubated at different constant temperatures between 5 and 50 °C under dry, oxygen-reduced conditions. The germination rates were assessed every two weeks as described above.

Semi-field trials

Semi-field trials were conducted at the field station of the GTZ in Akjoujt, Mauritania. Under standardised conditions, nymphs of *Schistocerca gregaria* (L_3/L_4) were treated with spray-dried blastospores corresponding to 5×10^{12} and 2×10^{13} blastospores per hectare, respectively. For application, a Micro-ULVA (Manufacturer: Micron) was used. Spray-dried blastospores were applied in three different formulations: a water-based formulation (20% molasses and 80% water), an emulsion containing 60% Telmion (85% vegetable oil + 15% emulsifier; manufacturer: Temmen, FRG) and 40% water, and an oil formulation (70% diesel fuel and 30% peanut oil). During the applications, the humidity ranged between 10 and 20% and the temperature between 25 and 30 °C. Treated larvae were transferred to field cages of $2 \times 2 \times 2$ m which had been erected in the natural habitat of the locusts. The trials were monitored daily over a period of 19 days. Three to five replicates with each 25 larvae were carried out. Hoppers which died within the first day after treatment were discarded. During the trials, the relative humidity ranged from 15 to 30% and the temperature from 10 to 35 °C.

Results

The germination rates of spray-dried and freshly produced blastospores of various *Metarhizium* spp. isolates are listed in Table 1. The viability of spray-dried blastospores was nearly the same, compared with those of freshly produced. Only in Ma 131 was the germination rate of spray-dried blastospores 25% lower. In bioassays with nymphs of *L. migratoria,* spray-dried blasto-spores of Mfl 5 caused high mortality after 14 days, but the time to kill 50% of locusts was two days longer compared with fresh blastospores (Fig. 1).

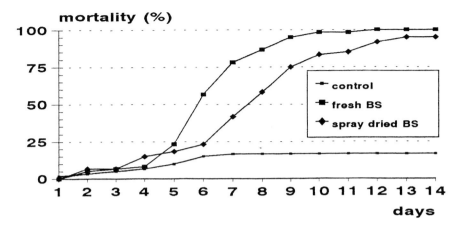

Figure 1. Bioassay using freshly produced and spray-dried blastospores (BS) against L3 of *Locusta migratoria.*

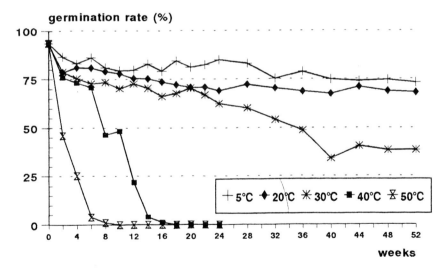

Figure 2. Viability of spray-dried blastospores of *M. flavoviride* Mfl 5 at constant temperatures after incubation for 24 h at 25 °C.

Table 1. Germination rate of spray-dried and freshly produced blastospores of various *Metarhizium* spp. strains after an incubation of 8 h

Isolate	Freshly produced blastospores(± sem)	Spray-dried blastospores (± sem)
Ma 97	98.7 (±0.71)	90.3 (±2.19)
Ma 106	97.4 (±0.59)	88.2 (±4.77)
Ma 131	97.1 (±0.98)	73.4 (±7.50)
Mfl 5	94.2 (±1.50)	90.6 (±1.40)
Mfl 6	94.3 (±2.52)	90.4 (±2.21)

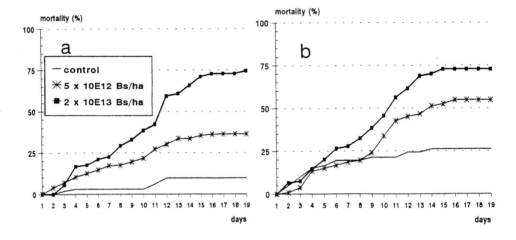

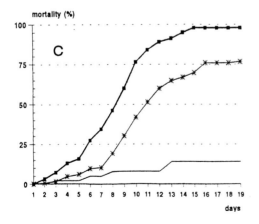

Figure 3. Comparison of different ULV formulations of spray-dried blastospores of *M. flavoviride* Mfl 5 in semi-field trials in Mauritania:
(a) 70% diesel fuel + 30% peanut oil,
(b) 40% Telmion + 60% water,
(c) 20% molasses + 80% water.

After 52 weeks of storage at 5, 20 and 30 °C, the germination rate was 73.1, 68.0 and 38.3%, respectively. Storage at 40 and 50 °C for about eight and two weeks, respectively, resulted in a loss of viability of 50% (Fig. 2). Short-term heating up to 70 °C could be tolerated for four hours.

In semi-field trials, three different formulations of spray-dried blastospores were compared. Mortalities up to 100% were observed after application of the water-based formulation containing 20% molasses and 80% water. Formulation in oil or in the oil-water emulsion resulted in mortalities up to 70% (Fig. 3).

Discussion

The spray-drying of blastospores of *Metarhizium* spp. may lead to a slightly slower germination, but the viability is comparable to freshly produced blastospores. These findings indicate a reduction of activity of blastospores by drying, but not an inactivation. Correspondingly, in bioassays with *L. migratoria* the efficacy of spray-dried blastospores was retarded but not reduced.

For practical use of *M. flavoviride* blastospores, long-term storage at high temperatures without loss of viability is needed. The shelf-life of biopreparations has to be 12–18 months (Couch and Ignoffo 1981). Our results have shown that storage at 5 and 20 °C is possible for at least one year. However, permanent storage temperatures of 30 °C and higher are not suitable for long-term storage. These findings correspond to the results of Stathers et al. (1993).

Conidia of the genus *Metarhizium* have a lipophilic cell wall. Therefore, it is easy to suspend them in oil-based formulations (Prior et al. 1988). When formulated in oil, conventional ULV application machinery can be used. In contrast, blastospores have a hydrophilic cell wall and generally cannot be suspended in oil. However, after spray-drying, blastospores can be suspended in both water- and oil-based formulations. The results of the semi-field trials indicate that spray-dried blastospores formulated in a water-based formulation (20% molasses, 80% water) are able to kill desert locusts under arid conditions. Treatments with blastospores formulated in the oil-based formulation or the oil-water emulsion resulted in lower mortality. An interpretation can be that the molasses may act as a protectant against desiccation and ultraviolet-radiation. Prior et al. (1988) assumed that water formulations do not adhere to the lipophilic cuticle and, therefore, that spores might be lost before they could germinate and penetrate. However, molasses can also be used as an adhesive. Therefore, the droplets could stick on the cuticle of the insect, and the germination of blastospores could follow.

One advantage of a molasses-based formulation is environmental safety. Furthermore, molasses is cheap and easy available. However, information on the stability of this formulation after mixing the individual components molasses, blastospores and water is still lacking.

The results of this paper demonstrate that a biopreparation based on blastospores of *M. flavoviride* may be implemented in integrated locust control programmes in the future.

Acknowledgements
We would like to thank D. Gloege for technical assistance. We are also grateful to Dr H. Wilps and his team for logistic support in Mauritania. The isolates Mfl 6 (= IMI 330189) and Ma 106 (= ARSEF 324) were provided by Dr C. Prior, IIBC, Ascot, UK, and Dr R. Humber, USDA, Ithaca, USA, respectively.

References

Couch TL, Ignoffo CM (1981) Formulation of insect pathogens. Pages 621–634 in Burges HD (ed) Microbial control of pests and plant diseases 1970–1980. New York: Academic Press

Fargues J, Reisinger O, Robert PH, Aubart C (1983) Biodegradation of entomopathogenic hyphomycetes: influence of clay coating on *Beauveria bassiana* blastospore survival in soil. J Invert Pathol. 41: 131–142

Fargues J, Robert PH, Reisinger O (1979) Formulation des productions de masse de l'hyphomycète entomopathogène *Beauveria* en vue des applications phytosanitaires. Annales de Zoologie Ecologie Animale 11: 247–257

Kleespies RG, Zimmermann G (1994) Viability and virulence of blastospores of *Metarhizium anisopliae* (Metch.) Sorokin after storage in various liquids at different temperature. Biocontrol Science and Technology 4: 309–319

Lomer CJ, Bateman RP, Godonou I, Kpindou D, Shah PA, Paraïso A, Prior C (1993) Field infection of *Zonocerus variegatus* following application of an oil-based formulation of *Metarhizium flavoviride* conidia. Biocontrol Science and Technology 3: 337–346

Prior C, Jollands P, le Patourrel G (1988) Infectivity of oil and water formulations of *Beauveria bassiana* (Deuteromycotina: Hyphomycetes) to the cocoa weevil pest *Pantorhytes plutus* (Coleoptera: Curculionoidea). J Invert Pathol 52: 66–72

Stathers TE, Moore D, Prior C (1993) The effect of different temperatures on the viability of *Metarhizium flavoviride* conidia stored in vegetable and mineral oils. J Invert Pathol. 62: 111–115

New Strategies in Locust Control
S. Krall, R. Peveling and D. Ba Diallo (eds)
© 1997 Birkhäuser Verlag Basel/Switzerland

Metarhizium flavoviride: recent results in the control of locusts and grasshoppers

C.J. Lomer with LUBILOSA project staff and collaborators[1-7]

International Institute of Tropical Agriculture, Plant Health Management Div., B.P. 08–0932, Cotonou, Benin,
[1] *CAB International Institute for Biological Control, Silwood Park, Buckhurst Road, Ascot SL5 7TA, UK*
[2] *CILSS/AGRHYMET-Département de Formation en Protection des Végétaux, B.P. 12625, Niamey, Niger*
[3] *Service Protection des Végétaux, B.P. Box 58, Porto Novo, Benin*
[4] *Département de Protection des Végétaux, B.P. 323, Niamey, Niger*
[5] *Service National de Protection des Végétaux, B.P. 1560, Bamako, Mali*
[6] *Plant Protection Research Institute, P. Bag X134, Pretoria, South Africa*
[7] *CSIRO, Black Mountain, Canberra, ACT 260, Australia*

Summary. The LUBILOSA project produces *Metarhizium flavoviride* in a di-phasic system with rice or millet substrate at IITA Cotonou and AGRHYMET Niamey. Yields of up to 100 g/kg are obtained. Spores are extracted dry and are stable in storage. Spores are readily suspended in different oils to make ultra low volume (ULV) formulations. We usually apply 100 g/ha in 2 l of oil, approximately 5×10^{12} spores/ha. Field population reductions following spore application have been observed in three systems. For *Zonocerus variegatus* in southern Benin, counts of fifth instar or young adult insects were observed to decline by 90% 10 days after application. *Hieroglyphus daganensis* at Malanville, northern Benin, was also controlled by ULV application of *Metarhizium* spores; however, the denser vegetation reduced the direct impact of the spray. This was compensated to some extent by pick-up of spores from the vegetation, resulting in 70% control 14 days after application. Similar results were obtained against *Oedaleus senegalensis* and *Kraussella amabile* in Mourdiah. However, results tend to be much more variable in the Sahelian grasslands, possibly owing to predator pressure. Application to desert locust hopper bands in Mauritania resulted in the destruction of treated bands; predator pressure again accounted for much mortality, and seemed to be enhanced by the fungal infection.

Résumé. Le projet LUBILOSA produit *Metarhizium flavoviride* selon un système à deux phases sur un substrat de riz ou de mil à l'IITA de Cotonou et à l'AGRHYMET de Niamey. Les rendements atteignent 100 g/kg. Les spores séchées supportent bien le stockage. Elles sont facilement utilisables en suspension dans différentes huiles pour constituer des formulations ULV. Nous faisons généralement des applications de 100 g par hectare dans deux litres d'huile, soit approximativement 5×10^{12} spores à l'hectare. Des réductions de population ont été observées en plein champ après l'épandage de spores dans trois systèmes. Dans le sud du Bénin, les comptages de larves au 5ème stade et de jeunes adultes de *Zonocerus variegatus* ont montré une diminution de 90% de la population dix jours après le traitement. *Hieroglyphus daganensis* a également été traité à Malanville dans le nord du Bénin par des épandages en ULV de spores de *Metarhizium*, mais la densité de la végétation a réduit les effets de l'application. Toutefois, le recyclage des spores sur la végétation traitée a permis une certaine compensation puisque 70% de la population a été anéantie en 14 jours. Des résultats similaires ont été obtenus contre *Oedaleus senegalensis* et *Kraussella amabile* à Mourdiah. Les résultats varient toutefois plus fortement dans les herbages sahéliens en raison probablement de la pression exercée par les prédateurs. L'application à des bandes de Criquet pèlerin en Mauritanie a provoqué leur destruction. La prédation a provoqué une grande mortalité parmi les criquets et a semblé se renforcer sous l'effet de l'infection fongique.

The potential of mycopesticides for acridid control

The possibilities for using biological agents to replace chemical pesticides were considered by Prior and Greathead (1989) and van Huis (1992). Of the various agents considered, pathogens seemed the most promising. In particular, the use of deuteromycete fungal spores as mycopesticides offered the best prospect for rapid implementation for the following reasons: (i) they are known insect pathogens and isolates are already available, (ii) host range data and mammalian safety data are already available for some isolates, (iii) production *in vitro* is possible on simple media and (iv) infection occurs via the cuticle, allowing their use as contact pesticides. Many deuteromycete fungi have lipophilic conidia, making their formulation as oil-based ultra low volume (ULV) suspensions an attractive possibility.

Incidence of fungal genera of interest as biocontrol agents

The principal genera of interest are *Metarhizium* and *Beauveria* (Hyphomycetes: Deuteromycetes). Both have been recorded from Orthoptera, although *Metarhizium* is more commonly found in Africa (see elsewhere in this volume).

Observations have been made on *Metarhizium* occurrence under epizootic and enzootic conditions. An epizootic of *Metarhizium flavoviride* Metschn. Sorokin. was observed affecting *Hieroglyphus daganensis* Krauss in Malanville, northern Benin, in 1991 (author's observations). Post-epizootic incidence of *M. flavoviride* in the Malanville area is reported by Shah et al. (1994). Epizootics have been also observed affecting *Diabolocatantops axillaris* (Thunberg) in Chad (C. Kooyman, personal communication) and *Ornithacris cavroisi* (Finot) near Niamey, Niger (H. van Groot and M. LeCoq, personal communication).

In the Ouémé province in Benin, isolations of *M. flavoviride* from *Zonocerus variegatus* (L.) were frequently made, and fungus incidence in field trial plots was 15% before application (Douro-Kpindou et al. 1995); this may represent an enzootic situation.

Most commonly, records of *M. flavoviride* consist of chance finds of individual specimens, either as cadavers or as a low incidence in live insects collected and kept in cages.

Mass production of *Metarhizium flavoviride*

M. flavoviride is produced at the International Institute of Tropical Agriculture (IITA) Cotonou and the Département de Formation en Protection des Végétaux (DFPV) AGRHYMET, Niamey, in a two-phase system, modified from similar systems in use in Brazil (Mendonça 1992). The first, liquid, phase is grown in shaker flasks in a sucrose/brewer's yeast medium inoculated with spores. After three days, the broth is transferred under sterile conditions to autoclaved rice or millet substrate in nylon bags, in plastic basins. Ventilation in the basins is increased during the incubation period by opening the bags, and after 10 to 14 days the spores are separated from the remaining substrate by sieving. Spores are further dried to $< 5\%$ moisture content, then sealed in plastic boxes or aluminium foil sachets with silica gel. Spores in this condition will keep $12-18$ months at temperatures of around 12 °C, and for two to three months at moderate tropical temperatures ($25-32$ °C) (Moore et al. 1996). Current cost of production is estimated at US$ 8 per hectare, including all capital, labour, substrate and overhead costs (D. Swanson, personal communication) under the particular conditions examined at IITA in 1995.

Application and formulation

Throughout the LUBILOSA field-testing programme from 1992 to 1994 a range of formulations, application rates and application equipment was tested. The formulation initially used consisted of 50% kerosene and 50% peanut oil. Experiments at Malanville in 1992 showed that the kerosene component could be increased to 70% without problems. Reducing the vegetable oil content to 30% reduced the cost of the formulation, and allowed an increase in the concentration of spores while keeping the viscosity to an acceptably low level. Fifty percent Ondina oil and 50% Shellsol T is also recommended when available.

The spore concentration initially used was 2×10^9 spores/ml. At application rates of $1-1.5$ litre/ha, (2×10^{12} spores/ha), adequate mortality of *Z. variegatus* was obtained. However, experience from Malanville in 1992 showed that a higher rate was preferable for Sahelian grasshoppers; in particular, a higher volume application rate was preferred. A concentration of 2.5×10^9 spores/ml, applied at 2 l/ha (5×10^{12} spores/ha) was adopted as a standard rate for the 1993 and 1994 trials.

The Micro-Ulva hand-held spinning disk sprayer (Micron, UK) was used in the trials. Ulva-Plus sprayers became available in 1993, and these were used interchangeably with the Micro-Ulva; they were found to be superior in several respects, and largely replaced the Micro-Ulva in the 1994 trials. The Ulva-Mast vehicle-mounted sprayer was used where conditions permitted, but both in Mourdiah (Mali) and in southern Benin, operational difficulties with the Ulva-Mast led to the use of the hand-held sprayers. These difficulties have been addressed by the manufacturer (Micron).

The Micronex spinning cage attachment for air-assisted sprayers was also tested; air-assisted spraying has the advantage that it is not dependent on wind, and may be able to penetrate vegetation. However, more work on droplet size control with this system is needed.

The active ingredients for all formulations were isolates of *M. flavoviride*. For *Z. variegatus* work the isolate I91–609, found on *Z. variegatus* in southern Benin, was used. For Sahelian grasshoppers, the 'standard' isolate, IMI 330189, found on *Ornithacris cavroisi* in Niger was used, except for one trial in Mali where an indigenous isolate (IIBC I92–794) from *Harpezocatantops stylifer* (Krauss) from Mourdiah was used.

Arena trials

The arena trial, or field bioassay format, is reported in Bateman et al. (1992b). It consists of a field laid out with 1-m^2 cleared arenas at 10- or 5-m intervals. At each arena, a pot of maize seedlings or a cassava cutting can be placed along with petri dishes, oil-sensitive papers and any other monitoring devices. Locusts or grasshoppers can be released onto the foliage just before spraying (with their wings pegged in the case of adult insects, or in large-mesh cages); after spraying, they are recaptured and incubated in cages. The advantage of this experimental format is that the spraying itself takes place outside under natural conditions, but the insects can be kept under close observation in cages during the incubation period. As well as being a useful training technique, the arena trial format allows the comparison of doses and strains, different formulations and different sprayers. The format allows calibration of optimum walking speed, flow rates and swathe widths. Before the importance of incubation conditions was fully appreciated, caged locusts were incubated in the laboratory. Later trials used field cages for incubation, as there can be differences between laboratory and field incubation (Langewald et al. 1997).

Field trials against *Zonocerus variegatus*

Small (0.25 ha) field trials with cage incubations were carried out in 1992 in the Lama forest, Zou province, Benin (Lomer et al. 1993). Further trials were carried out in 1993 on 1-ha plots in farmers' fields in Mono and Ouémé provinces in southern Benin. Two litres of formulation containing 2.5×10^{12} spores/l was applied to the plots. Samples of grasshoppers were taken at weekly intervals for cage incubations, and searches were made for cadavers. A counting procedure was developed based on sampling precision curves (Wilson and Room 1983). In each plot, four sub plots of 25 1-m^2 quadrats arranged in a 5 × 5 square were marked and the insects counted, always using the same observer for each sub plot.

The trial in Mono province clearly demonstrated population reductions of ~90% (Douro-Kpindou et al. 1995). Although the trial had been designed around the use of analysis of covariance, the mortality in the field was sufficiently convincing that a simple ANOVA of the combined means gave significant results. The second trial in the Ouémé was less clear-cut, as the adult grasshoppers were more mature and started to emigrate from the treated cassava fields to oviposition sites outside the fields.

Several aspects which were noted for further study in these trials were (i) the possibility of using the insects' natural migration pattern to disperse the fungus and (ii) the extent of secondary infection of live grasshoppers from cadavers sporulating in the field. Finally, it was observed that the counting would probably be better in straight transects than in square grids.

Field trials in northern Benin against *Hieroglyphus daganensis*

The 1992 trials in Malanville, northern Benin, were intended to replicate the format of the small field trials against *Z. variegatus*. However, results were considerably less convincing, with very shallow mortality curves and final mortalities of 50–70% after 21 days (Shah 1994). Trials focused on the evaluation of different field doses of spores, different formulations, sampling methods and sprayer types in 0.1- to 0.25-ha plots. Several problems were identified for resolution before the 1993 season. Firstly, the *M. flavoviride* formulations, while satisfactory for transportation and use within the same day, were found to be rather unstable when they had to be carried 750 km to northern Benin and stored until needed. Secondly, the vegetation and grasshopper behaviour in Malanville were such that fewer of the applied fungus spores impacted directly on the hoppers; there were, however, preliminary indications that some secondary pickup of spores was occurring. Thirdly, there was a suspicion that the *M. flavoviride* strain being used, IMI 331089, was less virulent to *Hieroglyphus daganensis* than I91-609 was to *Z. variegatus*.

Progress between the 1992 and 1993 field seasons in Malanville was made on formulation stability (Moore et al. 1996), but not on application or strain selection.

Work in Malanville in 1993 focused initially on selecting a good trial site of sufficiently uniform vegetation, and then on developing a sampling/counting procedure based on experience with *Z. variegatus*. Both the spore dose rate and the volume application rate were increased so that 5 × 10^{12} spores were applied in 2 l of 70:30 kerosene: peanut oil formulation to 4-ha plots.

H. daganensis nymphs migrated from short to long grasses, but remained within the plots during the incubation period, and the populations were reduced by about 70% (Fig. 1). Evidence for recycling of the fungus was observed (Lomer et al. 1997).

In 1994, trials focused on detailed measurements of secondary pick-up, which was found to be more important than direct impact in this system (Thomas et al., 1997).

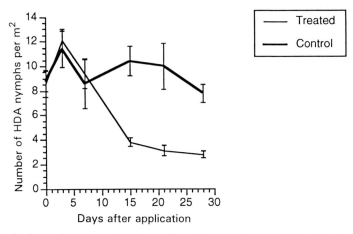

Figure 1. Reduction in grasshopper counts following *Metarhizium* application at Malanville, July 1993. Counts of *Hieroglyphus daganensis* nymphs in FT93/1, Madekali, Malanville, Benin, July 1993. *Metarhizium flavoviride* IMI 330189 conidia were applied to three replicate 4-ha plots at 4×10^{12} conidia/ha with Micro-Ulva spinning disk sprayers in 2 l of 70:30 kerosene:peanut oil per hectare. Conidia were 90% viable. Counts were made in two subplots in high reed vegetation, each of 4×5 m^2 in three replicate plots per treatment.

Field trials against grasshoppers in Niger

There were two trials of *M. flavoviride* in Niger in 1992. One trial, at Katanga, was similar to the work in Malanville and gave similar results, although the initial impact rate was better. For nymphs of *Cataloipus fuscocoeruleipes* (Sjöstedt) and *Tylotropidius gracilipes* (Brancsik), corrected mortalities of 90% were observed after five days of cage incubation in the day 0 sample and 45% seven days after treatment in the day 3 sample. For *Hieroglyphus daganensis* and *Homoxyrrhepes punctipennis* (Walker) the corresponding figures were 75 and 70%. The nymphs were grouped in this way because it is difficult to distinguish between the species in early instars. Clearly *Hieroglyphus daganensis* and *Homoxyrrhepes punctipennis* are less mobile than the other two species, but all four species were susceptible to *M. flavoviride* (Kooyman et al.; Lomer et al., LUBILOSA unpublished reports).

The second 1992 trial was a preliminary test with the vehicle-mounted Ulva-Mast sprayer. In this trial, the mortality in the initial day 0 sample was only 30%, and the mortality in the day 3 sample was 60%, indicating the importance of secondary pick-up in this system. The principal grasshopper species present in this trial were *Oedaleus nigeriensis* (Uvarov), *Pyrgomorpha cognata* (Olivier), Catantopinae spp. including *Catantops stramineus* (Walker), *Diabolocatantops axillaris* (Thunberg) and *Harpezocatantops stylifer* (Krauss).

In 1993 a larger Ulva-Mast trial was carried out, on 9-ha plots against a mixture of Sahelian grasshoppers, mainly *Acrotylus blondeli* (Saussure) and *Oedaleus senegalensis* (Krauss). The application rate was 5×10^{12} spores/ha in 2 l of formulation. Examination of vegetation showed that droplet coverage was good. Cage incubations showed very good mortality (>90% after eight days in the day 1 sample, 80% after 10 days in the day 3 sample), but a preliminary analysis of the insect counts showed no significant reduction, probably because of migration out of the plots. However, a more detailed analysis including observer as a factor, and initial quadrat counts as co-factor, showed differences in the counts between treatment and control plots. Problems with settling of spores in the suspension, which had been made up in the laboratory, and subsequent resuspension led to the conclusion that dry spores should be carried to the field and suspended before application (Bateman and Kooyman, LUBILOSA unpublished report).

The principal matters needing further attention in this ecozone are (i) increasing plot size to 20–50 ha, (ii) emphasising grasshopper counting procedures and (iii) following spore load to check for secondary recycling of *M. flavoviride*.

Field trials against grasshoppers in Mali

In 1992, trials were carried out to investigate the possibility of using a barrier treated with 5 l/ha of neem oil to reduce grasshopper migration in and out of *M. flavoviride*-treated plots. In the first trial, 0.25-ha plots were treated with 2×10^{12} spores/ha of IMI 330189 in 1 l/ha. *Oedaleus senegalensis* was the principal species present; samples were incubated in field cages, and cages kept under shelter at base. Field cages gave incubation conditions closer to those likely to be experienced by uncaged grasshoppers, but recovery of cadavers for sporulation was impossible. Very little difference was observed between the two cage types. Mortalities in each were around 80% after 10 days. The movement of nymphs in and out of the plots was monitored by including an ultraviolet (UV)-tracer (Lumogen) in the formulation, and counting the number of insects with droplets under UV light. The 10-m-wide neem-treated border was insufficient to reduce the movement of insects in and out of the plots; in both treated and control plots, numbers fell from 12/m^2 to between 2 and 4/m^2.

In a second experiment, the width of the neem oil-treated border was increased to 15 m and the application rate increased to 10 l/ha; the test insect in this case was *Kraussella amabile* (Krauss). However, the viability of the *M. flavoviride* spores had fallen to 70% by the time this second experiment was carried out, and only low fungus-induced mortalities were observed in the cage samples. Nevertheless, a significant second-order interaction was observed, indicating that the neem oil and the *M. flavoviride* spores acted synergistically to reduce grasshopper movement (Langewald et al., LUBILOSA unpublished report).

In 1993, grasshopper populations at Mourdiah were very low, and site selection posed a problem. Three trials were carried out. In the first trial, the standard *M. flavoviride* isolate from Niger (IMI 330189) was compared with the Mali isolate discovered at Mourdiah in 1992 on *Harpezocatantops stylifer* (I92-794), both applied at 2×10^{12} spores/ha on 1-ha plots. The Mali isolate was consistently and significantly better at all sampling dates. The mean mortality for samples on days 0, 3 and 7 was 85% compared with 57% for IMI 330189, and gave 60% sporulation compared with 30% for IMI 330189.

A second trial, on 1-ha plots, examined the effect of the addition of 1% UV-protectant *p*-hydroxybenzone to the formulation on the persistence of *M. flavoviride* spores. No significant effects were observed.

The third trial was carried out on nymphs of *Oedaleus senegalensis*, *Acrotylus blondeli* and *Cryptocatantops haemorrhoidalis* (Krauss) in 6-ha plots. Spores of IMI 330189 were applied at 10^{13} spores/ha; cage mortalities were good (100% in nine days with 75% sporulation). Cages in the field were damaged by livestock. Owing to low numbers of insects, the counting procedures were not sufficiently precise to show a population reduction in the field (Ciba-Geigy, unpublished report).

The 1994 results showed a reduction in grasshopper counts following treatment (Douro-Kpindou 1996).

South Africa

No isolates have yet been screened from Southern Africa, but small field tests have been carried out with the Niger isolate IMI 330189 in the Republic of South Africa, in collaboration with the Plant Protection Research Institute, Pretoria, against *Locustana pardalina* (Walker) and *Nomadacris septemfasciata* (Audinet-Serville). Ground application of 6×10^{12} spores/ha of

IMI 330189 gave good mortality; five out of six treated bands showed mortalities >95% in 7 to 14 days (Bateman et al. 1994).

Australia

Commonwealth Scientific and Industrial Research Organisation (CSIRO) (in collaboration with LUBILOSA, Australian Plague Locust Commission and New South Wales Department of Agriculture) have completed a total of seven field trials in Australia using *Metarhizium flavoviride* isolate ARSEF 324 against the two most important acridid pests in that country, Australian plague locust, *Chortoicetes terminifera* (Walker), and the wingless grasshopper, *Phaulacridium vittatum* (Sjöstedt). A variety of spray equipment ranging from a Cesna-fixed wing aircraft fitted with AU5000 micronair nozzles to a ground-based boom sprayer have been used successfully. Dose rates have ranged from 1.8×10^{12} to 7×10^{12} per ha, with plot size ranging from 0.25 to 50 ha. Formulations have all included at least 20% mineral oil and have been either a pure oil ULV at 2 l/ha or oil/water emulsion at up to 30 l/ha. Due to the recent severe drought all (including the aerial) but one of the field trials have been against wingless grasshoppers. All trials have demonstrated population reductions in the field usually of 60 to 90% after three weeks. Live grasshoppers from treated plots sampled on the day of spraying normally give over 90% mortality. It is possible that under very hot conditions the fungus is unable to establish in field insects but is able to infect insects brought back and incubated under protected conditions in the laboratory. In other cases, the apparently lower efficacy in the field is due to migration of untreated grasshoppers into the trial plots (Baker et al. 1994; Milner et al. 1994; Milner and Prior 1994).

Desert locust

Trials on desert locust have been carried out in Pakistan and Mauritania.

In Pakistan, conditions were very hot, and adults were already fledging at the time of application. Most treated insects flew away from the treated plots within three days of treatment. Cannibalism in the cage incubation samples was a problem, but the final number of survivors was significantly lower in the treated than in the control samples (Moore, LUBILOSA unpublished report).

In Mauritania, third to fourth instar hopper bands were treated; cage samples were taken and bands were followed in the field. Experimental difficulties included cannibalism in the cage samples, and erratic behaviour of the bands in the field. Treated bands split up when some moulted while others moved on; and treated bands would sometimes merge with untreated bands. The biggest problems concerned predation in the field, principally by birds (*Passer luteus* and weaver birds). Treated bands were particularly heavily attacked, and some bands completely destroyed despite attempts to protect the bands. Cage mortalities were good (90% in nine days), but it was difficult to be confident about the field results. Clearly, treated bands were weakened and became susceptible to increased attack by predators, but quantification of this effect was not possible (Kooyman and Godonou, LUBILOSA unpublished report).

Conclusions

M. flavoviride in ULV formulation shows great promise as a mycopesticide. The occurrence of the fungus in all African countries where surveys have been undertaken should avoid undue concerns about introduction of exotic isolates. Nevertheless, impact assessment of actual myco-pesticide applications will be needed. Work is in progress in collaboration with LOCUSTOX, GTZ and the Universities of Saarbrücken and Göttingen. Field trial results are promising, although more research is needed for desert locust. Pathogen recycling has been demonstrated in the case of *Z. variegatus* and *H. daganensis*. Work on grasshoppers in a wide variety of ecosystems has shown that the use of *M. flavoviride* as a biocontrol agent of locusts and grasshoppers is probably ready to move on to the next stage of development.

Increased spore production, improvements to packaging and progress with satisfying registration requirements mean that *M. flavoviride* is now available for further field testing in collaboration with national programmes and other organisations. A series of farmer participatory trials in collaboration with non-government organisations is planned for 1995. Requests for spores for testing should be made to any LUBILOSA staff. In the future, LUBILOSA will be seeking partners for increased scale of spore production.

Acknowledgements
The LUBILOSA (LUtte BIologique contre les LOcustes et SAuteriaux) programme is funded by the governments of Canada (CIDA), Netherlands (DGIS), Switzerland (SDC) and UK (ODA). The enthusiastic support of all project members, collaborators and institute directors is gratefully acknowledged.

References*

Baker GL, Milner RJ, Lutton GG, Watson, D (1994) Preliminary field trial on the control of *Phaulacridium vittatum* (Sjöstedt) (Orthoptera: Acrididae) populations with *Metarhizium flavoviride* Gams and Rozsypal (Deuteromycotina: Hyphomycetes). J Australian Entomol Soc 33: 190–192

Bateman RP, Price RF, Müller EJ, Brown HD (1994) Controlling brown locust hopper bands in South Africa with a myco-insecticide spray. Paper presented at Brighton Crop Protection Conference, UK, November 1994

Douro-Kpindou OK, Godonou I, Houssou A, Lomer CJ, Shah PA (1995) Control of *Zonocerus variegatus* with ULV formulation of *Metarhizium flavoviride* conidia. Biocontrol Science and Technology 5: 131–139

Douro-Kpindou OK, Langewald J, Lomer CJ, van der Paauw H, Shah PA, Sidibé A (1996) Field trials conducted on a biopesticide (*Metarhizium flavoviride*) for grasshopper control in Mali from 1992 to 1994. This volume

Langewald J, Thomas MB, Lomer CJ, Douro-Kpindou OK (1997) Use of *Metarhizium flavoviride* for control of *Zonocerus variegatus*: a model, relating mortality in caged field samples with disease development in the field. Entomologia Appl Exp, in press

Lomer CJ, Bateman RP, Godonou I, Kpindou D, Shah PA, Paraiso A, Prior C (1993) Field infection of *Zonocerus variegatus* following application of an oil based formulation of *Metarhizium flavoviride* conidia. Biocontrol Science and Technology 3: 337–346

Lomer CJ, Thomas MB, Godonou I, Shah PA, Douro-Kpindou OK, Langewald J (1997) Control of grasshoppers, particularly *Hieroglyphus daganensis,* in northern Benin using *Metarhizium flavoviride.* Memoirs of the Entomological Society of Canada, in press

Mendonça AF (1992) Mass production, application and formulation of *Metarhizium anisopliae* for control of sugarcane froghopper, *Mahanarva posticata,* in Brazil. Pages 239–244 in Lomer CJ, Prior C (eds) Biological control of locusts and grasshoppers. Wallingford, UK: CAB International

Milner RJ, Hartley TR, Lutton GG, Prior C (1994) Control of the wingless grasshopper *Phaulacridium vittatum* (Sjöstedt) (Orthoptera: Acrididae) in field cages using an oil-based spray of *Metarhizium flavoviride* Gams and Rozsypal (Deuteromycotina: Hyphomycetes). J Australian Entomol Soc 33: 165–167

Milner RJ and Prior C (1994) Susceptibility of Australian plague locust, *Chortoicetes terminifera,* and the wingless grasshopper, *Phaulacridium vittatum,* to the fungi, *Metarhizium* spp. Biological Control 4: 132–137

Moore D, Douro-Kpindou OK, Jenkins NE, Lomer CJ (1996) Storage of *Metarhizium flavoviride* Gams and Rozsypal for use as a mycopesticide against locusts and grasshoppers. J Invertebrate Pathol, in press

Prior C, Greathead DJ (1989) Biological control of locusts: the potential for the exploitation of pathogens. FAO Plant Prot Bull 37: 37–48

Shah PA (1995) Field studies on the development of *Metarhizium flavoviride* Gams and Rozsypal as a microbial insecticide for locust and grasshopper control. PhD thesis. University of London, 199 pp

Shah PA, Godonou I, Gbongboui C, Lomer CJ (1994) Natural levels of fungal infections in grasshoppers in Northern Benin. Biocontrol Science and Technology 4: 331–342

Thomas MB, Wood SN, Langewald J, Lomer CJ. (1997) Persistence of biopesticides and consequences for biological control of grasshoppers and locusts. Pesticide Science, in press

van Huis A (1992) New developments in desert locust management and control. Proc Exper Appl Entomol, N.E.V. Amsterdam 3: 2–18

Wilson LT, Room PM (1983) Clumping patterns of fruit and arthropods in cotton with implications for binomial sampling. Environmental Entomology 12: 50–54

*Submitted, in press or unpublished articles may be requested from the author

New Strategies in Locust Control
S. Krall, R. Peveling and D. Ba Diallo (eds)
© 1997 Birkhäuser Verlag Basel/Switzerland

Small-scale field trials with entomopathogenic fungi against *Locusta migratoria capito* in Madagascar and *Oedaleus senegalensis* in Cape Verde

F.X. Delgado, J.H. Britton[1], M.L. Lobo-Lima, E. Razafindratiana[2] and W. Swearingen

Department of Entomology, Montana State University, Bozeman, MT 59717, USA
[1] *Mycotech Corporation, Butte, MT 59701, USA*
[2] *GTZ/Crop Protection Biocontrol Laboratory, Antananarivo, Madagascar*

Summary. In a field trial in Madagascar in 1994, two isolates of *Metarhizium flavoviride* Gams and Rozsypol, SP3 and SP9, and an isolate of *Beauveria bassiana* (Balsamo) Vuillemin, SP16, were tested as formulated mycopesticides against the Malagasy migratory locust, *Locusta migratoria capito* Sauss. In a separate field trial in Cape Verde in 1994, SP9 was tested as a mycopesticide against *Oedaleus senegalensis* Krauss. In both field trials, SP9 caused 100% mortality in the treated *L. migratoria capito* and *O. senegalensis* populations. *L. migratoria capito* from plots treated with SP9 died sooner than locusts from plots treated with SP3 or SP16. Total locust mortality did not differ significantly between SP3 and SP9. However, both isolates caused higher locust mortality than SP16. All three isolates caused significantly greater mortality than that in the untreated control plots.

Résumé. Dans un essai sur le terrain mené à Madagascar en 1994, deux isolats de *Metarhizium flavoviride* Gams et Rozsypol, SP3 et SP9, et un isolat de *Beauveria bassiana* (Balsamo) Vuillemin, SP16, ont été testés comme formulations mycopesticides sur le criquet migrateur malgache *Locusta migratoria capito* (Sauss). Au cours d'un autre essai conduit dans l'Archipel du Cap-Vert en 1994, SP9 a été testé comme mycopesticide contre *Oedaleus senegalensis* (Krauss). Au cours de ces deux essais, SP9 a tué 100% des populations de *L. migratoria capito* et d'*O. senegalensis*. Les populations de *L. migratoria capito* se trouvant sur des parcelles traitées au SP9 ont été décimées plus rapidement que celles se trouvant sur des parcelles traitées au SP3 ou au SP16. La différence au niveau du taux de mortalité totale était insignifiante entre SP3 et SP9, ces deux derniers isolats ont toutefois causé une mortalité plus forte que SP16. La mortalité due à ces trois isolats a été plus forte que celle constatée sur les parcelles témoins non traitées.

Introduction

In response to the outbreak of the Malagasy migratory locust, *Locusta migratoria capito* Sauss, in Madagascar in 1993, Montana State University's Africa Grasshopper/Locust Biocontrol Program was given a grant by the US Agency for International Development to survey that locust population for natural pathogens, identify these pathogens, and evaluate their potential for biocontrol of locusts in Madagascar.

In May 1993, researchers from Montana State University (MSU) and Mycotech Corporation surveyed approximately 10,000 locusts for naturally occurring pathogens (Delgado et al. 1996). Thirty-three fungal isolates of *Metarhizium flavoviride* Gams and Rozsypol, *M. anisopliae* (Metschikoff) Sorokin, and *Beauveria bassiana* (Balsamo) Vuillemin were identified for further testing. Additionally, two species of protozoa and a virus were collected for further evaluation.

The 33 fungal isolates were screened using a matrix developed by Mycotech Corporation. Tests included bioassays for virulence and evaluations of heat tolerance and spore production. Five strains underwent further testing, including mammalian toxicological studies and laboratory bioassays to evaluate their virulence to beneficial insects. Two of the tested strains showed some adverse toxicological effects on mammals and received no further consideration. None of the three remaining strains caused any significant negative effects on the four beneficial insects used in the laboratory bioassays, which included honey bees and three lepidopterans.

These three strains, *M. flavoviride* SP3 and SP9 and *B. bassiana* SP16, were subsequently evaluated in a field trial against *L. migratoria capito* in Madagascar. *M. flavoviride* SP9 was also tested in a separate field trial against *Oedaleus senegalensis* in Cape Verde. These field trials are discussed in the remainder of this paper.

Materials and methods

Formulated conidia of isolates SP3, SP9 and SP16 in oil suspensions were provided by Mycotech Corporation, Butte, Montana, USA. All three fungal strains had been previously isolated by the project researchers from naturally infected *L. migratoria capito* in Madagascar. Prior to application of the treatments, viability of the conidia was checked by plating dilutions of the formulations on Saboraud dextrose agar. Plates were incubated at 25 °C and germinated conidia were counted at 16 h.

Field test against migratory locust

Field tests were conducted during November and December 1994 in Madagascar. The three fungal isolates, SP3, SP9 and SP16, were compared for mortality effects against *L. migratoria capito*. Locusts were predominantly third and fourth instars. The test site was in a recession area naturally infested by migratory locusts. Plots measuring 50 m^2 were enclosed by cloth netting, approximately 0.5 m high, to minimize locust migration. Density of the locusts in the area was 0.5 nymphs per square metre. Before spraying, third and fourth instar nymphs were collected from areas near the plots and held overnight to minimize bias due to handling. Immediately before treatment, approximately 100 nymphs were placed in each enclosed plot to insure that adequate locust numbers were available for subsequent sampling. Formulations were applied at a rate of 2.5×10^{13} conidial spores in 5 l of oil per ha. Plots were arranged following a complete randomized design with four replicates. Controls were untreated. Treatments were applied with Mini-Ulva sprayers (Micron Sprayers, Bromyard, Herefordshire, UK).

Approximately three hours after treatment, 20 nymphs from each plot were collected and transferred to the laboratory. Each locust was isolated in a 177-ml dish with perforated lid for 10 days. Locusts were fed daily with native untreated vegetation. Mortality was assessed daily, and cadavers were maintained in the dishes with moistened cotton plugs added to promote hyphal growth in the case of fungal infection. Data were analyzed with a general linear model program and orthogonal contrasts.

Field test against Senegalese grasshopper

The field trials in Cape Verde tested the effect of formulated *M. flavoviride* SP9 against *O. senegalensis* when nymphs were predominantly third instars. The experimental design was a randomized complete block with four replicates. Individual plot size was 5000 m^2. The formulated SP9 was applied at a rate of 2.5×10^{13} spores at 5 l of oil per ha with Micro-Ulva sprayers. Control plots were untreated.

To assess treatment effects, two evaluation methods were used. The first method involved samples of 100 grasshoppers, collected three hours post-treatment, which were handled as described for the previous trial. The second evaluation method involved samples of 40 grasshoppers equally divided into eight bottomless cages (10 l volume), which were placed over natural vegetation within each plot area. Data were analyzed as described previously.

Results and discussion

Field test against migratory locust

Locusts from plots treated with SP9 died more quickly than did locusts from other treatments (Fig. 1). Locust mortality was 100% with SP9 at day 8 post-treatment, versus 89% with SP3 and 56% with SP16 at day 10. Overall mortality in locusts exposed to SP3 and SP9 did not differ significantly by the end of the trial. Both *M. flavoviride* strains caused significantly higher overall mortality than did *B. bassiana* SP16. However, the mortality of locusts treated with SP16 was statistically greater than that in the untreated control plots by day 7 post-treatment.

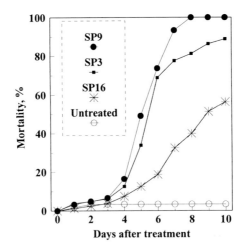

Figure 1. Cumulative mortality of *Locusta migratoria capito* nymphs from field plots treated with formulated conidia of two isolates of *Metarhizium flavoviride*, SP3 and SP9, and an isolate of *Beauveria bassiana*, SP16, and untreated controls in Madagascar, 1994. Locust samples from each field plot were held in the laboratory.

Field test against Senegalese grasshopper

Grasshopper densities in the test area in Cape Verde were estimated at $30/m^2$ when treatments were applied. By four days post-treatment, mortality among grasshoppers exposed to SP9 and

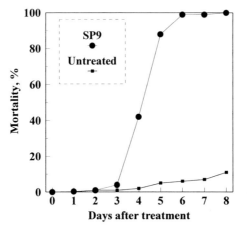

Figure 2. Cumulative mortality of *Oedaleus senegalensis* nymphs from field plots treated with formulated conidia of *Metarhizium flavoviride* isolate SP9 and untreated controls in Cape Verde, 1994. Grasshopper samples were held in the laboratory following collection from field plots.

held in the laboratory was significantly greater than that in grasshoppers from the untreated control plots (P<0.01) (Fig. 2). At eight days post-treatment, grasshopper mortality was 100% in the group treated with SP9 versus 11% in the control population.

For grasshoppers held in field cages, mortality by five days after treatment with SP9 was significantly greater than that in the untreated control plots (P<0.05) (Fig. 3). At eight days post-treatment, grasshopper mortality was 90% in the population treated with SP9 versus 35% in the control population. The more rapid mortality and higher mortality levels among treated grasshoppers held in the laboratory, compared with those held in field cages, may be related to the ability of grasshoppers to thermoregulate in field cages but not in the laboratory. Thermoregulation for increased body temperature provides survival advantages to grasshoppers because many entomopathogens are not heat tolerant (Carruthers et al. 1992).

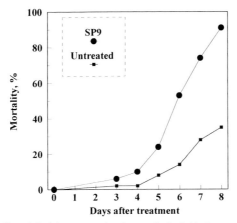

Figure 3. Cumulative mortality of *Oedaleus senegalensis* nymphs in field plots treated with formulated conidia of *Metarhizium flavoviride* isolate SP9 and untreated controls in Cape Verde, 1994. Grasshopper samples were held in cages in the field plots.

Conclusions

Results from the field tests summarised in this paper demonstrate that one or more of the fungal isolates tested have significant potential for development as mycopesticides for biocontrol of Madagascar's migratory locust population. More generally, these results suggest that the approach followed – involving entomopathogen survey, isolation, identification, screening, bioassays and field testing – has promise as a relatively inexpensive and expeditious way to develop cost-effective and environmentally friendly alternatives to synthetic pesticides for locust and grasshopper control.

Acknowledgements
Funding was provided by USAID as Grant # 687-0517-G-00-3109-00 from USAID/Madagascar for the
Madagascar research and Grant # AOT-0517-G-00-4119-00 from AELGA, AID/Washington for the Cape Verde
research.

References

Carruthers RI, Larkin TS, Firstencel H (1992) Influence of thermal ecology on the mycosis of a range-
    land grasshopper. Ecology 73: 190–204
Delgado FX, Britton JH, Lobo-Lima ML, Razafindratianna E, Swearingen W (1996) Field and laboratory
    evaluations of leading entomopathogenic fungi, isolated from *Locusta migratoria capito* Sauss in
    Madagascar. *In*: Microbial Control of Grasshoppers and Locusts. MS Goettel, DL Johnson (eds).
    Memoirs Entomological Society of Canada. In press

New Strategies in Locust Control
S. Krall, R. Peveling and D. Ba Diallo (eds)
© 1997 Birkhäuser Verlag Basel/Switzerland

Development of a mycoinsecticide for the Australian plague locust

R.J. Milner[1], G.L. Baker[2], G.H.S. Hooper[3] and C. Prior[4]

[1] CSIRO, Division of Entomology, Canberra, ACT 2601, Australia
[2] New South Wales Department of Agriculture, Rydalmere, NSW 2116, Australia
[3] Australian Plague Locust Commission, GPO Box 858, ACT 2601, Australia
[4] International Institute of Biological Control, Ascot, Berks. SL5 7TA, UK

Summary. In Australia, the most serious acridid pest is the Australian plague locust, *Chortoicetes terminifera*, which has the potential to cause substantial damage to crops and pastures during periodic outbreaks. Other acridid pests include the wingless grasshopper, *Phaulacridium vittatum*, which regularly causes economic damage to pastures, crops and trees in cooler districts from New South Wales to Western Australia. Control of the Australian plague locust is generally by aerial spraying of bands and swarms with fenitrothion. This is primarily undertaken by the Australian Plague Locust Commission. Recent laboratory experiments have shown that both these pests are susceptible to the same acridid isolates of *Metarhizium flavoviride* from Australia or Africa. The initial field trial against the Australian plague locust gave promising results despite evidence of toxicity to the conidia of the formulating emulsifying oil. Further studies on the formulation showed that conidia freshly suspended in water were less effective than those suspended in peanut oil or the emulsifying mineral oil. A field trial showed that the problem with the emulsifying oil could be overcome by mixing the conidia in the oil immediately prior to spraying. It is now known that conidia can be stored for many months in the same mineral oil free of the emulsifying agent. The Australian plague locust is a particularly attractive target given that control is often directed at nymphs which occur in high density bands with very sparse cover of vegetation. In addition, public opinion in Australia is favourably disposed towards non-chemical methods of pest control.

Résumé. En Australie, le locuste *Chortoicetes terminifera* constitue le fléau acridien le plus redoutable. Il peut causer de graves dommages aux cultures et pâturages pendant les périodes d'invasion. Parmi les autres acridiens ravageurs d'Australie, on compte le sauteriau aptère, *Phaulacridium vittatum*, qui inflige régulièrement des dégâts aux pâturages, aux cultures et aux arbres dans les districts plus froids de la Nouvelle-Galles du Sud à l'Australie-Occidentale. La stratégie de lutte employée contre *C. terminifera* consiste généralement en épandages aériens de fénitrothione sur les bandes larvaires et les essaims. Ces épandages sont généralement réalisés par la Australian Plague Locust Commission. De récents essais en laboratoire ont montré que ces deux ravageurs sont sensibles aux mêmes isolats de *Metarhizium flavoviride* d'Australie ou d'Afrique. Le premier essai mené sur le terrain contre *C. terminifera* a donné des résultats prometteurs bien que l'huile émulsifiante de la formulation se soit révélée toxique pour les conidies. D'autres études sur la formulation ont montré que les conidies venant d'être mises en suspension dans de l'eau étaient moins efficientes que les conidies en suspension dans de l'huile d'arachide ou dans l'huile minérale émulsifiante. Un essai effectué sur le terrain a démontré que le problème de l'huile émulsifiante pouvait être résolu en mélangeant les conidies à l'huile juste avant de procéder aux pulvérisations. *C. terminifera* représente une cible particulièrement sensible aux applications à base de spores fongiques, ce qui est d'autant plus intéressant que les opérations de lutte sont souvent dirigées contre les larves qui constituent des bandes de forte densité dans les zones ayant une végétation très clairsemée. De plus, l'opinion publique australienne est favorable aux méthodes de lutte antiacridienne non-chimique.

Introduction

The Australian plague locust, *Chortoicetes terminifera* (referred to hereafter as "locusts"), is a major, though sporadic, pest of crops and pastures which if not controlled would have caused over $100 million damage in 1984 alone (Wright 1986). Control of populations which pose an interstate threat is the responsibility of the Australian Plague Locust Commission and such populations are generally treated by ultra low volume (ULV) spraying of fenitrothion from the air to nymphal bands and adult swarms. Another acridid, the wingless grasshopper, *Phaulacridium vittatum* (referred to hereafter as "grasshoppers"), is a serious pest of pastures in Western Australia and parts of South Australia, Victoria and New South Wales. It is estimated that, on average, damage to pastures is worth over $10 million per year. There is a need, and a demand, for an environmentally benign method for control for both pests.

In 1993, a program of research commenced at the Commonwealth Scientific and Industrial Research Organisation (CSIRO) Division of Entomology in Canberra aimed at evaluating the potential value of oil-based sprays of *Metarhizium flavoviride* which had shown promise against locusts and grasshoppers in Africa (Lomer et al. 1993). Isolate FI985 from *Austracris guttulosa* was selected for field trials as it was highly pathogenic under laboratory conditions to both acridids and is an isolate native to Australia (Milner and Prior 1994). Field trials have mostly been against wingless grasshopper (Baker et al. 1994; Milner et al. 1994), because the locust outbreak of 1993 was abruptly ended by the severe drought in 1994. However, a single field trial, undertaken against locusts in October 1993, gave promising results (Hooper et al. 1995). The spray killed up to 41% of nymphs in samples taken one day after spraying, even though spore viability was found to be < 1%. The low viability was shown to be due to the emulsifying oil (DC Trate made by Ampol) used in the formulation. Initial laboratory studies had shown this oil to be non-toxic when tested for one week at room temperature prior to the field trial; however, under the higher temperature experienced in the field, a slow toxicity became apparent. DC Trate was selected because it was non-toxic in our initial screen and is registered in Australia for use on crops. The present paper describes a laboratory experiment and field experiment to test the hypothesis that this slow toxicity could be avoided by mixing the conidia with the DC Trate on the day of spraying.

Materials and methods

Screening of formulating agents

The efficacy of a recently prepared suspension of conidia in DC Trate was compared with aqueous (Tween 80) and peanut oil suspensions in the laboratory. Conidia of FI985, produced on rice, were mixed with each of the formulating agents to give a concentration of 2×10^9 conidia/ml (equivalent to that used for field application at 2 l/ha). This dose 1 concentrate was then diluted with the appropriate substrate to give five decimal dilutions. A hand-held pressurised paint sprayer was then used to deposit a fine mist of droplets of each of these suspensions, including water and oil controls, onto short pieces of cut grass. The treated pieces of grass were then placed with 4th instar locust nymphs and the insects incubated for seven days at 30 °C. Fresh food was provided as needed, and dead insects were removed daily and placed in moist chambers to assess sporulation.

Field trial

In March 1994, a field trial was undertaken at Tarago, New South Wales, to test the efficacy of a DC Trate spore suspension prepared immediately prior to spraying. Two plots of 5 ha, about 1 km apart, were selected as having reasonably high populations of mostly adult wingless grasshoppers. One plot was left untreated, and the other was treated with FI985 in pure DC Trate at 4 l/ha using a vehicle-mounted Micronair AU8000 rotary atomiser set to deliver droplets averaging 70 µm in diameter. The dose applied was 3.1×10^{12} conidia/ha. The population was assessed weekly, using a standard sweep-net, in two predetermined areas near the centre of the treated plot and one area of the untreated controls. Live grasshoppers were taken back to the laboratory and incubated to determine the incidence of *Metarhizium* in the populations.

Results

Screening of formulating media

There was no mortality of any control locusts during the five days of the experiment. The oil formulations killed one day or more faster than the water formulation and also gave high levels of mortality at a 1000-fold dilution of the field rate, while the water formulation gave just 20% mortality at 100-fold dilution of the field rate (Fig. 1 A–C). At the highest dose, DC Trate gave the fastest kill, but at lower doses the peanut oil formulation was better.

Field trial

The weather during the three weeks following treatment was cool and dry with day time temperatures of 20–22 °C and night time temperatures of 10–12 °C. Probably because of these cool conditions there was very little evidence of movement of grasshoppers in or out of either plot.

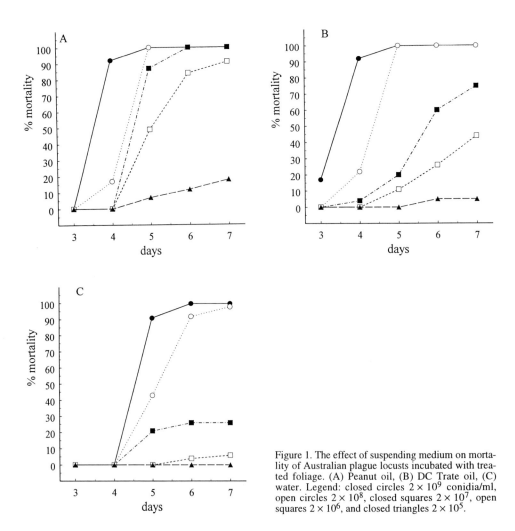

Figure 1. The effect of suspending medium on mortality of Australian plague locusts incubated with treated foliage. (A) Peanut oil, (B) DC Trate oil, (C) water. Legend: closed circles 2×10^9 conidia/ml, open circles 2×10^8, closed squares 2×10^7, open squares 2×10^6, and closed triangles 2×10^5.

The control population remained stable at about 2 grasshoppers/m^2 (the actual population was probably much higher, but the efficiency of the sampling was reduced by the cool weather), while the treated population showed a decline from 4.5–6.2 to about 1 (Fig. 2). This decline was most marked between 12 and 21 days post-spraying. Seventy percent of the treated insects sampled in the field on day 21 and incubated in the laboratory died after four days of incubation, suggesting that a greater level of control might have been achieved had the field population been sampled longer. After 21 days post-treatment, the weather became very cold and wet-resulting in a sharp decline in population in both treated and control plots.

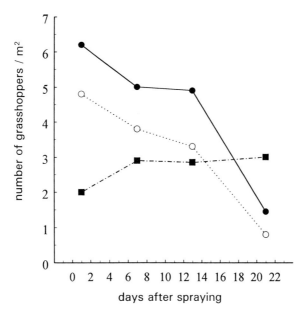

Figure 2. Effect of spraying *Metarhizium flavoviride* conidia suspended in DC Trate oil on population density of the wingless grasshopper at Tarago, New South Wales, March 1994. Legend: circles – treated sampling sites 1 and 2; closed squares-control

Discussion

FI985 has been shown to be virulent for both the major acridid pests in Australia in the laboratory and in the field (Milner and Prior 1994; Baker et al. 1994; Hooper et al. 1995). Laboratory experiments have shown that locusts become infected when fed pieces of grass sprayed with conidia of FI985 formulated in water, peanut oil or DC Trate. Since it is known that *Metarhizium* does not infect locusts per os (Charnley 1982), it is likely that the infection takes place on the external mouthparts and buccal cavity. Under field conditions, this secondary pickup from vegetation is likely to be an important factor in determining efficacy of a mycoinsecticide. The comparison between water- and oil-based sprays have confirmed that, under laboratory conditions, conidia in oil reduces the median lethal time by about one day (Bateman et al. 1993). In addition, doses down to 100-fold below field rate caused 100% mortality which was delayed by two days from the highest dose. While this is under ideal laboratory conditions with high humidity, no ultraviolet radiation, optimum temperature and forced contact with the target, nevertheless, given these results, the promising field trial result (Hooper et al. 1995) and the low

LD50 (Milner and Prior 1994), it is possible that field doses of below 10^{12} conidia/ha could be effective for the Australian plague locust. In the experiment reported here, peanut oil was more effective than DC Trate. This may be due to the greater viscosity of the peanut oil resulting in more conidia remaining on the locust cuticle rather than being ingested. The ingested conidia probably are passed out in the faeces, still viable. It is not known if conidia in the faeces are likely to be a source of infection in healthy locusts. However, it is known that the emulsifying agent in DC Trate causes slow deterioration of conidia such that conidia are mostly non-germinable after seven days in DC Trate at 37 °C (Milner, unpublished). This could also have reduced the efficacy of the conidia in DC Trate in comparison with peanut oil, which is not toxic to the conidia (Stathers et al. 1993).

The Tarago field trial showed that a ULV spray of 3.1×10^{12} conidia/ha in 4 l oil can reduce wingless grasshopper populations by 80–90% after three weeks under cool conditions. Other trials have shown that FI985 can be effectively applied at 2 l/ha from a fixed-wing aircraft as well as at much higher volume with oil/water emulsions and produce good levels of control after one to three weeks depending on the prevailing weather conditions (Milner and Baker unpublished). Field trials against Australian plague locust, planned for 1994/5, were abandoned due to the severe drought in Australia. Some locust hatchings were reported, but the nymphs were not able to survive as there was no green food.

In Australia, as in many other countries, there is concern about the hazards of aerially sprayed chemical pesticides. We have found that the Australian plague locust is particularly susceptible to *Metarhizium* and have laboratory and field data to suggest that ULV application of conidia in oil could be effective against hopper bands where rapid control is not required. In addition, the same isolate of *Metarhizium* could be used for control of wingless grasshoppers to protect pastures, crops and trees from defoliation. Further work is needed to develop the most effective strategies for application in terms of dose, formulation, timing and method of application as well as studying the effects on non-targets and the economics of production and commercialisation.

Acknowledgements
The authors would like to thank Mr George G. Lutton, Mr Tom R. Hartley and Mr Peter A. Spurgin for their expert technical assistance during this study. The field site at Tarago was kindly provided by the owner, Mr David Pockley.

References

Baker GL, Milner RJ, Lutton GG, Watson DM (1994) Preliminary field trial on the control of *Phaulacridium vittatum* (Sjostetd) (Orthoptera: Acrididae) populations with *Metarhizium flavoviride* Gams and Rozsypal (Deuteromycetina: Hyphomycetes). J Aust Entomol Soc 33: 190–192

Bateman RP, Carey M, Moore D, Prior C (1993) The enhanced infectivity of *Metarhizium flavoviride* in oil formulations to desert locusts at low humidities. Ann Appl Biol 122: 145–152

Charnley AK (1982) Physiological aspects of destructive pathogenesis in insects by fungi: a speculative review. Pages 665–706 in Anderson JM, Rayner, ADM, Walton DWH (eds) Invertebrate microbe interactions. London: Cambridge University Press

Hooper GHS, Milner RJ, Spurgin PA, Prior C (1995) Initial field assessment of *Metarhizium flavoviride* Gams and Rozsypal (Deuteromycetina: Hyphomyctes) for control of *Chortoicetes terminifera* (Walker) (Orthoptera: Acrididae). J Aust Entomol Soc 34: 83–84

Lomer CJ, Bateman RP, Godonou I, Kpindou D, Shah PA, Paraiso A, Prior C (1993) Field infection of *Zonocerus variegatus* following application of an oil-based formulation of *Metarhizium flavoviride* conidia. Biocontr Sci Technol 3: 337–346

Milner RJ, Hartley TF, Lutton GG, Prior C (1994) Control of the wingless grasshopper, *Phaulacridium vittatum* (Sjostedt) (Orthoptera: Acrididae) in field cages using an oil-based spray of *Metarhizium flavoviride* Gams and Rozsypal (Deuteromycetina: Hyphomycetes). J Aust Entomol Soc 33: 165–167

Milner RJ, Prior C (1994) Susceptibility of the Australian plague locust, *Chortoicetes terminifera*, and the wingless grasshopper, *Phaulacridium vittatum*, to the fungi *Metarhizium* spp. Biol Contr 4: 132–137

Stathers TE, Moore D, Prior C (1993) The effect of different temperatures on the viability of *Metarhizium flavoviride* conidia stored in vegetable and mineral oils. J Invertebr Pathol 62: 111–1115

Wright DE (1986) Economic assessment of actual and potential damage to crops caused by the 1984 locust plague in south-eastern Australia. J Environ Manag 23: 293–308

New Strategies in Locust Control
S. Krall, R. Peveling and D. Ba Diallo (eds)
© 1997 Birkhäuser Verlag Basel/Switzerland

Melia volkensii: a natural insecticide against desert locusts

H. Rembold

Max-Planck-Institut für Biochemie, D-82152 Martinsried, Germany

Summary. In search of a soft chemistry for desert locust control, botanical insecticides have been shown to be highly effective against locusts and to be non-toxic to mammals and birds. They are environmentally friendly due to their complete degradation in the soil. Biologically interesting limonoids have been identified in tropical Meliaceae, like *Azadirachta indica* (neem) or *Melia volkensii*. The latter has only been found in East Africa. Each tree is capable of yielding 100 kg of dry fruits per season, from which about 1 kg of a highly active powder can be produced. Field tests have shown that the crude powder in a dose of about 10 g ha^{-1} gave effective control. The effect results from acute toxicity (28%), retarded growth and an 80% rate of malformations. First results from a technical-scale production of *M. volkensii* powder are presented.

Résumé. Parmi les substances chimiques «douces» utilisables dans la lutte contre le Criquet pèlerin, les insecticides végétaux se sont avérés être fort efficaces contre les locustes et être non-toxiques pour les mammifères et les oiseaux. Se dégradant complètement dans le sol, ils ne sont pas néfastes pour l'environnement. Des limonoïdes biologiquement intéressants ont été identifiés sur des méliacées tropicales, telles que *Azadirachta indica* (neem) et *Melia volkensii*, ce dernier croissant uniquement dans l'Est de l'Afrique. Par saison, chaque arbre donne environ 100 kg de fruits secs à partir desquels on peut extraire environ un kilo d'une poudre extrêmement active. Les essais sur le terrain ont montré que la poudre brute dosée à environ 10 g/ha^{-1} donnait de très bons résultats: forte toxicité (mortalité de 28%), retardement de la croissance et 80% de malformations. Cet article présente les premiers résultats d'une production à l'échelle technique de poudre de *M. volkensii*.

Introduction

Before searching for new strategies in locust control, we have to explain why we are not satisfied with the present organophosphates, carbamates, pyrethroids and other well-accepted synthetic insecticides. Why alternative methods of controlling locust populations? The reasons are well known: the type of highly industrialised agriculture practised today in the first world favours the establishment of a few well-adapted pests which have developed increasing resistance against many synthetic insecticides. All their undesirable side-effects makes their further application an impending threat to ecology and human health.

Some specialists already favour an Integrated Pest Management (IPM) approach with an extreme reduction or even go so far as to question the use of synthetic insecticides. However, we still do not have a really practicable and economically acceptable alternative to the cheap and highly effective modern synthetics, which admittedly have become environmentally safer than their prototypes. For these reasons, more target-specific methods of insect control are constantly being sought worldwide. Instead of using neurotrophic insecticides with their potential mammalian toxicity, the manipulation of insect-specific endocrine systems offers an attractive alternative.

During coevolution of plants and insects chemical defence strategies have developed, and botanical growth inhibitors may have resulted from this process of coevolution. The tropical Meliaceae, primarily, the neem tree, *Azadirachta indica*, has proved a treasury of excellent insect growth inhibitors. The present paper will concentrate on *Melia volkensii* (*Mv*), which is widespread in East Africa (Ethiopia, Somalia, Kenya, Tanzania). Its high yields of fruits, with up to 100 kg dry weight per season, and its highly prized timber, makes it an interesting candidate for developing new and more environmentally friendly locust control methods.

Material and methods

Mv fruits were collected in the Embu District of Kenya, dried in the shade and finally ground in a stone mill, using 1-mm width mesh. About 800 kg (37% yield) of dry powder, made up in 100-kg batches, was extracted with a 6:4 mixture of ethanol-water (v:v), and the alcohol removed in vacuo (2% dry matter). The water phase was collected, and the precipitate plus a thin oil layer were separated. The water phase was extracted with ethyl acetate, and after washing the organic phase with water, the polar components then precipitated with petroleum ether. The precipitate from the concentrated aqueous ethanol extract was washed with water and finally dried. The combined precipitates gave a total yield of 0.4% (7 kg) of *Mv* powder. For application, the powder was either dissolved in polar solvents (alcohols, ketones, esters) or applied in an oil formulation through a Micron ULVA sprayer.

Results and discussion

The process of producing a stable dry powder with insect growth-inhibiting properties from *M. volkensii* fruits is shown in Figure 1. It follows the method described by Mwangi and Rembold (1986) and makes use of the both lipophilic and hydrophilic characters of the active compounds. The ripe, yellow fruits have to be dried at a temperature not exceeding 40 °C. The hulled brown dry fruits with their extremely hard kernel must be pulverized in a hammer mill and the whole sieved meal consequently used for extraction. Unlike neem seeds with their high oil contents, *Mv* seeds are almost without oil, which makes them much less susceptible to fungal infection and production of mycotoxins. Consequently, their processing is much easier than that of neem

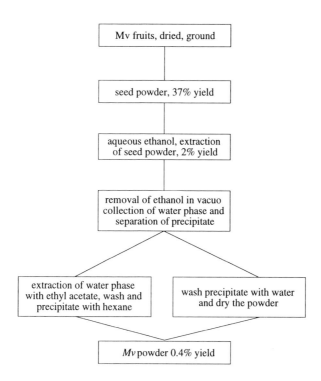

Figure 1. Flow chart for extraction of *Melia volkensii* powder.

seeds. The crude powder makes up less than half a percent from the fresh *Mv* fruits. The material can be further purified by dissolving it in organic solvents of different polarity and even further by open column chromatography, as already described in detail (Mwangi and Rembold 1988)

Mv extract induces mortality, reduction in fitness and up to 100% death as overaged nymphs due to the high rate of almost 80% malformations in hoppers and adults of *Schistocerca grega-ria* under field conditions (Wilps and Nasseh 1994). *Mv* extract also showed growth-inhibiting plus strong anti-feedant activity against the locust larvae in laboratory tests (Mwangi 1982).

In a pilot field test, application of an oil-based formulation of *Mv* powder to larvae in a dose of 10 g/ha caused 28% mortality and 100% retarded growth. Of even greater significance for the survival of *S. gregaria* populations, however, was the fact that *Mv* extracts delayed the attainment of sexual maturity. Nasseh et al. (1993) found that untreated insects were fertile by 30 days at latest after adult molting. Only 14% of females treated with *Mv* extracts were sexually mature after 53 days and most of them, if they survived, attained sexual maturity not until after roughly 70 days. This reduces the reproductive period by approx. 30 to 40 days, which means that the number of progeny of *Mv*-treated locusts is reduced by 500 to 600 larvae per female! This calculation does not take into account the general decline in egg production in aging insects and the serious effects on the physiological and hormonal performance of the treated locusts. The authors also observed phase shifts from gregarious to solitary locusts. About 80% of laboratory-reared insects treated with *Mv* extract showed changes in coloration. This speaks in favour of an effect on hormonal control systems which needs to be studied in more detail.

From practical considerations this is an interesting finding. Larval growth is slowed down by two to three weeks, which is equivalent to one reproduction cycle of the desert locust. A concomitant reduction in fitness and migration of the hopper bands leads to a deficit in food resources. This is because the most important host plant, *Schouwia thebaica*, only temporarily occurs in the recession areas. One may speculate that *Mv* application even affects the following two to three generations, due to larval starvation, population reduction and reduced reproduction of the surviving adults. A considerable prolongation of larval development after *Mv* treatment was also ascertained by other authors (Rembold and Mwangi 1989; Al-Sharook et al. 1991).

Besides interference with reproduction and physiological performance, *Mv* extracts exhibit a dose-dependent effect against *S. gregaria* adults with 95 to 100% mortality within 24 h (Wilps et al. 1993). The same authors demonstrated that flight performance was affected, with the result that treated locusts were unable to mobilise sufficient energy for long-distance flights. They exhibited a reduced hyperlipemic response to injection of adipokinetic hormone (AKH) which occurred when adult locusts were treated in the larval stage. Obviously some of the *Mv* compounds interfere with the neuroendocrine hormonal system, which accords with results obtained with *Locusta migratoria* after injection of the active ingredients of neem extract, which comprises a whole group of limonoids with azadirachtin A being the main representative (Fig. 2). Radiolabelled azadirachtin A adheres on the membranes of the corpora cardiaca and on the membranes of the nerves innervating these organelles. Furthermore, the synthesis of neuroendocrine granules is impaired in the corpora cardiaca, which are responsible for *de novo* synthesis of several neuropeptides involved in hormonal control (Rembold et al. 1989; Subrahmanyam and Rembold 1989; Subrahmanyam et al. 1989). The decreased hyperlipemic response following *Mv* application could thus indicate similar or identical interaction of the biologically active *Mv* compounds with the hormonal control of flight. Reduced hyperlipemic competence is also found in adults that have been treated with *Mv* extracts, while larvae exhibited no morphogenetic effects. Although these larvae have undergone a normal adult molt, they are nevertheless damaged at the physiological level. Why this happens is not clear. Either the active compounds

Figure 2. Chemical structure of the main active ingredient of neem seeds, azadirachtin A. Its ED50 in the *Epilachna varivestis* assay (Rembold et al. 1980) is at 1.66 ppm.

in *Mv* extract, which are not azadirachtins (Rembold and Mwangi 1989), have a much higher biological activity than the neem components and therefore produce a higher residual effect, or morphogenetic programmes are altered (activated or inhibited) at the larval stage. This would support the fact that both adult phase transformation and sexual maturity are influenced by *Mv* treatment at the larval stage.

No molecules have yet been identified which could explain why the biological activity of crude *Mv* extract is about 10% that of pure azadirachtin. Several limonoids were isolated and structurally elucidated from *M. volkensii* fruits (Rajab and Bentley 1988), but only volkensin has shown some feeding inhibition and had no effect on insect growth and development (Rajab et al. 1988). It will be an interesting challenge for future chemical work to unravel the structure of those compounds which, present in about 10 g of crude *Mv* powder per hectare, are sufficient for locust control (Wilps and Nasseh 1994). It is also possible, however, that a series of biologically avtive compounds in 10–50 ppm quantities have a highly synergistic effect. It is well known that the individual compound often exhibits the same activity at much lower concentration when present in crude extract as when it is applied in its pure state.

Conclusion

Up to now natural products have not entered the commercial pesticide market. Of the known total, only about 1% are used in this niche market. One reason is their unpredictable production, which depends on climate, soil exhaustion and consequent high cost. Natural products can offer interesting new lead structures, but examples are rare and industrial research still relies on mass screening of 20,000 to 30,000 synthetic compounds per company per annum. There is an opportunity here for developing countries, with their rich sources of bioactive botanicals, to play a more important role in pest control. The tropical Meliaceae appear to be ideal candidates for penetrating this market. Even though neem is well researched (Schmutterer 1995) and is readily available, it has not been commercially exploited.

How can we explain this? Firstly, there are problems of harvesting, logistics and quality control and, secondly, its limited shelf-life and high costs detract from its value. At harvest, fruits must be carefully dried to avoid fungal infection and subsequent contamination. Enormous quantities are required for processing, and this is only possible on a co-operative farming basis. Final production necessitates strict quality control following ISO standards before it can enter the synthetic insecticide market. However, these conditions will never be met unless a market is created for these botanical insecticides.

What are the advantages of using botanical pesticides? They would save on hard currency if produced in their country of origin; no or at least smaller amounts of synthetic pesticides would be imported; the chance of entering the international pesticide market, in niche areas at least, would be possible. Both neem and *Mv* can be cultivated on poor soils, which would help in afforestation programmes, production of timber and would provide jobs in many fields. More important, botanicals are non-toxic to mammals and, according to preliminary studies, have shown no evidence of adverse side-effects on epigeal arthropods (Peveling et al. 1994).

Acknowledgements
Our own research has been partially supported by Max-Planck-Gesellschaft, the German Academic Exchange Program (DAAD) and last, but not least, by the Bundesministerium für wirtschaftliche Zusammenarbeit und Entwicklung (BMZ) and the Deutsche Gesellschaft für Technische Zusammenarbeit (GTZ) within its program on Integrated Biological Control of Grasshoppers and Locusts. All this support is gratefully acknowledged.

References

Al-Sharook Z, Balan K, Jiang Y, Rembold H (1991) Insect growth inhibitors from two tropical Meliaceae. J Appl Ent 111: 425–430
Mwangi RW (1982) Locust antifeedant activity in fruits of *Melia volkensii*. Entomol Exp Appl 32: 277–280
Mwangi RW, Rembold H (1986) Growth-regulating activity of *Melia volkensii* extracts against the larvae of *Aedes aegypti*. Pages 669–681 in Schmutterer H, Ascher KRS (eds) Proc 3rd Int Neem Conf, Nairobi
Mwangi RW, Rembold H (1988) Growth-inhibiting and larvicidal effects of *Melia volkensii* extracts on Aedes aegypti larvae. Entomol Exp Appl 46: 103–108

Nasseh O, Wilps H, Rembold H, Krall S (1993) Biologically active compounds in *Melia volkensii*: Larval growth inhibitor and phase modulator against the desert locust *Schistocerca gregaria* (Forskal) (Orth., Cyrtacanthacrinae). J Appl Ent 116: 1–11
Peveling R, Weyrich J, Müller P (1994) Side-effects of botanicals, insect growth regulators and entomopathogenic fungi on epigeal non-target arthropods in locust control. Pages 147–176 in Krall S, Wilps H (eds) New trends in locust control. GTZ Schriftenreihe 245. Rossdorf: TZ-Verlag
Rajab MS, Bentley MD (1988) Tetranortriterpenes from *M. volkensii*. J Nat Prod 51: 168–171
Rajab MS, Bentley MD, Alford AR, Mendel MJ (1988) A new limonoid insect antifeedant from the fruit of *Melia volkensii*. J Nat Prod 51: 168–171
Rembold H, Sharma GK, Czoppelt Ch, Schmutterer H (1980) Evidence of growth disruption in insects without feeding inhibition by neem fractions. J. Plant Dis Prot 87: 290–297
Rembold H, Mwangi RW (1989) Compounds from Melia volkensii and their growth inhibitory effect on Aedes aegypti larvae. Pages 3–8 in Borovsky D, Spielman A, (eds) Host regulated developmental mechanisms in vector arthropods.
Rembold H, Müller T, Subrahmanyam B (1989) Tissue-specific incorporation of azadirachtin in the malpighian tubules of *Locusta migratoria*. Z Naturforsch 476: 903–907
Schmutterer H (1995) The Neem Tree *Azadirachta indica* A. Juss. and other meliaceous plants. Weinhein: VCH, 696 pp
Subrahmanyam B, Rembold H (1989) Effect of azadirachtin A on neuroendocrine activity in *Locusta migratoria*. Cell Tissue Res 256: 512–517
Subrahmanyam B, Müller T, Rembold H (1989) Inhibition of turnover of neurosecretion by azadirachtin in *Locusta migratoria*. J Insect Physiol 35: 493–500
Wilps H, Nasseh O, Rembold H, Krall S (1993) The effect of *Melia volkensii* extracts on mortality and fitness of adult *Schistocerca gregaria* (Forskal) (Orth., Cyrtacanthacrinae). J Appl Ent 116: 12–19
Wilps H, Nasseh O (1994) Field tests with botanicals, mycocides and chitin synthesis inhibitors. Pages 51–79 in Krall S, Wilps H (eds) New trends in locust control. GTZ Schriftenreihe 245. Rossdorf: TZ-Verlag

New Strategies in Locust Control
S. Krall, R. Peveling and D. Ba Diallo (eds)
© 1997 Birkhäuser Verlag Basel/Switzerland

193

Potential for *Melia volkensii* fruit extract in the control of locusts

R.W. Mwangi[1], J.M. Kabaru[1] and H. Rembold[2]

[1]*University of Nairobi, P.O. Box 30197, Nairobi, Kenya*
[2]*Max-Planck Institute of Biochemistry, D-82152 Martinsried, Germany*

Summary. Fruits from the East African tree, *Melia volkensii* (Gurke) contain terpenoid compounds with well-established insecticidal activity. At high doses a concentrated *M. volkensii* extract (*Mv*) causes death or lack of physical fitness in locusts by irreversible paralysis of the locust skeletal muscles, without affecting the malpighian tubules or the pulsation of the dorsal heart. This effect is temperature related, with lower doses becoming more effective as the temperature increases. This action favours *Mv* toxicity against locusts in hot desert areas. Mammalian toxicological studies showed that *Mv* does not present any acute or chronic toxicity effects when orally administered to laboratory mice. It was thus not possible to establish an oral LD_{50} for the product in mice. *Mv* production in bulk and shelf-life are discussed with a view to demonstrating its advantages as a possible locust control product.

Résumé. Les fruits de l'arbre de l'Afrique de l'Est *Melia volkensii* (Gurke) contiennent des composés terpinoïdes dont l'action insecticide est bien établie. Des extraits concentrés de *M. volkensii* (*Mv*) appliqués à fortes doses causent la mort des locustes ou diminuent leur forme physique en provoquant une paralysie de leurs muscles squelettiques sans toutefois affecter les tubes de Malpighi ou la pulsation du coeur dorsal. Les effets obtenus varient en fonction de la température ambiante. Les doses réduites sont d'autant plus efficaces que la température est élevée, d'où une meilleure efficacité de *Mv* contre les locustes dans les zones désertiques chaudes. Des études toxicologiques mammaliennes ont montré que *Mv* administré oralement à des souris de laboratoire n'avait pas d'effets toxiques aigus ou chroniques. Il n'a par conséquent pas été possible de déterminer une DL_{50} par voie orale pour les souris. Cette étude apporte des informations sur la production de *Mv* en grandes quantités et sur sa durée de conservation. Il expose également les perspectives de l'utilisation du produit dans la lutte antiacridienne.

Introduction

In the course of evolution, plants have acquired the ability to biosynthesise compounds that have insecticidal or insect repellent properties. Such compounds naturally protect the plant from insect damage. Plants of the family Meliaceae produce such compounds that are primarily terpenoids, also commonly known as limonoids. One of the well-known limonoid compounds that has insect growth-disrupting activity is azadirachtin, from the neem tree, *Azadirachta indica*, of the family Meliaceae. Some other Meliaceae also contain azadirachtin, but its occurrence is not universal throughout the family. One plant which has terpenoid compounds, but no azadirachtin, is *Melia volkensii* (Gurke) (Mwangi and Rembold 1988).

Melia volkensii is a tall woody tree that bears large olivelike fruits. It is found in Kenya, Tanzania, Ethiopia and Somalia. It normally thrives well in the dry savannahs, especially in abandoned cultivations. Local farmers grow it for its termite-resistant timber and for livestock fodder. It is also planted as a shade tree. On average, it takes five years from germination to fruiting. A tea prepared from the bark of the tree is used in traditional healing to alleviate pain (Kokwaro 1976). *Mv* was reported to contain anti-feedant activity against the desert locust, *Schistocerca gregaria*, for the first time by Mwangi in 1982. Over the past decade much data evaluating its potential for the control of locusts and other insects has been accumulated.

Isolation and identification of the limonoid compounds in *Mv* have been carried out by Rajab et al. (1988), Rajab and Bentley (1988) and by Balan (1993). The limonoid compounds have been identified as volkensin, the well-known salannin, 1-tigloyl-trichilinin, 1-cinnamoyl-trichilinin, meliacin and ohchinin-3-acetate. Volkensin and salannin (Fig. 1) are both found in large amounts in *Mv*. Using the *Aedes* mosquito bioassay method, Mwangi and Rembold (1988) showed that some of these compounds were found to exhibit high biological activity at between less than an LD_{50} (median lethal dose) of $50-100$ ppm within 48 h (Balan 1993). However, up to now no single compound from *Mv* has been identified as the principal biological component. The possibility exists that this is due to a mixture of different compounds, the so-called cocktail effect of biological activity.

Formulated *Mv* has undergone limited field tests in Mauritania to evaluate its efficacy against the desert locust. The results of these field trials (Wilps and Nasseh 1994a,b; Peveling et al. 1994) look promising and indicate that *Mv* is even more effective than azadirachtin. The main effects observed in field and semi-field trials are, primarily, death, a shift in phase to the solitary status, retarded development, reduced physical fitness and inhibition of moulting in the nymphal stages.

The effect of temperature on insects treated with different doses of *Mv* is also addressed. Although many reports on the biological activity of *Mv* exist, thus far no attempt has been made to carry out mammalian toxicological studies to verify its safe use for locust control operators. Adult African migratory locusts (*Locusta migratoria migratorioides* R. & F.) were used for

Figure 1. Chemical structure of volkensin (i) and salannin (ii) found in *M. volkensii* fruit.

determining the temperature responses of locusts treated with *Mv*, while adult mice were used for measuring mammalian toxicology.

Materials and methods

A crude *Melia volkensii* extract was obtained by extraction of the dry fruit powder using a 6:4 ethanol:water solvent (v:v). The extract was dried, redissolved in absolute ethanol, and the ethanol-insoluble precipitate was discarded. The ethanol-soluble extract was precipitated in water, and the precipitate was dried out. This fraction was used in the experiments on the dose-temperature response relationships and those on the locust treatments.

Adult locusts were injected with the *Mv* test material suspended in 30% ethanol in a volume not exceeding 10 µl of the test solution, while controls received 10 µl of 30% ethanol. To assess temperature responses, batches of adult *Locusta* ($n = 16$) were first acclimatised for one hour and then maintained at six different constant temperatures (15, 20, 25, 30, 35 and 40 °C) after treatment with *Mv*. Oxygen consumption was estimated using a mercury manometer.

The dried ethanol-soluble supernatant, which contains all the insecticidal activity, was also used for the mouse toxicology tests. Adult mice were force-fed the *Mv* solution in 50% ethanol using a cannula introduced into the stomach through the mouth for the oral toxicity tests. Another group of adult mice was injected with the solution intraperitoneally using a hypodermic syringe, while a third group received treatment by spraying of the diluted *Mv* suspension in water on the area of skin to be tested.

Results

Figure 2 shows that temperature significantly influenced the response of locusts to *Mv* toxicity. At 15 °C adult migratory locusts injected with 3 µg of *Mv* per gram of body tissue remained outwardly unaffected for 2 h, while at 40 °C the onset of paralysis was 30 min and all were paralysed within 1 h. There was thus a progressive increase in the sensitivity of *Mv*-treated locusts with increasing temperature. Other experimental results indicate that the temperature response was dose related, with lower doses required to achieve the LD_{50} level at temperatures of 30 °C as compared with higher doses required at temperatures below 25 °C.

Topical application of *Mv* to the arthrodial membrane beneath the pronotum gave similar results (Fig. 3), except that it took longer and required a higher *Mv* (10 µg) dose as compared

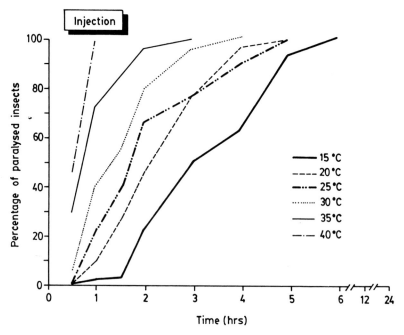

Figure 2. Effect of different constant temperatures on percentage paralysis of *Locusta* adults (n = 16) after *Mv* injection.

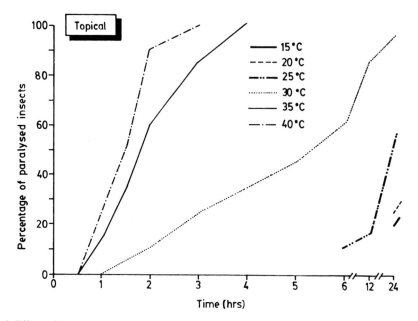

Figure 3. Effects of constant temperature on percentage of *Locusta* adults (n = 16) after topical application of *Mv*.

Table 1. Relationship between mean oxygen consumption and dose of *Mv*-injected *Locusta* adults ($n = 16$ in each case)

Mv Dose µg/g	Mean oxygen consumption µl/g/min/±SE
0 (control)	21.9 ± 0.69
0.5	18.6 ± 1.64
1.0	14.1 ± 0.85
2.0	3.0 ± 0.30
3.0	2.0 ± 0.16
4.0	1.4 ± 0.21

with the earlier injection method in Figure 2. The higher dose required for topical application is not unexpected, since only a small fraction of the *Mv* penetrates into the insect. The fact that higher temperatures favour locust immobilisation is advantageous, since locust control operations generally occur in deserts where temperatures rise from 30 to 40 °C during the day. Physical and meteorological factors are then favourable for ultra low volume (ULV) sprays.

Locust paralysis with *Mv* is non-reversible, with death occurring within 24 h of exposure. It is important to note, however, that the dose causing skeletal muscle paralysis in locusts is greater than the field dose. Only a small quantity is known to impair flight performance, reduce physical fitness and reverse the gregarious phase in the desert locust. Also, it is likely that paralysis represents the maximum manifestation of the physical impairment caused by *Mv* doses. We have data which show that injecting *Mv* at 4 µg/g reduces the amplitude of abdominal contractions from 2.5 to 0.5 mm without affecting the frequency of the contractions which at 25 °C remain at 19 cycles per minute.

This implies that although the frequency of ventilation remains more or less constant after adult *Locusta* are treated with sub-lethal doses of *Mv*, the amplitude of each ventilation cycle is significantly reduced. This decreases the oxygen tension and raises the CO_2 tension in the tissues and contributes to the reduced physical fitness observed in treated locusts. Data shown in Table 1 confirm the significant reduction in oxygen consumption after *Mv* treatment, which is

Table 2. The dorsal heart in *Locusta* adults after topical treatment and injection with *Mv* ($n = 16$ in each case)

Mv Treatment	Control (Pulsations/min)	Treated (Pulsations/min)
Bait (1% solution)	70.0 ± 7.9	66 ± 5.5
Injection (3.0 µg/g)	81.8 ± 2.3	78 ± 2.1
Topical (10.0 µg/g)	86.8 ± 2.1	80 ± 2.3

Table 3. Effects of *Mv* mice after oral administration and intraperitoneal injection (*n* = 10)

Mode of exposure	Dosage	% mortality	Average time to die (min)
Intraperitoneal injection (mg/kg)	Control	0	–
	20	0	–
	50	0	–
	100	0	–
	200	0	–
	300	2	60
	400	5	45
Oral intubation (g/kg)	Control	0	–
	3	0	–
	6	0	–
	10	0	–

dose related. Spiracles remain closed in those locusts which show reduced ventilation movements after *Mv* treatment.

The locust skeletal muscle neuromuscular junction is glutamate mediated, while the dorsal heart and the smooth muscles of the gut, including those of the malpighian tubules, are mediated by acetylcholine. From the results shown in Table 2 it is apparent that after skeletal muscle paralysis has occurred, there is no significant change in the pulsation of the dorsal heart. It was also observed that the malpighian tubules, as well as the gut, still contract at more or less the same frequency as untreated controls. These observations therefore point to a target specificity of the skeletal muscles in relation to muscular paralysis.

Results obtained by treating adult mice (Tab. 3) show that *Mv* is non-toxic to mice when administered orally. The maximum possible dose was 10 g/kg of body weight. No change in behaviour, appearance or function was observed using this oral dose. However, a dose of 500 mg/kg of *Mv* injected intraperitonially proved fatal within 40 min, although the mice could survive without any observable effects after injection of doses as high as 200 mg/kg of body weight. Mice that died exhibited vigorous convulsions and muscular spasms before they finally died. Post-mortem observations of the carcasses showed massive haemorrhage of the erythrocytes. Mice that survived after treatment with *Mv* at 300–400 mg/kg exhibited symptomatic fits for 3 h but recovered completely after 24 h. Continuous oral treatment of mice with 10 g of *Mv* per kilogram daily for two weeks did not result in any adverse changes. These mice were dissected every week over a two-month period, but no histological changes were detected in the blood, lungs, liver or kidney tissues.

Application of *Mv* at a concentration of 1% in water did not elicit any adverse effects either on the skin or eyes. A spray of 1% *Mv* to saturation level in a humidity chamber resulted in no change to mice exposed for a period of 24 h.

Discussion

It is apparent that *Mv* is a product whose margin of safety for the environment and for the operator is better than most conventional chemicals currently recommended for locust control.

Shelf-life of *Mv* has been estimated to be more than three years. *Mv* has been kept as an 80:20 methanol/water solution at room temperature of 22 °C in one of our laboratories now for eight years. Loss of biological activity was only 15%. Its stability would thus seem to indicate that *Mv* material can be processed, transported, formulated and stored for years without loss of biological activity.

More recently, we have perfected a method of bulk isolation of the active fraction without retaining many of the inactive components of the *M. volkensii* fruit kernel. This procedure involves precipitation of the total biological activity in water after extraction in 60% ethanol. Using this procedure, we have been able to reduce the mass of the active fraction to 10% of the ethanolsoluble fraction. The yield of this fraction is more than 10 kg of dry active powder per ton of dry *M. volkensii* fruit.

This material is currently undergoing field testing, with results indicating that ±10 g/ha is an optimum field dose for desert locust control when using the *Mv* powder formulated in a vegetable oil and applied by ULV drift spraying. At this rate *Mv* control is expected to be reasonably affordable and competitive.

References

Balan K (1993) Das Wachstum der Gelbfiebermücke – Naturstoffe aus *Melia volkensii*. Ph.D. thesis. University of Munich
Kokwaro JO (1976) Medicinal plants of East Africa. East African Literature Bureau. Nairobi, Kenya,157–158
Mwangi RW (1982) Locust antifeedant activity in fruits of *Melia volkensii*. Enotomol Exp Appl 32: 277–280
Mwangi RW, Rembold H (1988) Growth-inhibiting and larvicidal effects of *Melia volkensii* extracts on *Aedes aegypti* larvae. Entomol Exp Appl 46: 103–108
Peveling R, Weyrich P, Müller P (1994) Side-effects of botanicals, insect growth regulators and entomopathogenic fungi on epigeal non-target arthropods in locust control. Pages 147–155 in Krall S, Wilps H (eds) New trends in locust control. GTZ Schriftenreihe no 245. Rossdorf: TZ-Verlag
Rajab MS, Bentley MD (1988) Tetranortriterpenes from *Melia volkensii*. J Natural Products 551: 840–844

Rajab MS, Bentley MD, Ashford AR, Mendel MJ (1988) A new limonoid insect antifeedant from the fruit of *Melia volkensii*. J Natural Products 551: 168–171

Wilps H, Nasseh O (1994a) Field tests with botanicals, mycocides and Chitin synthesis inhibitors. Pages 52–79 in Krall S, Wilps H (eds) New trends in locust control. GTZ Schriftenreihe no 245. Rossdorf: TZ-Verlag

Wilps H, Nasseh O (1994b) Current status and future prospects of natural products for locust control. Pages 24–33 in Rembold H, Benson JA, Franzen H, Weickel B, Schulz FA (eds) New strategies for locust control in natural-product and receptor research. Proceedings of the CEC workshop held in Hamburg, Germany, 10–11 June 1993. Bonn: ATSAF

Field trials with neem oil and *Melia volkensii* extracts on *Schistocerca gregaria*

B. Diop[1] and H. Wilps[2]

[1]*Division Protection des Cultures (DRAP), PB 180-Nouakchott, Mauritania*
[2]*Integrated and Biological Control of Locusts and Grasshoppers, PB 5180, 65726 Eschborn, Germany*

Summary. From 1990 to 1995 different neem and *Melia volkensii* products were tested against hoppers of *Schistocerca gregaria*. Because of the limited occurrence of locusts, these investigations consisted only of field-cage trials until 1992. Thereafter, hoppers were increasingly treated. Depending on the amount of active ingredients applied, mortality rates of up to 100% were achieved after 14 days. Equally significant was reduced fitness, as a rule appearing 1–2 days after treatment in the form of a nearly complete loss of mobility. As a result, the hoppers became easy prey for predators.

Résumé. De 1990 à 1995, l'efficacité de certains produits à base de Neem et de *Melia volkensii* a été testée dans la lutte contre le criquet pèlerin *Schistocerca gregaria*. Compte tenu d'invasions réduites de locustes, ces recherches se sont jusqu'en 1992 limitées à des essais en cage. Par la suite, les traitements contre les criquets ont été intensifiés. Selon les quantités de matière active appliquées, des taux de mortalité allant jusqu'à 100% ont été atteints au bout de 14 jours. La détérioration de l'état de santé physique, apparaissant généralement 1 à 2 jours après le traitement sous forme de perte quasi complète de la mobilité, était également significative. Les criquets devenaient ainsi des proies faciles pour les prédateurs.

Introduction

Insecticides prepared from the seeds of Meliaceae have been used for many years against insect pests (Schmutterer 1995). The effects of these products differ between insects and are – as a rule – dose dependent. In the desert locust, *Schistocerca gregaria* (Forskål), both lethal and sub-lethal effects such as feeding repellency and fitness reduction have been reported (Nasseh et al. 1992, 1993; Wilps et al. 1992a, b, 1993). The latter includes reduced food consumption, decreased mobility (loss of walking and flying ability), retarded development and reduced fecundity (Wilps 1989; Nicol and Schmutterer 1991; Wilps and Nasseh 1994). The basis for the decline in fitness remains largely unknown, but some investigations indicate interactions of the triterpenoids found in the Meliaceae, known as the essential group of active substances, with the hormonal regulation of reproduction and locomotion (Rembold and Sieber 1981; Schlüter et al. 1985; Rembold et al. 1987, 1989; Subrahmanyam et al. 1989; Wilps et al. 1992a, b; 1Wilps and Nasseh 1994a, b).

This paper summarises the results of field and semi-field (cage) test applications of neem oils of different origins, and with varying contents of active ingredients, as well as extracts of *Melia volkensii* formulated in vegetable oil, against *S. gregaria* hoppers. These experiments were carried out from 1990 to 1995 in the Tamesna desert in the Niger and in the desert regions of Inchiri, Mauritania. In the first years (1990–1992), emphasis was laid on semi-field trials, due to the generally limited availability of locusts. Thereafter, treatments were directed against third to fifth instar hopper bands in the field.

Materials and methods

Insects, treatments and controls

The hoppers tested in the semi-field trials (second to fourth instars) were collected in the field and acclimatised for 3–5 days in field cages (2 × 2 × 2 m) which were mounted on natural vegetation. The vegetation was composed of preferred plants of *S. gregaria*, mainly *Schouwia thebaica, Fagonia olivieri,* and *Hyoscyamus muticus*. In these trials group size varied between 30 and 100 individuals per cage. All products were directly applied onto the target, using hand-held spinning disk sprayers suitable for ultra low volume (ULV) application. In the semi-field trials, hoppers were sprayed in open arenas of 16 m², enclosed by a plastic fence, and transferred to cages immediately after treatment. In the field, applications were directed against hoppers (fourth to fifth instars) in their roosting sites. The size of the hopper bands varied between 40,000 and 200,000 insects. Treatments were generally carried out between 7 and 9 a.m. Control insects were untreated or treated with vegetable oil only.

Products

Botanicals prepared from Meliaceae contain a cocktail of active substances. Triterpenoids have been identified as the principal substances, the best known being azadirachtin, which is found in the seeds of *Azadirachta indica*, but not in those of *M. volkensii*. Because of this complexity, the effects of these products cannot be assigned to one single active component, but rather to the total content of various active ingredients. Preparation, chemical extraction of seeds and product design were all done as previously described (Nasseh et al. 1993; Schmutterer 1995). The various neem products were supplied by Prof. Schmutterer (University of Giessen, Germany), Dr. Langewald (IITA, Cotonou, Benin) and Dr. Kleeberg (Trifolio Corp., Lahnau, Germany). *M. volkensii* extracts were provided by Prof. Mwangi (University of Nairobi) and Prof. Rembold (Max-Planck Institute, Munich, Germany). The dose rates used in the individual experiments are cited in the text or in the tables and figures. Cage trials were replicated three or four times. In the field, five hopper band treatments were carried out.

Quantitative evaluation of experiments

The cage trials were evaluated on a daily basis. The effects assessed were (1) mortality, (2) malformation (of antennae, eyes, legs and wings) and (3) retardation of development. Treated hopper bands were observed daily, and their displacement was recorded. The number of dead insects was estimated as accurately as possible (but see text for problems in quantifying these effects). In some cases, hopper samples were collected from the bands immediately before and after treatment and transferred to field cages for controlled observation.

Results and discussion

Over the five-year period of these investigations, depending on the concentrations of the *M. volkensii* and neem active ingredients in the formulations tested, mortality in the semi-field trials ranged from 28% (minimum) to 100% until 14 days post-application (Tab. 1). In 60% of all

Table 1. Mortality rates of third to fifth instar *S. gregaria* hoppers after ULV application of botanicals (semi-field trials)

Treatment	Test site and year	Dose rate (g a.i./ha)	Mortality (%) after	
			7 days	14 days
Neem oil	Tamesna 1990	<0.1	10	28
Neem oil	Inchiri 1992	0.3	20±4	38±8
Neem oil	Inchiri 1995	0.6	30±6	48±2
Neem oil	Tamesna 1991	0.8	41±3	92±3
Neem Azal F	Tamesna 1991	2.5	36±5	70±6
Neem Azal F	Tamesna 1991	5	58±3	100
M. volkensii	Inchiri 1992	1	18±4	40±3
M. volkensii	Inchiri 1993	5	46±8	51±9
M. volkensii	Inchiri 1993	10	73±9	80±6
M. volkensii	Inchiri 1994	10	55±6	91±8
Control, untreated	1990–1995	-	≤6	≤10
Control, veg. oil	1990–1995	1–3 1	≤15	≤22

Values are the mean ±SD of three to six trials for each variant. Control values are the highest observed in individual treatments from 1990 to 1995.

tests mortality was >50%. However, no dose-response relationship could be established. This was due to the fact that azadirachtin A was the only active ingredient whose concentration in the neem oils tested was known, while other insecticidal components having an insecticidal activity such as salannin and equally active dehydro forms have not been quantified. Additive and/or synergistic effects of these different compounds are likely, but they have not been unequivocally demonstrated so far. The active ingredients of *M. volkensii* also belong to the class of the tetraterpenoids, and here the total concentration of three different terpenoids is calculated as the amount of active ingredient. All these botanicals, unlike many synthetic insecticides, lack a knock-down effect. The slow rate of response up to 14 days and longer is, however, comparable to chitin synthesis inhibitors (Nasseh et al. 1992; Wilps and Diop 1995), which may also take 14 days to cause an effect.

Apart from lethal effects, malformations and delayed development (Tab. 2), as well as an overall reduction of fitness were equally important. These sub-lethal effects were expressed as a nearly complete loss of mobility. At higher doses, fledglings were not able to fly and nymphs – while still able to walk – stopped hopping (Wilps et al. 1992a, b, 1993). As a consequence, these locusts could not escape from predators (Wilps and Peveling 1995), and about 30% even fell victim to conspecifics (Wilps, unpublished data). This cannibalism can be explained by the gregarious behaviour. When roosting, hoppers climb up into trees and bushes, and are tightly packed in close proximity to each other. A minimum distance is maintained by defensive movements of their hind legs. Without this defence mechanism, other hoppers often start feeding on the abdomen, especially during or immediately after moulting.

In the case of attacks by predators, especially birds (e.g. *Cursoris cursor, Passer luteus, P. simplex*), sphecoid wasps (e.g. *Prionyx* sp.) and carabids (e.g. *Calosoma* sp.), hoppers were an easy prey. In five cases the complete elimination of treated hopper bands was observed (Fig. 1

Table 2. Malformation and delayed development of late instar *S. gregaria* hoppers after application of botanicals

Treatment	Dose rate (g a.i./ha)	Malformation (%)	Development delay relative to control (days)
Neem oil	≤0.1	8% n.s.*	0
Neem oil	0.3	38%	≤6 n.s.
Neem Azal F	2.5	95%	0
Melia volkensii	5	58%	18
Control, veg. oil	1 l/ha	6%	–

All effects are statistically significant unless marked with n.s. Malformations of survivors were determined one day after successful completion of the adult moult. Only cases with less than 80% mortality included.
* non-significant as compared to the control

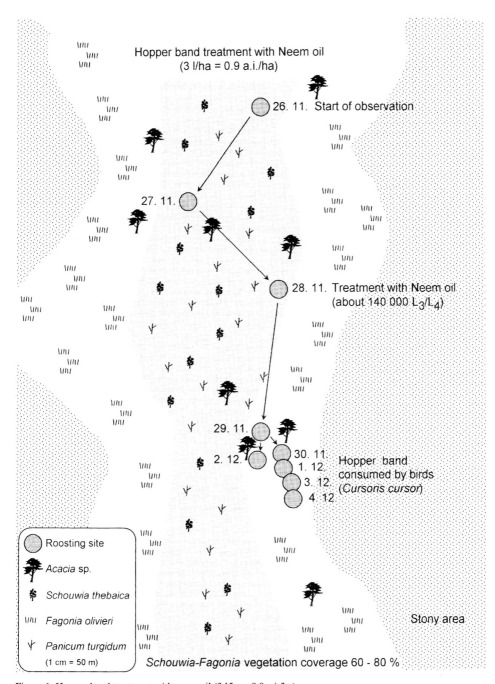

Figure 1. Hopper band treatment with neem oil (3 l/ha = 0.9 a.i./ha).

presents one example). In this regard, the methodological difficulties in hopper band quantification should be mentioned. Some of the treated bands split up or merged with immigrating untreated bands. The assessment of hopper mortality due to predators was equally difficult, because cadavers were quickly consumed by scavengers whose activities were only indicated by the fragments of heads, thoraces and piles of extremities lying about.

On the grounds that lethal and sub-lethal effects add to an overall sufficient control efficacy, botanicals may present an environmentally acceptable alternative to synthetic pesticides (Peveling et al. 1994). However, the following reservations must be made: (1) So far no standardised product is available in adequate amounts for operational use, although in India some very promising commercial products have become available, and (2) these botanicals are relatively slow acting and can therefore not be used for the direct protection of crops actually threatened.

Acknowledgements
We would like to express our gratitude to Sani Moudi and his co-workers at the Centre Antiacridienne in Agadez and Cheikh ould Dih and co-workers of the DRAP in Nouakchott for their repeated assistance and ongoing support. We also thank the GTZ (Deutsche Gesellschaft für technische Zusammenarbeit) team leaders Dr Pantenius and J. Haag in Niamey, as well as Volkhard Leffler in Nouakchott, and their co-workers. We are also grateful to Eberhard Dorow for his exact applications, as well as the suppliers of the various botanicals, as already mentioned above. Last but not least, we offer a hearty thank you to the co-workers at our stations in In-Abangharit (Tamesna, The Niger) and Akjoujt (Inchiri, Mauritania).

References

Nasseh O, Wilps H, Krall S (1992) Neem products – effective biocides for combating the desert locust *Schistocerca gregaria* (Forskål) – Report on investigations carried out on field and laboratory-reared locusts under natural conditions in the Tamesna desert (Republic of the Niger). Zschr Pflkr Pflsch 100: 611–621

Nasseh O, Wilps H, Rembold H, Krall S (1993) Biologically active compounds in *Melia volkensii* – Larval growth inhibitor and phase modulator against the desert locust *Schistocerca gregaria* (Forskål). J Appl Ent 116: 1–11

Nicol CMJ, Schmutterer H (1991) Kontaktwirkungen des Samenöls des Niembaumes *Azadirachta indica* (A. Juss) bei gregären Larven der Wüstenheuschrecke *Schistocerca gregaria* (Forskål). J Appl Ent 111: 197–205

Peveling R, Weyrich J, Müller P (1994) Side-effects of botanicals, insect growth regulators and entomopathogenic fungi on epigeal non-target arthropods in locust control. Pages 147–176 in Krall S, Wilps H (eds) New trends in locust control. GTZ "Schriftenreihe" publication. Rossdorf: TZ-Verlags-Gesellschaft

Rembold H, Müller T, Subrahmanyam B (1989) Tissue-specific incorporation of azadirachtin in the malpighian tubules of *Locusta migratoria*. Z Naturforsch 476: 903–907

Rembold H, Sieber K-P (1981) Inhibition of oogenesis and ovarian ecdysteroid synthesis in *Locusta migratoria migratorioides* (R. & F.). Z Naturforsch 43c: 903–907

Rembold H, Uhl M, Müller T (1987) Effect of azadirachtin A on hormone titers during the gonadotrophic cycle of *Locusta migratoria*. Proc 2nd Int Neem Conference, Nairobi, 1986. Eschborn: GTZ, 289–298

Schlüter U, Bidmon HJ, Grewe S (1985) Azadirachtin affects growth and endocrine events in larvae of the tobacco hornworm, *Manduca sexta*. J Insect Physiol 31: 773–777

Schmutterer H (ed) (1995) The neem tree. Weinheim: Verlag Chemie

Subrahmanyam B, Müller T, Rembold H (1989) Inhibition of turnover of neurosecretion by azadirachtin in *Locusta migratoria*. J Insect Physiol 35: 493–500

Wilps H (1989) The influence of neem seed kernel extracts (NSKE) of the neem tree *Azadirachta indica* on flight activity, food ingestion, reproduction rate and metabolism in the Diptera *Phormia terraenovae* (Diptera, Muscidea). Zool Jb Physiol 93: 271–282

Wilps H, Diop B (1996) Barrier spraying and sleeping place treatment of *Schistocerca gregaria* hopper bands. Trop Pest Management. in press

Wilps H, Nasseh O (1994) Field tests with botanicals, mycocides and chitin synthesis inhibitors. Pages 51–79 in Krall S, Wilps H (eds) New trends in locust control. GTZ "Schriftenreihe" publication. Rossdorf: TZ-Vlgs-Ges

Wilps H, Kirkilionis E, Muschenich K (1992a) The effects of neem oil and azadirachtin on mortality, flight activity and energy metabolism of *Schistocerca gregaria* Forskål – a comparison between laboratory and field locusts. Comp Biochem Physiol 102c: 67–71

Wilps H, Nasseh O, Krall S (1992b) The effect of various neem products on the fitness of adult *Schistocerca gregaria*. Pages 337–346 in Lomer CJ, Prior C (eds) Biological control of locusts and grasshoppers. Proceedings of a Workshop held at the International Institute of Tropical Agriculture, Cotonou, Republic of Benin, 29 April–1 May 1991

Wilps H, Nasseh O, Rembold H, Krall S (1993) The effect of *Melia volkensii* extracts on mortality and fitness of adult *Schistocerca gregaria* (Forskål). J Appl Entomol 116: 12–19

Wilps H, Peveling R (1995) Short report of the GTZ field component 1993–1995. GTZ, PN 89.2031.6, 40 pp

Locust control by means of selective baiting

R.E. Price and H.D. Brown

Plant Protection Research Institute, Agricultural Research Council,
P. Bag X134, Pretoria, 0001, South Africa

Summary. Renewed research into baiting as an alternative method of locust control was recently initiated by the Plant Protection Research Institute, Pretoria, South Africa. This technique was reexamined in the light of increasing environmental concern over the repeated use of broad spectrum ultra low volume (ULV) pesticide sprays for the control of the brown locust, *Locustana pardalina*, in the Karoo. Screened first in the laboratory to establish optimal dose rates, preliminary field trials in the Karoo with silafluofen 80 EC (Neophan), applied at a concentration of 2000 ppm in a bran bait formulation, demonstrated that rapid and effective control of nymphal bands could be consistently achieved. Rates of 2 – 10 kg of moistened bait/band, simply broadcast by hand around roosting bands (n = 13) in the early morning, averaged 91% (range 67 – 100%) control. Median lethal time was 4.6 h in summer. Broadcasting the bait in a ±1-m-wide barrier around the roost before the insects completed their morning descent to the ground was the most effective method of dose transfer. Baiting at other times of the day was less successful. It was equally effective in summer and autumn and was successfully applied in both Karoo scrub and mixed grass biotopes favoured by the brown locust. Being a simple method of locust control, this technique could also provide employment for economically disadvantaged rural communities in the Karoo.

Résumé. De nouvelles recherches sur l'appâtage comme moyen alternatif de lutte contre les locustes ont été récemment entreprises par le Plant Protection Research Institute de Pretoria en Afrique du Sud. La technique de l'appâtage a été revue à la lumière de l'inquiétude croissante en matière d'environnement suscitée par l'épandage à large échelle de pesticides par pulvérisateur en ULV (à très bas volume) pour lutter contre le Criquet brun *Locustana pardalina* dans le Karoo. Précédés d'études en laboratoire pour déterminer les doses optimales, des essais ont été menés sur le terrain dans le Karoo avec des appâts à base de silafluofen 80 EC (Neophan) à une concentration ajustée à 2000 ppm et mélangé à du son de céréales. Ces essais ont montré que l'appâtage était un moyen efficace de lutte contre les bandes larvaires. Des appâts mouillés de 2 à 10 kg par bande larvaire, déposés simplement à la main protégée par un gant tôt le matin autour des bandes perchées (n = 13), ont anéanti en moyenne 91% des locustes (variation de 67 à 100%). Le temps létal moyen était de 4,6 heures en été. Une barrière d'appâts de ± 1 m de large disposée autour des perchoirs avant que les insectes n'en descendent le matin s'est avérée être la méthode la plus efficace de transmettre la dose biocide. Les appâtages effectués à d'autres heures du jour se sont montré moins efficients. Les taux de réussite ont été équivalents en été et en automne, ainsi que dans les broussailles ou la végétation herbacée mixte du Karoo qui constituent les biotopes préférés des locustes bruns. Ce procédé simple de lutte antiacridienne pourrait également générer des emplois pour les communautés rurales démunies du Karoo.

Introduction

The brown locust, *Locustana pardalina* (Walker), has its outbreak areas located in the semi-arid Karoo regions of South Africa and southern Namibia (Faure and Marais 1937). Posing a threat to some nine countries in southern Africa, it exhibits the highest outbreak frequency of any African plague locust: over the past 48 years, for example, there have only been five seasons in which no chemical control was required in the Karoo.

Current preventive control strategy relies on applying broad spectrum insecticides to control brown locust outbreaks in the Karoo. Standard application practice is to deliver the insecticide by means of ULV sprays, applied mainly by ground equipment. However, repeated spraying of pesticides in this environmentally sensitive ecosystem is now being increasingly questioned by landholders and conservationists. How to reduce the insecticide load and yet at the same time exercise appropriate control of a serious agricultural pest has become a controversial issue.

Thus far there is no substitute for fast-acting pesticides for locust control. However, one way of reducing the environmental risk is to modify the mode of application and deliver the insecticide in a more target-specific manner. Baiting offers one method of presenting a toxic dose to a pest, which at the same time limits the number of non-target organisms coming in contact with the pesticide. In search of more environmentally acceptable alternatives, we have therefore been re-examining the role of baits for locust control.

Bait formulation, where the insecticide is mixed with an edible carrier such as wheat or maize bran, was a common form of locust control in the past (Steedman 1990). But logistical problems encountered with transport and storage proved problematic, with the result that baits have largely been phased out in modern control operations. In their place oil-based ULV and aqueous sprays have largely taken over. However, baits with chemical insecticides (e.g. carbaryl) are still used for the control of rangeland grasshoppers in the western USA (Onsager et al. 1980) and in certain other situations.

Bran bait containing 2–3% sodium arsenite was used extensively in South Africa for control operations against brown locust and red locust, *Nomadacris septemfasciata* (Serville), during the 1930s. It was applied at rates of 70–135 kg/ha (60–120 lbs/acre) until replaced by the organochlorine BHC (HCH) in the late 1940s. At the time, extensive field testing on the suitability of various bait carriers, such as wheat bran, maize meal, oats, sawdust, and even dung (e.g. Du Plessis and Botha 1939) showed that bran was the most acceptable carrier. Additives such as sugar, salt or vegetable oils made no difference.

The present paper describes small-scale field testing with silafluofen 80 EC or Neophan, a recent non-ester pyrethroid product of Hoechst Schering Agrevo (Pty) Ltd., formulated in bran bait for the control of the brown locust. Neophan is a broad spectrum stomach and contact insecticide with an acute oral LD_{50} (median lethal dose) >5000 mg/kg for rats and >2000 mg/kg for birds. Since control of late instar nymphal bands is the main method of outbreak prevention applied by the South African locust control organisation, we targeted these stages for our work. In addition, because locust control operations in the Karoo carry on into autumn, we also compared baiting under both summer and autumn conditions.

Material and methods

Dose rate

Silafluofen (760 g a.i./l EC, Batch #33675), supplied by Hoechst Schering Agrevo (Pty) Ltd., South Africa, was mixed into dry wheat bran to produce bait concentrations of 1000, 1500, 2000 and 4000 ppm and first assayed against gregarious 5th instar brown locust nymphs in the laboratory to establish a suitable field dose.

Targets

Targets selected for baiting comprised individual bands of gregarious 4th to 5th instar brown locusts in the Hopetown (29°47'S; 24°10'E) and Victoria West (30°55'S; 22°38'E) districts of the northern Cape Province. These marched throughout most of the day, strung out in characteristic columns, covering a kilometre or more a day, before concentrating to roost at sunset in tightly packed aggregations on the canopies of prominent bush clumps. Bands ranged up to ±0.3 ha in size and were readily located for baiting in the early morning by their conspicuous red coloration. The predominant behaviour and preferred feeding times in summer and autumn were first identified before treatments commenced. Air (AT) and soil surface temperatures (SST) were continuously recorded with data loggers, while light intensity (lux) was measured with a Hagner EC1 light meter.

Bait mixing

Bait was made up on site prior to application by dissolving 12.5 ml of silafluofen 80 EC in 5 l of water and admixing it with 5 kg of wheat bran using a wooden paddle. Moisture content was important; moist crumbly bait, from which a drop or two of water could still be squeezed when compressed between the fingers, proved ideal. Dry bait tended to blow away in the wind, while sodden bait could not be evenly broadcast.

Application

Two methods of applying the bait were tested: either by broadcasting it by hand or placing it out in small heaps. Access to heaped bait was found to be restricted by the first arrivals, which crowded out subsequent nymphs when these attempted to feed. It was therefore broadcast over the ground in all subsequent trials to maximise exposure.

Baiting of marching bands proved unsuccessful; their mobility made uptake difficult. We therefore focused on the roosting bands as possible targets for control. The most effective method was to treat a ±1-m-wide strip around the band, with a coverage of ±20–25 g bait particles per square metre of surface area, from which nymphs picked up a lethal dose. The bait was laid down as close as possible to the base of the bushes on which the band roosted, because this proved to be the preferred zone for basking and crawling about. Nymphs favoured the east side of the bushes for basking, which was therefore more liberally treated.

Mortality assessment

Mortality was assessed at 24 h post application by marking out the area containing dead hoppers and then determining their density by means of quadrats (75 × 75 cm). The extent of the area strewn with dead nymphs multiplied by the mean density per unit area was then used to estimate the number of individuals found in a band. Any survivors from the baiting were followed and subsequently sprayed with a heavy dose of deltamethrin UL and their number added. Mortalities were then calculated for the total sample.

Results

Dose

A rate of 2000 ppm silafluofen 80 EC produced >90% mortality within 72 h and was the minimum effective dose. Bait containing 4000 ppm was not consumed, while the 1000 and 1500 ppm concentrations produced <50% mortality. The laboratory bioassay showed the bait had a strong stomach (LD_{50} = 3.85 mg/nymph and LD_{90} = 11.2 mg/nymph) and contact action (90% mortality within 72 h). Bait with 2000 ppm silafluofen 80 EC was then tested against gregarious nymphal bands in the field.

Target behaviour

We first observed the daily behaviour of bands closely, so as to gain insight in to how best to apply the bait. Daily behaviour fell into the following categories: roosting, basking, walking, marching and feeding. The typical daily behaviour pattern shown by 5th instar brown locust nymphs in summer is given in Figure 1 and the details for both seasons are discussed below.

In summer, descent from the roost commenced at ±07h15 when AT reached 20 °C and SST was 21 °C and light intensity measured 260 × 100 lux. The majority of nymphs were down on the ground basking by 08h00, when the above measured 23 and 26 °C respectively and light was 481 × 100 lux. Following basking, which lasted for ±30 min, nymphs typically started to crawl about, nibbling and feeding around the roost. Peak feeding occurred between 08h15 and 08h45, when temperatures reached 24 and 30 °C respectively. By 09h00 (AT > 25 °C) concerted marching commenced, and the nymphs then all vacated the roosting site.

The rest of the day was spent marching with occasional halts to feed; bands roosted between 12h30 to 14h00, perching on the tops of individual bushes over a wide area, when AT was >31 °C and SST > 50 °C. Marching progressively intensified during the afternoon and continued up to ±17h30, when temperatures measured 25 and 40 °C respectively; thereafter bands slowed down and milled about, alternatively pausing to feed and bask in the setting sun, before finally climbing into the larger bushes to roost for the night (lux = 312 × 100). Sunset was at 19h00.

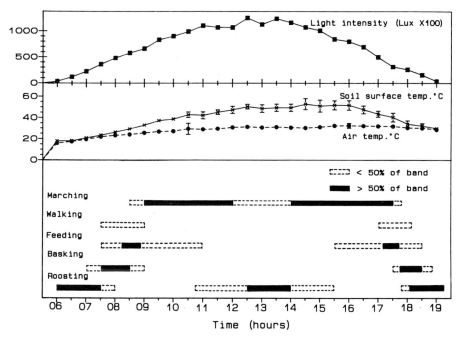

Figure 1. Typical diurnal behaviour pattern of 5th instar brown locust bands in relation to air temperature (AT), soil surface temperature (SST) and light intensity during summer at Hopetown; a solid bar denotes when >50% of nymphs within the band exhibited a specific behaviour pattern, and a broken line denotes <50%.

In autumn, owing to the shorter, cooler days, nymphs only descended from their roosts between 07h45 and 09h00 with AT of 13 to 16 °C and SST of 11 to 17 °C and 215 to 350 × 100 lux. Basking time increased, sometimes to mid-morning (10h30), when AT reached 20 °C and SST was >25 °C. Marching was also less intense, and there was no midday roosting period; recorded maxima of 20.4° and 35.1 °C, respectively, were evidently within their thermal tolerance limits. Nymphs ceased marching after 16h00, when AT dropped below 20 °C and light intensity to <400 × 100 lux, and commenced basking around the bases of bushes. By 17h00, when AT and SST measured ±18 and <25 °C respectively and lux was 110 to 150 × 100, >50% of nymphs were on their roost. Sunset occurred at 17h30 in autumn.

Bait trials

The Hopetown bait site in summer supported an abundance of lush green grass on which locusts could feed. Plant cover was estimated at 25 to 30% and comprised mixtures of grass and dwarf Karoo scrub. AT ranged from 10 to 35 °C (mean max. 31.7 °C), while SST ranged from 12 to 63 °C (mean max. 48.7 °C). Relative humidities averaged >90% at night and 40% during the day.

The Victoria West site in autumn was dry and cool. Vegetation was predominantly dwarf scrub, with little to no grass present, forming a 19% plant cover. AT ranged from 6 to 23 °C (mean max. 20.4 °C) while SST ranged from 5 to 40 °C (mean max. 35.1 °C). Relative humidity (R.H.) averaged 86% at night and 29% by day.

Baiting was best carried out in the early morning in summer after first light, from ±06h00 to 08h00, at air temperatures <20 °C, which is a time when the locusts were not readily disturbed. This also made for efficient dose transfer, since the nymphs retained their cohesive gregarious behaviour following descent from the roost, and their density per unit area thus remained high. Also, a proportionately smaller area (50–60%) needed to be treated. Under summer conditions, nymphs remained in contact with the bait for ±1 h, which nevertheless gave effective control (see Table 1), whereas in autumn exposure increased to 3 h, favouring the baiting technique. Fifth instar nymphs fed more readily on the bait than did 4th instars and were therefore more susceptible to baiting. Practically no bait particles remained on the site after contact with the locusts.

Toxicity

First symptoms appeared within 1 h of contact with the bait; nymphs thereafter became progressively disorientated. Trembling movements, interspersed with frequent grooming of anten-

Table 1. Band size, habitat and measured mortality of 5th instar brown locust nymphal bands after 24 h when treated with different rates of Neophan bait in summer (Hopetown)

Band no.	Band size	Habitat	Bait rate (kg)	$n =$	% Mortality
1	small	scrub	2.0	26000	90.0
2	small	grass	1.0	43648	66.8
3	small	scrub	2.0	32000	98.0
4	medium	grass	4.0	104426	100.0
5	medium	scrub	4.0	94102	99.0
6	medium	grass	3.0	95208	98.1
7	large	scrub	5.0	345000	85.0

nae with the forelegs, soon developed. Prior to falling over, they typically raised the anterior parts of the body up to an almost vertical position. Dose transfer appeared to be by both contact and ingestion. No recovery was observed.

Percentage mortalities, achieved by baiting variously sized 5th instar bands in summer and autumn, showed that rapid and very effective control (91%: range 67–100%) was achieved within 24 h during both seasons (Tabs 1, 2). Where there was poor control (e.g. band 2, Tab. 1), this was due to underdosing and misjudging the size of the band.

In summer, median times for knock-down and mortality of bands were 1.8 h and 4.6 h respectively. LT_{90} for these parameters occurred at 3.0 h and 7.6 h respectively.

Band targets were classed as small (10 m^2), medium (50 m^2) and large (1000 m^2) in size. The recommended dosage rates for these are:

- 2 kg for small bands
- 3–4 kg for medium bands
- 5–10 kg for large bands

Table 2. Band size, habitat and measured mortality of 5th instar brown locust nymphal bands after 24 h when treated with different rates of Neophan bait in autumn (Victoria West)

Band no.	Band size	Habitat	Bait rate (kg)	$n =$	% Mortality
1	small	scrub	2.0	32454	82.5
2	small	scrub	2.0	21609	96.5
3	medium	scrub	3.0	222234	75.0
4	medium	scrub	4.0	148202	99.5
5	large	scrub	7.5	259137	99.0
6	large	scrub	10.0	616155	97.0

On occasion, groups of survivors which had escaped picking up a dose and had marched off were observed circling back into the target zone, where they acquired a secondary dose, which now killed them. It was also observed that where a part of the band had somehow escaped treatment, migratory behaviour diminished, and the survivors hung around the treated band nucleus without marching further.

Discussion

Neophan bran bait gave effective control of gregarious nymphal bands of brown locusts in the Karoo. The level of control achieved with this product in a bait formulation equalled that obtained with any of the ULV-applied insecticides in current use in the Karoo. There was also no recovery of affected insects, as can occur with some compounds.

When applied in a manner that ensured direct interaction with the band target, such as by exploiting the basking and aggregation behaviour of locusts coming off their roost in the morning, so as to maximise uptake and kill per unit area, rapid and effective control consistently resulted. Furthermore, because only a relatively small strip was treated with bait, with no fallout of spray in the adjacent downwind area, there was also the additional benefit of reduced environmental contamination.

Exposure time, i.e., the length of time spent by the nymphs in basking and crawling about on the ground adjacent to the roost where the bait was broadcast, was crucial for successful control. Ambient temperature determined exposure time, and dose transfer was therefore maximised in autumn when up to 3 h was spent around the roost. Nevertheless, equally effective control with bait was achieved in summer, when kills of up to 99% resulted from a ±1-h exposure time.

Although baiting was expected to be more successful under dry conditions, when food was in short supply, it proved equally effective in lush areas (Hopetown) where alternative food was abundant. Baiting also proved effective in both summer and autumn. The characteristic high-density nature of brown locust bands, which roost as tightly packed, discrete targets on the canopy of bushes, lend themselves to spot treatment with baits. Furthermore, during the incipient stage of locust outbreaks in the Karoo, the majority of bands are generally of a manageable size (±0.3 ha) and present ideal targets for baiting.

Simply prepared and applied at low cost, baits containing silafluofen 80 EC offer a practical and ecologically attractive alternative to ULV sprays for dealing with small to medium-sized outbreaks and probably also for direct crop protection by farmers. Although labour intensive, baiting by locust control officers, hired on a temporary basis, could additionally involve local communities in sparsely populated areas, such as the Karoo, and thereby provide jobs in economically disadvantaged rural areas. Small-scale hopper band control by means of such a baiting technique could complement the mainstream ULV ground spray operations in South Africa and be successfully integrated into the present locust control strategy.

Acknowledgements
Without the support of Bill Goodwin, formerly of Hoechst Schering Agrevo (Pty) Ltd., Halfway House, Johannesburg, this project would not have got off the ground. Thanks go to the Directorate of Resource Conservation of the South African Department of Agriculture for locating targets and to our colleagues in PPRI, Lizel Seesink for field assistance and Margaret Kieser and Elizabeth Müller for fine-tuning the report and presentation. Financial support for one of us (HDB) to attend the GTZ Bamako Conference came from Messrs R. Smelt and S. Smolikowski of Hoechst Schering Agrevo; the Secretary General, Southern African Regional Commission for Conservation and Utilisation of the Soil (SARCCUS); and from the Agricultural Research Council to whom thanks are due.

References

Du Plessis C, Botha DH (1939) Preliminary field experiments on the attractiveness of certain chemicals and bait carriers to the hoppers of the brown locust. J Ent Soc Sth Afr 2: 74–92
Faure JC, Marais SJS (1937) The control of *Locustana pardalina* (Walk.) in its outbreak centres. Fourth International Locust Conference, Cairo 1936, Appendix 37, 5 pp
Onsager JA, Henry JE, Foster RN, Staten RT (1980) Acceptance of wheat bran bait by species of rangeland grasshoppers. J Econ Ent 73: 548–551
Steedman A (1990) Locust handbook. 3rd ed. Chatham: Natural Resources Institute, vi + 204 pp

New Strategies in Locust Control
S. Krall, R. Peveling and D. Ba Diallo (eds)
© 1997 Birkhäuser Verlag Basel/Switzerland

Neurotransmitter-receptors as targets for new insecticides

T. Roeder, J. Degen, C. Dyczkowski and M. Gewecke

Universität Hamburg, Zoologisches Insitut, Neurophysiologie, Martin-Luther-King-Platz 3, D-20146 Hamburg, Germany

Summary. The locust neuronal octopamine receptor is believed to be an ideal target for highly specific insecticides. In our study we characterized a number of high affinity agonists of this receptor subtype. Using structure-activity relationships, we were able to optimize the structure of these compounds in terms of their affinities. A variety of these compounds show a high degree of specificity for insect octopamine receptors versus vertebrate adrenergic receptors. The high affinity together with the high degree of specificity makes compounds such as the phenyliminoimidazolidines ideal starting points for the development of new insecticides.

Résumé. Le récepteur neuronal à l'octopamine des locustes est considéré comme étant une cible idéale pour des insecticides hautement spécifiques. Nous présentons dans notre étude plusieurs agonistes de haute affinité de ce sous-type de récepteur. Nous avons pu en utilisant la relation structure-activité optimiser la structure de ces composés sur le plan de l'affinité. Un certain nombre de ces composés montre une spécificité très élevée pour les récepteurs à l'octopamine des insectes par rapport aux récepteurs adrénergiques des vertébrés. La haute affinité et le degré élevé de spécificité font des composés tels que les phényliminoimidazolidines des substances idéales pour la mise au point de nouveaux insecticides.

Introduction

Most insecticides interact with targets within the central nervous system. Among them are the receptors for neurotransmitters. They are believed to be ideal targets for insecticides because they are responsible for communication within the central nervous system. Among the receptors that are targets for currently used insecticides are the GABA receptor (γ-amino-butyric acid) and the nicotinic acetylcholine receptor. The latter is the target of imidacloprid, which is a new, commercially available insecticide with low vertebrate toxicity. The neuronal octopamine receptor of insects is another very interesting target for new insecticides. Octopamine receptors are restricted in their occurrence to invertebrates. Substances that interact specifically with insect octopamine receptors have no counterpart in vertebrates and should therefore be characterized by low vertebrate toxicity. Octopamine is involved in the modulation of most peripheral organs and sense organs in invertebrates, especially in insects (see Orchard 1982). In addition, it has a very important role within the central nervous system of insects. It is vital for the generation and maintenance of various rhythmic activities such as walking and flight (Sombati and Hoyle 1984; Claassen and Kammer 1986). Other behaviours, such as learning and memory, are also under the control of octopamine (Bicker and Menzel 1989). This multi-potent neuroactive amine is believed to be the main switch for control of the mood and the arousal of the animal. Dishabituating effects of octopamine were reported from some insect preparations (Sombati and Hoyle 1984). Sub-lethal concentrations of octopaminergic insecticides such as chlordimeform have effects that could easily be interpreted as an interaction with the octopaminergic system. Hyperactivity and subsequent leaf walk-off is one major effect that is caused by application of sub-lethal concentrations of these compounds.

The target of octopaminergic insecticides, the neuronal octopamine receptor, that transmits the known effects of octopamine in the central nervous system such as control of rhythmic behaviors or the regulation of the activity of the insect, was characterized using various methods. Especially the radiolabelled ligands ^{3}H-octopamine and ^{3}H-NC-5Z are ideally suited for this purpose (Roeder and Nathanson 1993). Using this approach, a number of different high-affinity agonists and antagonists were characterized (Roeder 1990; Roeder 1995).

Material and methods

Adult desert locusts (*Schistocerca gregaria*) of either sex were used for most experiments. They were fed with a diet of grass and bran and held at 35 °C with a light/dark cycle of 12 h/12 h. The nervous tissue was dissected and stored frozen in incubation buffer (10 mM Hepes/NaOH pH 7.4, 5 mM $MgSO_4$, 200 µM PMSF) until use. The nervous tissue was homogenized and centrifuged, and the resulting pellet resuspended in the original volume. This procedure was repeated twice. The washed pellets were stored frozen until use.

The incubation was performed in a total volume of 100 µl with approximately 0.5 mg/ml protein and 10 nM ^{3}H-octopamine or 1 nM ^{3}H-NC-5Z as the radioligand and the indicated concentrations of the compounds tested. It proceeded for 1 h and was stopped by filtration through prewetted glass fibre filters that were washed subsequently with ice-cooled incubation buffer. The filters were scintillation-counted and evaluated using the LIGAND program (Munson and Rodbard 1980).

Further experimental details are given elsewhere (Roeder and Gewecke 1990).

Results and discussion

Both ligands, ^{3}H-octopamine and ^{3}H-NC-5Z label the neuronal octopamine receptor with high affinity and specificity. NC-5Z is better suited because of its higher affinity ($K_I = 1.05$ nM) compared with the K_I of octopamine (7 nM). In addition, NC-5Z is not substrate of endogenous degrading enzymes such as monoamine oxidase.

To study the pharmacological characteristics of the neuronal octopamine receptor, that is, the target of octopaminergic insecticides, the affinity of numerous agonists and antagonists derived from different classes of compounds was estimated. We were able to find at least four antagonists with very high affinity for the locust octopamine receptor, all characterized by a tetracyclic structure. Substances such as mianserin and maroxepine have affinities in the lower nanomolar range. Unfortunately, our attempts to detect insecticidal activity at reasonable concentrations failed. This result is in close agreement with our knowledge about the physiological rationale of octopaminergic insecticides. Sub-lethal concentrations of these insecticides, such as the well-known chlordimeform, lead to hyperactivity with leaf walk-off. Octopamine appears to control the motivational state of the animal (see Roeder 1994). Therefore, inhibition of octopaminergic neurotransmission using reversible antagonists calms the animal down but has no insecticidal relevance.

Agonists of the neuronal octopamine receptor are much better suited. They activate the octopamine-stimulated adenylcyclase and lead to the known insecticidal effects of octopaminergic compounds. To study the structural requirements of high-affinity agonists, the affinity of numerous substances was estimated. As a first step, different substituents at position 1 of the phenolic ring were studied. The most promising structural feature was a heterocyclicring system spaced by at least one group. Interestingly, small changes in the structure resulted in a dramatic drop in affinity. If the spacing group is omitted, the affinity is at least four orders of magnitude lower. The so-called phenyliminoimidazolidines (PIIs) were chosen for a detailed analysis of structure-affinity relationships. Compounds with different substitutions at the phenolic ring system had strongly different affinities. Among the compounds tested, the 4-chlor, 2-methyl-PII is the one with highest affinity for the locust neuronal octopamine receptor (K_I value = 0.3 nM). One structural feature of most high-affinity compounds is the substitution pattern at the phenolic ring system. Especially positions 2 and 4 of the phenolic ring lead to substances with higher affinity. Substitutions at other positions such as positions 3 and 6 all resulted in lowering affinity. This is in contrast to peripheral-type octopamine receptors, where positions 2 and 6 are of greatest importance. Position 4 could be of major interest, because even bulky substitutions such as the azido group are tolerated without significant reduction in affinity (Tab. 1). At this position, the introduction of side chains that increase the ability of the compound to reach its target should be possible. A further improvement of the structural features that are necessary for high-affinity agonists of the locust neuronal octopamine receptor is possible by the introduction of other, structurally related classes of compounds. Other heterocycles spaced by at least one or even two

Table 1. Affinity of phenyliminoimidazolidines (PIIs) for the locust neuronal octopamine receptor

Substance	Substitution	K_I (nM)
NC 7	4-chloro-2-methyl	0.30±0.04
St 92	2,4,6-triethyl	0.56±0.14
NC 8	2,4-dichloro	0.81±0.18
NC 5	2,6-diethyl	0.87±0.32
NC 9	2,4-dimethyl	1.02±0.42
NC-5Z	4-azido-2,6-diethyl	1.05±0.47
NC 3	2,4,5-trichloro	2.27±0.89
NC 13	2,4,6-trimethyl	4.38±1.30
NC 12	4-bromo	14.90±3.30
NC 11	2,4,6-trichloro	18.70±3.00
NC 4	2,6-dimethyl	19.80±6.50
NC 10	-	23.40±4.70
p-azidoclonidine	4-azido, 2,6-dichloro	44.50±7.10
clonidine	2,6-dichloro	47.40±17.50
p-aminoclonidine	4-amino, 2,6-dichloro	58.00±16.20
NC 20	2,6-diisopropyl	132.00±35.60

groups from the phenolic ring system were tested. Among them are, for example. the S-benzyl-aminothiazolines or the aminooxazolines, which are as effective as the PIIs. In addition to high affinity, other properties of these compounds are of great importance. One of the main advantages of new octopaminergic insecticides should be their low activity in corresponding vertebrate

Table 2. Relative potencies of octopamine agonists in comparison with mammalian a-adrenoreceptors substance

	$K_I (\alpha2)/K_I$ (OAR$_3$ locust)	$K_I (\alpha1\ A)/K_I$ (OAR$_3$ locust)
octopamine	197.000	1392.000
tyramine	114.000	445.000
adrenaline	0.014	1.420
noradrenaline	0.036	2.100
NC 5	33.500	-
NC 8	2.780	-
NC 9	5.500	-
clonidine	0.120	9.070
p-aminoclonidine	0.015	-

$K_I (\alpha2)$ and $K_I (\alpha1\ A)$ are the K_I values of the listed substances for the vertebrate $\alpha2$- and $\alpha1$ A-adrenergic receptors respectively. K_I (OAR$_3$) means the K_I value of the listed substances for the locust neuronal octopamine receptor. The quotient of the values for the vertebrate receptor in comparison with the locust receptor is a measure of the specificity of the compounds for the insect receptor.

systems, since vertebrates do not have octopamine receptors, and the respective insecticides have no target in vertebrates. We compared the affinities of several compounds measured in the locust preparation with data obtained from experiments using adrenergic receptors, which are the homologous receptors in vertebrates (Tab. 2). The most specific compounds are octopamine and tyramine, with specificity up to 200 times that for the insect receptors. Nevertheless, both substances are, due to other reasons, not suit as insecticides. Among the high-affinity agonists some compounds reach values of approximately 30 (30 times higher affinity for the locust neuronal octopamine receptor than for the corresponding vertebrate adrenergic receptors), which is a very good starting point for the further improvement of octopaminergic insecticides. The quantification of the insecticidal activities of the different classes of compounds is currently in progress. Using this wide variety of high-affinity octopaminergic agonists, the study of the structural requirements for specific insecticides should be clarified in the near future.

Acknowledgements
This work was supported by the Gesellschaft für Technische Zusammenarbeit as a part of the project Integrated Biological Control of Grasshoppers and Locusts.

References

Bicker G, Menzel R (1989) Chemical codes for the control of behaviour in arthropods. Nature 337: 33–39

Claassen DE, Kammer AE (1986) Effects of octopamine, dopamine and serotonin on production of flight motor output by thoracic ganglia of *Manduca sexta*. J Neurobiol. 17: 1–14

Munson PJ, Rodbard D (1980) LIGAND: a versatile computerized approach for characterization of ligand-binding systems. Anal Biochem 107: 220–239

Orchard I (1982) Octopamine in insects: neurotransmitter, neurohormone and neuromodulator. Can J Zool 60: 659–669

Roeder T (1990) High-affinity antagonists of the locust neuronal octopamine receptor. Eur J Pharmacol 191: 221–224

Roeder T (1994) Biogenic amines and their receptors in insects. Comp Biochem Physiol 107C: 1–12

Roeder T (1995) Pharmacology of the octopamine receptor from locust central nervous tissue (OAR3). Br J Pharmacol 114: 210–216

Roeder T, Gewecke M (1990) Octopamine receptors in locust nervous tissue. Biochem Pharmacol 39: 1793–1797

Roeder T, Nathanson JA (1993) Characterization of insect neuronal octopamine receptors (OA$_3$ receptors). Neurochem Res 18: 921–925

Sombati S, Hoyle G (1984) Generation of specific behaviours in a locust by local release into neuropil of the natural neuromodulator octopamine. J Neurobiol 15: 481–506

Control agents and methods

Poster contributions

New Strategies in Locust Control
S. Krall, R. Peveling and D. Ba Diallo (eds)
© 1997 Birkhäuser Verlag Basel/Switzerland

Mass production of *Metarhizium flavoviride* in submerged culture using waste products

D. Stephan and G. Zimmermann

Federal Biological Research Centre for Agriculture and Forestry, Institute for Biological Control, Heinrichstraße 243, D-64287 Darmstadt, Germany

Introduction

Metarhizium flavoviride is a well-documented pathogen of locusts and a promising candidate for biocontrol of these pests. Commercial utilisation as a biopesticide necessitates the production of large amounts of the fungus at low cost. A submerged culture technique was developed in order to produce high concentrations of blastospores (Bs) of *M. flavoviride* using extremely cheap media. The investigations were carried out within the framework of the Deutsche Gesellschaft für Technische Zusammenarbeit (GTZ)-project "Integrated Biological Control of Grasshoppers and Locusts".

Material and methods

Metarhizium flavoviride, strain Mfl 5, was isolated from *Locusta migratoria capito,* Madagascar. Blastospores were produced in 50-ml aliquots of the relevant, autoclaved liquid medium in 300-ml Erlenmeyer flasks on a rotary shaker (180 rpm) in 72 h at 25 °C. The flasks were inoculated with 5×10^7 blastospores. The concentration of blastospores was determined using a Thoma hemocytometer. All tests were replicated three times. Four parameters were tested:

- Nitrogen sources (8%): blood-, horn-, bone- and fish- meal, Naturpur (composted chicken droppings), Biosol (waste product of an antibiotic production) and a mixture of these six nitrogen sources;
- Carbohydrate sources (4%): molasses, sugar-beet syrup, glucose;
- Different concentrations of sugar-beet syrup and Naturpur;
- pH values of 5, 6, 7, 8, 9 (medium: 4% sugar-beet syrup + 8% Naturpur).

In order to mass-produce blastospores in a laboratory fermenter (Infors), 2 l of 8% Naturpur was boiled, filtered and mixed with 4% of sugar-beet syrup. After autoclaving, the medium was inoculated with 200 ml of a two-day-old liquid culture of *M. flavoviride* grown on the same medium. The blastospore concentration was determined at different intervals.

Results and discussion

All waste products tested were suitable as nitrogen sources for *M. flavoviride*. The highest number of blastospores were observed in media containing glucose and blood meal, Naturpur, Biosol or the mixture (Tab. 1). A further increase up to 5.16×10^8 Bs/ml was achieved after replacing glucose by sugar-beet syrup or molasses. The best concentration of sugar-beet syrup and Naturpur resulted in a maximum yield of 6.9×10^8 Bs/ml at a concentration of 4% and 8%,

Table 1. Influence of different waste products as nitrogen sources (8%) and glucose (8%) on the blastospore concentration of Mfl 5

nitrogen source	blastospores $\times 10^8$ ml^{-1} ($\pm$sem)
mixture	3.99 ($\pm$ 0.58)
Naturpur	3.90 ($\pm$ 0.74)
Biosol	2.97 ($\pm$ 0.14)
blood meal	2.88 ($\pm$ 0.54)
bone meal	1.57 ($\pm$ 0.45)
horn meal	1.29 ($\pm$ 0.16)
fish meal	0.86 ($\pm$ 0.26)

Table 2. Influence of different concentrations of sugar-beet syrup and Naturpur (S/N%) on the blastospore concentration of Mfl 5

S/N (%)	blastospores $\times 10^8$ ml^{-1} ($\pm$sem)
4:8	6.87 ($\pm$0.81)
4:12	6.85 ($\pm$0.67)
8:8	6.34 ($\pm$0.57)
2:12	4.89 ($\pm$0.29)
2:8	4.51 ($\pm$0.33)
2:4	3.93 ($\pm$0.23)
2:2	3.43 ($\pm$0.21)
4:2	3.22 ($\pm$0.26)

respectively (Tab. 2). This was about 2.5 times higher than in the formerly used standard medium described by Adamek (1963). Different pH values did not influence the yield of blastospores. In a laboratory fermenter, the maximum yield of blastospores rose to 1×10^9 Bs/ml after two days of fermentation using the waste-product medium. Corresponding to the results of Abu-Laban and Saleh (1992) and Dangar et al. (1991), waste products and especially animal manures are efficient nutrients for mass production of fungi.

References

Abu-Laban AZ, Saleh HM (1992) Evaluation of animal manures for mass production, storage and application of some nematode egg parasitic fungi. Nematologica 38: 237–244

Adamek L (1963) Submers cultivation of the fungus *Metarhizium anisopliae* (Metsch.). Folia Microbiologia (Praha) 10: 255–257

Dangar TK, Geetha L, Jayapal SP, Pillai GB (1991) Mass production of the entomopathogen *Metarhizium anisopliae* in coconut water wasted from copra making industry. J Plantation Crops 19 (1): 54–69

New Strategies in Locust Control
S. Krall, R. Peveling and D. Ba Diallo (eds)
© 1997 Birkhäuser Verlag Basel/Switzerland

Field trails conducted on a biopesticide (*Metarhizium flavoviride*) for grasshopper control in Mali from 1992 to 1994

O.-K. Douro Kpindou[1], J. Langewald[1], C.J. Lomer[2], H. van der Paauw[3], P.A. Shah[1] and A. Sidibé[4]

[1] Institut International d'Agriculture Tropicale (IITA) B.P. 08-0932, Cotonou, Bénin
[2] Institut International de Lutte Biologique (IIBC) Silwood Park, Ascot, Berkshire, UK
[3] Ciba-Geigy, CH 4002, Basel, Switzerland
[4] Service National de Protection des Végétaux (SNPV), B.P. 1560, Bamako, Mali

Metarhizium flavoviride was produced in diphasic culture, initially in a sucrose-yeast medium, with sporulation on rice. Spores were extracted in kerosene or sieved and dried. For application, the spores were formulated with a mixture of peanut oil and kerosene (30:70). The spore formulation was applied with spinning disk sprayers at ultra-low volume.

In 1992, field applications resulted in a mortality rate of 92% for *Oedaleus senegalensis* (Krauss, 1877) (Orthoptera: Acrididae, Oedipodinae) kept in field cages. In 1993, experiments compared two strains of *Metarhizium flavoviride,* the Niger strain IMI 331089 and one from Mali (I92-794). Mortality rates obtained for samples incubated in cages were between 31% and 93% respectively for IMI 330189 (day 0) and I92-794 (day 3) for *Kraussella amabile* (Krauss, 1877) (Orthoptera: Acrididae, Gomphocerinae). Higher mortality in the sample collected three days after application than in the day 0 sample is frequently observed, and seems to be due to secondary pick-up of spores from vegetation. Field applications in 1994 resulted in mortality rates between 50% and 97% for *O. senegalensis* and *K. amabile* respectively, and field counts showed a population reduction of 85% in one hectare-plots.

New Strategies in Locust Control
S. Krall, R. Peveling and D. Ba Diallo (eds)
© 1997 Birkhäuser Verlag Basel/Switzerland

LUBILOSA: a joint project for the biological control of locusts and grasshoppers in the Sahel

A. Paraïso[1], C. Lomer[2], O. Douro-Kpindou[2], C. Kooyman[1]

[1]IIBC/IITA/AGRHYMET Locust and Grasshopper Biocontrol, B.P. 12625 Niamey, Niger
[2]IITA-Bénin, B.P. 08-0932, Cotonou, Bénin

Locusts and grasshoppers are very serious crop pests, especially in the Sahel. Irregular invasions cause damage that is often difficult to control. Control campaigns are based mainly on the use of chemical insecticides. The joint IITA/IIBC/DFPV project for the biological control of locusts and grasshoppers (LUBILOSA) is aimed at exploiting the possibilities of using oil-based formulations containing fungal spores for microbiological control of acridoids.

In 1989 the CAB International Institute for Biological Control (CABI-IIBC) in Britain, jointly with the International Institute for Tropical Agriculture (IITA), the Plant Health Management Division, Programme for Biological Control, at Cotonou (Benin) and the Department for Training in Crop Protection, AGRHYMET, in Niamey (Niger) started the project Lutte Biologique contre les Locustes et les Sauteriaux (LUBILOSA) (Biological Control of Locusts and Grasshoppers).

The project began following results obtained in Britain concerning the possibility of using oil-based formulations of fungal spores pathogenic to insects and the advantages associated with these formulations. These advantages include good adhesion of the infective spores to the insect cuticle, the protection of spores in oil droplets against rapid desiccation at high temperature and low relative humidity and, finally, good viability of spores in oil-based formulations.

Following a series of studies carried out between 1989 and 1992, a comprehensive list was prepared of all known pathogens of acridoids. Early results indicated the feasibility of using pathogens of insects for the biological control of locusts and grasshoppers. Progress was also made in testing the efficacy of various strains under laboratory and field conditions, as well as developing medium-technology methods to produce spores of entomopathogenic fungi.

Trials with fungal spores pathogenic to acridoids were conducted against *Zonocerus variegatus* L. in southern Benin and against *Hieroglyphus daganensis* (Krauss, 1877) in northern Benin. A series of trials was carried out in Senegal, Niger and Burkina Faso, with the principal aim of investigating the possibility of using spores of a fungi pathogenic to acridoids, *Metarhizium flavoviride* Gams and Roszypal, for the control of the following grasshoppers: *H.*

daganensis, Kraussella amabile (Krauss, 1877), *Zacompsa festa* (Karsch, 1893) and *Oedaleus senegalensis* (Krauss, 1877). Further work of this type was carried out in Mali against *O. senegalensis* and in Mauritania against *Schistocerca gregaria* (Forskål, 1775).

New Strategies in Locust Control
S. Krall, R. Peveling and D. Ba Diallo (eds)
© 1997 Birkhäuser Verlag Basel/Switzerland

Application of an oil-based formulation containing spores of an entomopathogenic fungus, *Metarhizium flavoviride,* against grasshoppers in the Sahel

A. Paraïso, A. Beye, S. Djiba, S. Check, N. Abdoulaye, O. Diop, S. Gan Bobo, C.L. Otoïdobiga, A.K. Nadié, C. Kooyman, C. Lomer, O. Douro-Kpindou

IIBC/IITA/AGRHYMET Locust and Grasshopper Biocontrol Project (LUBILOSA), B.P. 12625, Niamey, Niger

A series of trials was carried out in Senegal, Niger and Burkina Faso with the principal aim of investigating the potential of an oil-based formulation of spores (conidia) of an entomopathogenic fungus, *Metarhizium flavoviride* Gams and Roszypal, for locust and grasshopper control. The acridian species to be controlled in our trials were *Hieroglyphus daganensis* (Krauss, 1877), *Kraussella amabile* (Krauss, 1877), *Zacompsa festa* Karsch, *Oedaleus senegalensis* (Krauss, 1877) and *Zonocerus variegatus* (Linnaeus).

In Senegal, the treatments were against *H. daganensis* and *K. amabile* at Kolobane Tchombane, a village 9 km from Thiès. The dose rate applied was 2.5×10^{12} spores/ha. Twenty five individuals of each species were sampled from every plot on the day of treatment and then 4, 8, 12, 16 and 20 days after treatment. These grasshoppers were placed in cages in groups of 25 in the laboratory and mortality was assessed. In both species, mortality exceeded 70% after 10 days. Seventeen days post-treatment, mortality varied between 90 and 95%. Samples taken at days 16 and 20 also had a mortality of over 70%. From these results it was deduced that fungal spores may persist for several weeks in agro-ecosystems inhabited by locusts and grasshoppers. At Ziguinchor, treatments were directed against *Z. festa* and *K. amabile*. Mortality was 80% in grasshoppers sampled from treated plots 12 days post-treatment.

The trials in Niger were carried out in the Gouré region and consisted of an application of spores of *M. flavoviride* at a dose rate of 5×10^{12} spores/ha against different stages of the Senegalese grasshopper, *O. senegalensis*. The level of mortality in these trials – over 70% at day 10 – confirmed previous results obtained in laboratory assays.

Comparison trials between several strains of the same fungus were carried out in Burkina Faso (Bobo-Dioulasso – the valley of the Kou and Léguéma) at a rate of 5×10^{12} spores/ha against the variegated grasshopper *Z. variegatus*. From this work it was clear that there was a significant difference between all the strains used and the control for the day of the treatment. Dead insects were incubated in petri dishes on filter paper lightly moistened with water to encourage sporulation of the fungus. The high level of sporulation – over 70% – shows clearly that most grasshoppers dying in the cages were indeed infected with *M. flavoviride*.

From these different trials we are able to state that a biopesticide, based on spores of *M. flavoviride*, has promising prospects in the context of integrated control strategies against locusts and grasshoppers in the Sahel.

New Strategies in Locust Control
S. Krall, R. Peveling and D. Ba Diallo (eds)
© 1997 Birkhäuser Verlag Basel/Switzerland

Biocontrol of locusts in Madagascar: developing indigenous pathogens

W.D. Swearingen

Montana State University, Entomology Department, Bozeman, MT 59717, USA

Since 1993, MSU, Mycotech, and Malagasy scientists have been evaluating indigenous entomo-pathogens in Madagascar for biocontrol of *Locusta migratoria capito*. Initial surveys isolated 39 fungal pathogens and 2 protozoa (one of which appears to have excellent potential for long-term suppression of locusts). The fungal strains were subjected to extensive evaluations for virulence and spore productivity and stability. The five most promising strains underwent standard toxicological testing involving rats and rabbits. Three of these strains (*Metarhizium flavoviride* SP3 and SP9 and *Beauveria bassiana* SP16) exhibited no adverse effects and were selected for laboratory biotests involving non-target insects, including honeybees and three lepidopteran species. None of the strains were significantly pathogenic to the non-target insects used in these tests.

The three strains were then tested in small-scale field trials in Madagascar in December 1994. Simultaneous biodiversity tests were conducted to evaluate impacts on non-target insects in the field. In the small-scale field trials, low-walled arenas (measuring 50 m^2) established in locust-infested areas were sprayed with fungal spores in oil-based formulations. Four arenas were treated with each of the three strains with 4 untreated arenas as controls (a total of 16 arenas). Simultaneously, 10 one-hectare nearby plots were treated as part of the biodiversity tests. Two plots were treated with each strain, 2 were treated with fenitrothion and 2 were untreated controls. In the small-scale field trials, *M. flavoviride* SP9 achieved 100% mortality in 8 days. *M. flavoviride* SP3 and *B. bassiana* SP16 were somewhat less effective, with 89 and 56% mortality, respectively, in 10 days. In the biodiversity studies, SP9 and SP16 showed no adverse effects. However, SP3 proved to be just as harmful as the fenitrothion. Procedures are now underway to increase the virulence of *B. bassiana* SP16. SP9 and SP16 are scheduled to be tested in large-scale field trials in January 1996. SP3 has been eliminated from further testing owing to its negative impacts on non-target insects in the biodiversity studies in the field.

New Strategies in Locust Control
S. Krall, R. Peveling and D. Ba Diallo (eds)
© 1997 Birkhäuser Verlag Basel/Switzerland

Preliminary investigations on the combination of *Metarhizium flavoviride* blastospores with botanicals (neem, *Melia volkensii*) for biological locust control

M. Welling[1], D. Stephan and G. Zimmermann

Federal Biological Research Centre for Agriculture and Forestry, Institute for Biological Control, Heinrichstraße 243, D-64287 Darmstadt, Germany
[1]Present address: Federal Biological Research Centre for Agriculture and Forestry, Messeweg 11/12, D-38104 Braunschweig, Germany

Introduction

Blastospores of the entomopathogenic fungus *Metarhizium flavoviride* Gams and Rozsypal have been proven to be effective against locusts. It takes several days to two weeks, however, until high mortalities are achieved. In order to enhance the speed of action and/or to reduce the concentration of fungus material, the suitability of a combination of *M. flavoviride* blastospores with low doses of botanicals (various neem products and an extract of *Melia volkensii*) was investigated. Possible synergistic effects of a combined application on locusts were studied.

The following investigations were carried out within the framework of the Deutsche Gesellschaft für Technische Zusammenarbeit (GTZ) project "Integrated Biological Control of Grasshoppers and Locusts".

Material and methods

First, the compatibility of *M. flavoviride* (Mfl 5, isolated from *Locusta migratoria*, Madagascar) with botanicals was investigated: The germination of blastospores and the growth of mycelium were recorded in petri dishes on potato-dextrose-agar (PDA) containing various concentrations of botanicals. The following botanicals were tested: cold-pressed neem oil (concentrations: 1, 5 and 10%), the Azadirachtin-enriched products NeemAzal-F and NeemAzal-T (concentrations: 0.02, 0.1 and 0.2%) and an ethanolic extract of seeds of *Melia volkensii* (concentrations: 0.2, 1 and 2%).

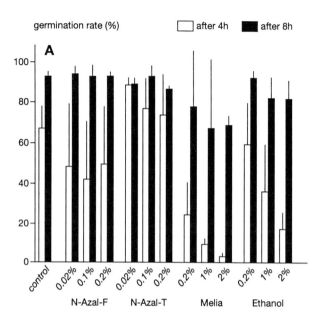

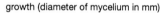

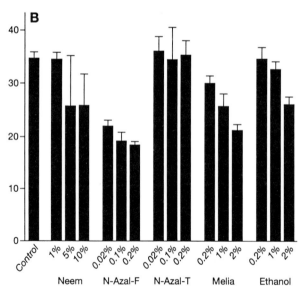

Figure 1. Effects of botanicals on the viability of *Metarhizium flavoviride* (bars = SD). (A) Germination rate of blastospores on PDA containing various concentrations of neem products and *M. volkensii* extract, respectively, after incubation at 25 °C for 4 and 8 h, respectively. (B) Growth on PDA containing various concentrations of neem products and M. *volkensii* extract, respectively, after an incubation period of 15 days at 25 °C.

In a second step, fourth instar nymphs of *L. migratoria* were sprayed with a water/oil emulsion containing either blastospores in two concentrations (2×10^7 and 2×10^6 ml^{-1}), neem oil (10 and 2%) or a combination of both.

Results

Compatibility tests

The ethanolic *M. volkensii*-extract was the only botanical causing a slight, concentration-dependent delay in the germination of blastospores which was still visible after 8 h (Fig. 1A, the germination rate in the neem regime was not assessable). The growth of the mycelium, however, was reduced by nearly all botanicals to a certain extent. Only NeemAzal-T did not influence the growth of the mycelium negatively (Fig. 1B).

Bioassays

After two weeks, blastospores alone had caused a mortality of 90% (2×10^7 ml^{-1}) and 70% (2×10^6 ml^{-1}) of locusts, whereas neem oil alone had caused mortalities of 40 and 16%, respectively. The combination of blastospores and neem oil did not result in an accelerated or higher mortality. Similar tests with the other botanicals still have to be done.

Discussion

In laboratory tests no severe side-effects of the botanicals on *M. flavoviride* could be detected. Although first experiments with a combination of *M. flavoviride* and neem against *L. migratoria* did not show a synergistic effect, synergism in tests with *Schistocerca gregaria* might occur, since this species is more susceptible to neem than *L. migratoria*. In addition, further tests with the other botanicals mentioned above will be carried out.

New Strategies in Locust Control
S. Krall, R. Peveling and D. Ba Diallo (eds)
© 1997 Birkhäuser Verlag Basel/Switzerland

Sorosporella sp., a fungal pathogen of the migratory locust, *Locusta migratoria capito*, in Madagascar

M. Welling[1] and G. Zimmermann

Federal Biological Research Centre for Agriculture and Forestry, Institute for Biological Control, Heinrichstraße 243, D-64287 Darmstadt, Germany
[1]*present address: Federal Biological Research Centre for Agriculture and Forestry, Messeweg 11/12, D-38104 Braunschweig, Germany*

Introduction

Fungi of the genus *Sorosporella* are little known entomopathogens. Up to now, the fungus was mostly described in eastern Europe and North America as a pathogen of curculionid beetles or larvae of Noctuidae (e.g. Speare 1920). Recently, *Sorosporella*-killed grasshoppers were found in Mali (Shah 1993) and, sporadically, in Benin (Shah et al. 1994).

The following investigations on a strain of *Sorosporella* sp. found in *Locusta migratoria capito* in Madagascar were carried out within the framework of the Deutsche Gesellschaft für Technische Zusammenarbeit (GTZ) project "Integrated Biological Control of Grasshoppers and Locusts".

Symptoms and incidence

The cuticle of infected locusts becomes pale and breaks up easily, releasing masses of reddish-brown resting spores which fill the whole cadaver. The thick-walled resting spores are globular with a diameter of 7.5 μm and agglutinated in units of tens to hundreds of spores.

Out of 309 dead *L. migratoria* collected in Madagascar in April 1992, 140 showed typical symptoms of a *Sorosporella* infection. Only two specimens were found which had been killed by *Metarhizium* sp. In 1993, *Sorosporella*-killed larvae (3rd to 5th instar) and adults were frequently found in several places in south-western Madagascar.

Cultivation and bioassays

On artificial media, growth of the fungus was extremely slow. Out of 11 solid media tested, rice malt extract agar (3% ground rice, 3% malt extract, 0.3% peptone and 1.5% agar) was the best. On this medium, white colonies were visible about two weeks after inoculation. Occasionally their colour changed into reddish-brown after several months of desiccation. On artificial medium, cylindrical conidia of 11×2.8 µm in shape were formed which could never be detected in dead locusts. Conidia were produced in clusters or clumps, not in chains.

Three types of bioassays with nymphs of *L. migratoria* were carried out: (1) Feeding trials with *Sorosporella*-contaminated wheat, (2) topical application of conidia and fragmented mycelium, (3) injection of resting spores and conidia, respectively, suspended in Tween 80 (nymphs in the control were injected with Tween 80 only).

In the first and second types of bioassays, no increased mortality compared with the control and no indications of a *Sorosporella* infection were observed. After injection of resting spores, the mortality increased rapidly within the first 4 days to nearly 60% (control: 9%). After injection of conidia, mortality increased remarkably between day 11 and 15 from 30% (control: 23%) to 90% (control: 33%). After three weeks, more than 90% of the nymphs treated with resting spores and 100% of the nymphs treated with conidia were killed, whereas the mortality rate of the control was 45%. Only 10% of the cadavers in the variant treated with resting spores and 42% in the variant treated with conidia showed symptoms of a *Sorosporella* infection.

Discussion

The findings in the field indicate that *Sorosporella* sp. is an important and frequently occurring locust pathogen in Madagascar. Although the bioassays in the laboratory did not reveal clear results, the fungus seems to have a high virulence to locusts in its natural habitat. Facing the fact that an efficient production method for *Sorosporella* sp. on artificial culture is still lacking, its implementation into integrated locust control programmes is unlikely at present.

A more comprehensive description of this fungus is given by Welling et al. (1995).

References

Shah PA (1993) Observations on a species of *Sorosporella* (Deuteromycotina: Hyphomycetes) infecting *Kraussaria angulifera* (Orthoptera: Acrididae) in the Republic of Mali. J Invert Path 62: 318

Shah PA, Godonou I, Gbongboui C, Lomer CJ (1994) Natural levels of fungal infections in grasshoppers in Northern Benin. Biocontrol Science & Technology 4: 331–341

Speare AT (1920) Further studies of *Sorosporella uvella*, a fungous parasite of noctuid larvae. J Agricult Res 18: 399–439

Welling M, Zelazny B, Scherer R, Zimmermann G (1995) First record of the entomopathogenic fungus *Sorosporella* sp. (Deuteromycotina: Hyphomycetes) in *Locusta migratoria* (Orthoptera: Acrididae) from Madagascar: Symptoms, morphology and infectivity. Biocontr Sci Technol 5: i465–474

New Strategies in Locust Control
S. Krall, R. Peveling and D. Ba Diallo (eds)
© 1997 Birkhäuser Verlag Basel/Switzerland

The problem of a replacement for dieldrin

M. Launois and T. Rachadi

CIRAD-GERDAT-PRIFAS, B.P. 5035, 34032 Montpellier Cedex 1, France

For more than 30 years the main strategy for preventive control of the desert locust *Schistocerca gregaria* (Forskål, 1775) has been based on the correct use of an organochlorine, dieldrin. This insecticide was used because it was effective at very low doses for locust control, activated both by contact and ingestion, had a long persistence, a long storage life and was relatively inexpensive.

In 1987, the use of this product for locust control was no longer recommended by the donor countries on the grounds of possible risks to the environment, including the human population. There are, in 1995, still more than 100,000 l of dieldrin to be destroyed on the African continent.

A very large number of active ingredients suitable for locust control have been put forward as replacements for dieldrin and organochlorines in general: organophosphates, carbamates, pyrethroids, biopesticides and insect growth regulators. This last category has a number of interesting potentials.

Trials were carried out in 1994 over a range of locust situations with fipronil, a pyrazole. These showed that this active ingredient could be a very good successor to dieldrin, as it has the same characteristics as the standard product without presenting the same potential risks for the environment in its widest sense.

New Strategies in Locust Control
S. Krall, R. Peveling and D. Ba Diallo (eds)
© 1997 Birkhäuser Verlag Basel/Switzerland

Locust control with deltamethrin

H.D. Brown and M.E. Kieser

Plant Protection Research Institute, Agricultural Research Council, P.Bag X134, Pretoria 0001, South Africa

Introduction

The brown locust, *Locustana pardalina* (Walker), is a chronic pest problem and a potential threat to the food security of some nine countries in southern Africa (Lea 1964). Intervention relies mainly on nymphal band control in the Karoo outbreak region of this locust species and involves the detection and direct spraying of bands with ground-based ultra low volume (ULV) spray technology.

Current insecticide research in the Locust Research Division of the Plant Protection Research Institute, Pretoria, is directed towards optimising and improving the chemical control of locusts in South Africa and also to evaluating environmentally safer compounds. Following the banning of the chlorinated hydrocarbon BHC (HCH) in South Africa (Anonymous 1981), for long the mainstay of locust control in the Karoo, and its replacement with organophosphates (OPs) such as fenitrothion and diazinon (Brown 1988), certain problems concerning the routine use of these insecticides for locust control surfaced:

- OPs act slowly in the Karoo during cool autumn conditions (March to April), when >60% of all brown locust control is undertaken.
- Such delayed mortality made it difficult for locust control operators, inexperienced in ULV spraying and used to applying highly visible persistent dust formulations, to assess their results. This in turn resulted in wasteful respraying of targets and needless environmental contamination. Bird toxicities resulted.
- The high mobility of brown locust targets enables sprayed insects to depart from spray sites before the chemical takes effect; dose uptake was therefore restricted to direct droplet impingement.

This work summarises the results of over 130 experimental spray treatments made with deltamethrin from 1986–89 in the Karoo, where the product was rigorously tested against brown locust nymphs and adults in an attempt to solve these problems.

Conclusions

Chemical control of locusts in South Africa today has become largely pyrethroid driven with deltamethrin playing a leading role. The OPs are gradually being phased out. Advantages flowing from the use of deltamethrin are:

- Its low avian and mammalian toxicity poses less environmental risk and also makes it safer for use by control operators. Certain beneficial insects such as the sarcophagid parasitic locust fly, *Wohlfahrtia pachytyli* Townsend, have been shown to successfully exploit deltamethrin-affected locusts as hosts and have thereby increased their abundance (Price and Brown 1993).
- The product proved effective in all seasons and habitat situations. Although death was delayed under cool autumn conditions, sub-lethal toxicity in fact increased. Locusts were knocked down and remained in a moribund state, with little to no recovery.
- At field doses between 12.5 and 17.5 g a.i./ha, deltamethrin rapidly immobilised nymphs and adult locusts and thereby kept them within the sprayed area, so that secondary pick-up of chemical from the vegetation was maximised.
- Control operators capitalised on the rapid toxicity and could thus make a snap judgement of their control results. Deltamethrin thus served as a useful chemical marker for measuring the results of ULV spraying, which was technically difficult for inexperienced locust officers. This eliminated the need for follow-up visits to spray sites to check on the outcome of control and resulted in significant savings on motor transport, thereby making locust control more cost-effective in South Africa.

Acknowledgements
This poster embodies an enormous amount of work undertaken over the years in the Karoo by the PPRI locust spray team, in particular Roger Price, Edwin Butler, Peter Napier Bax, Carel Kriel and others, to whom thanks are due for assisting with field trials. We are also grateful to the Directorate of Natural Resource Conservation of the South African Department of Agriculture for their assistance in locating spray targets.

References

Anonymous (1981) Proclamation no R928 by Minister of Agriculture. Govt Gazette no 7506. Pretoria: Govt Printer
Brown HD (1988) Current pesticide application: effectiveness and persistence. Pages 101–117 in B McKenzie and M Longridge (eds) Proceedings of Locust Symposium. S Afr Inst of Ecol Bull special issue
Lea A (1964) Some major factors in the population dynamics of the brown locust, *Locustana pardalina* (Walk.). Monog Biol 14: 269–283
Price REP, Brown HD (1993) An unusual case of a pesticide benefitting a natural enemy. Proceedings of the 9th entomological congress. Ent. Soc. Sth. Afr., Johannesburg: 90

Carbosulfan, an effective new product for locust control

C.J. Boase

Pest Management Consulting, Cowslip Pightle, Hazel Stub, Camps Rd., Haverhill, Suffolk CB9 8HB, UK

The 1986–89 desert locust plague highlighted the need for a greater range of locust insecticides with differing modes of action to be available. There are clear advantages to both donor and user in having such a choice, as it enables locusts at all stages and in all situations to be treated effectively and appropriately.

Carbosulfan (Marshal) is a fast-acting carbamate insecticide which is widely registered and sold in tropical countries for control of a range of agricultural insect pests. Up to 1994, about 35 well-documented trials with carbosulfan UL and EC were carried out by official organisations against nymphal and adult *Schistocerca gregaria* in Mali, Senegal, Sudan and Saudi Arabia. Treatments were applied using hand-held and vehicle-mounted Controlled Droplet Application (CDA) sprayers. Efficacy was assessed using transect counts, quadrats and cages.

At doses of 100 g a.i./ha, rapid knock-down of directly treated nymphs and adults occurred, with up to 92% knock-down occurring within 1 h. At 100 to 150 g a.i./ha, up to 96% mortality occurred within 24 h. Locusts subsequently feeding on treated vegetation were also controlled effectively, although the time taken to reach maximum mortality was rather longer. No recovery of knocked-down locusts was observed in any trial.

These data, together with other results against African migratory locusts and brown locusts, clearly demonstrate carbosulfan's activity against both nymphal and adult stages, at rates of about 100 g a.i./ha. Its fast knock-down and availability in DP, EC and UL formulations enables it to be used to protect crops against locust attack, as well as in a strategic plague prevention. Large-scale operational use of carbosulfan from both ground and air in Saudi Arabia has confirmed its effectiveness against large swarms of desert locusts.

Staurorhectus longicornis (Giglio Tos), a recently appearing pest species on pastures in the dry Chaco of Paraguay and semi-field tests for its control

F. Wilhelmi

Consultant, Albertstraße 28, D-67655 Kaiserslautern, Germany

In 1975, the Mennonite colonies in the Paraguayan Chaco reported the first severe outbreak of the grasshopper species *Staurorhectus longicornis* (Giglio Tos). The frequency of outbreaks and the scale of damage have increased during recent years, sometimes causing the complete destruction of pastures. The damaged grasslands are covered with two grass species only, *Cynodon plectostachys* (Estrella) and *Cenchrus ciliaris* (Buffalo grass), both of which are introduced.

The control efficiency of Nomolt (teflubenzuron, 50 g a.i./l), Alsystin 250 OF (triflumuron, 250 g a.i./l), enriched Neem-Azal F (5% azadirachtin plus 15% derivatives) and unpurified neem oil (0.04% azadirachtin, content of derivatives not specified) has been tested in semi-field tests. Trials were carried out during a four-week period in December–January 1991/92. Twenty 2 m × 2 m × 1 m sized test cages with 200 introduced nymphs each were used in a randomized block design. The grass cover of the cage plots was pruned and all superfluous plant material removed prior to spraying. The products were applied using a hand-held Micro-Ulva spinning disk sprayer. The application volume was 1 l/ha in all treatments, and the various formulations were diluted if necessary. The escape-proof cages were searched daily (about 1 h/cage) for dead or malformed nymphs. Changes in activity were measured by repeated counts of animals still able to hop to the wire mesh when flushed by a stick swept through the grass. Damage estimations and observations on grasshopper distribution and population density paralleled the trials.

Teflubenzuron and triflumuron yielded mortality rates up to 80% (ANOVA, $p < 0.05$). The two neem oils caused only about 30% mortality within a 14-day trial period ($p < 0.05$). All products, however, revealed very similar effects in depressing the activity of the hoppers by 90%. In additional trials, which also included adults, no anti-feedant effect of neem oils could be ascertained in choice or in no-choice situations, but 60% of the animals feeding on contaminated grass died within 10 days. The difference in mortality remains as yet unexplained.

Grasshopper infestation was unevenly distributed within the colony area. Pastures with high and low hopper densities were often in close vicinity. On the Estrella grasslands, *S. longicornis* dominated the arthropod fauna, whereas on indigenous grasslands hardly any were found.

The estimated loss of biomass (pasture consumed) on the 3.5-ha-large experimental site, caused by *S. longicornis* at a density of $10-20$ individuals/m^2 (equal number of nymphs and adults), was equivalent to 45 cattle grazing days. This figure considers the high nutrition value of grass leaves, which were the only plant parts the grasshoppers fed on. The real economic loss, however, can only be expressed in terms of milk and meat production.

The obviously manmade *S. longicornis* problem in the Chaco may not yet have reached its full extent. Continued field trials and observations are required to study the development of the pest situation and to evaluate its economic impact.

New Strategies in Locust Control
S. Krall, R. Peveling and D. Ba Diallo (eds)
© 1997 Birkhäuser Verlag Basel/Switzerland

Mechanical control of the desert locust *Schistocerca gregaria* (Forskål, 1775)

S.H. Han

IFAN B.P. 206, Université Cheikh Anta Diop, Dakar, Senegal

Summary. A mechanical control method for the detection of oothecae of *Schistocerca gregaria* by means of a portable airblast device is described. This technique can also be used for the destruction of larvae by burying them in trenches.

Introduction

Many methods of locust control have been used in the past (Duranton et al., 1987), such as beating, burning, trenching, mechanical control (through harrowing and tilling), biological, ecological and chemical control. Recently Djitteye (1993) used a natural locust control method, i.e., digging up oothecae. However, none of the mechanical locust control methods hitherto used have really achieved satisfactory results. We describe a new technique for the mechanical control of the desert locust using an airblast device.

Materials and methods

We used an airblast device (RYOBI Sweeper Vac RSV 3100E Model) on locust eggs and larvae which was tested in the Saint Louis region of Senegal in October 1993.

The method consists of:

• detecting locust eggs laid in the ground by blowing away the sand and exposing the froth plugs;

• destroying larvae by burying them in trenches 5 m long, 0.60 m wide, 1 m deep.

Results

Detection and localisation of eggs

Data provided by the ministry of agriculture and the information collected among farmers (places where they have seen mature locusts) enabled us to establish the existence of oviposition sites. It took one single operator 5 min to remove the sand over 1 m² with the airblast device. We were then able to locate oothecae by exposing the froth plugs. The operation was replicated in three other sites. The number of oothecae found varied between 40 and 50.

Destruction of larvae by burying them

After digging a trench with the help of farmers (which took 30 min), we pushed the larvae towards the trench using the same device, which enabled us to collect 300,000 to 400,000 larvae at the bottom of the trench in 20 min before burying them. Also to be noted is the fact that digging these sandy soils can be easily performed by two people, without the help of farmers.

Conclusion

This technique is novel but can only be used in sandy areas. Costs are reduced since the method consists of operating a very simple, portable device. The technique enables the detection of locust egg pods that may be destroyed on the spot with pesticides. It can also be used to destroy larvae by burying them alive. A further advantage of the technique is that it reduces chemical pollution to some extent.

References

Djitteye O (1993) Méthode de lutte contre les criquets: le déterrement des oothèques. Dakar: Ed. Enda. 83–84

Duranton JF, Launois M, Launois-Luong MH, Lecoq M, Rachadi T (1987) *Guide antiacridien du Sahel.* Ministère de la coopération et Cirad-Prifas 344 pp

Control agents and methods

Working groups

New Strategies in Locust Control
S. Krall, R. Peveling and D. Ba Diallo (eds)
© 1997 Birkhäuser Verlag Basel/Switzerland

Results and recommendations of the working group *Control agents and methods*

Working group 1

A.B. Bal (Chairman) and A. Hamadoun (Secretary)

The working group's discussions dealt first with locust control agents and their characteristics, including strategies and development stages to which they are best suited. In this context, preventive control should be understood to mean any strategy developed to avoid widespread infestation. The second part of the discussion concerned control methods, and concluded with a general recommendation.

Control agents: see table

Control methods

Crop management control methods

Techniques such as good crop establishment, crop care, and isolation of the plot from fallow land reduce the impact of pests in general and of grasshoppers in particular, and their adverse effects on the environment. Such cultural control practices should be encouraged by providing farmers with information and training.

Mechanical methods

Destruction of egg pods and of the young larvae of grasshoppers and locusts is recommended. Good knowledge of objectives and techniques is necessary to ensure that these measures are carried out properly.
• Drawbacks: sometimes arduous

Biological methods

The future of biological agents is promising, therefore their encouragement is recommended.
• Drawbacks: relatively slow acting

Chemical methods

The careful use of pesticides, highly recommended, is still relevant, but it requires that:
⇒ operators must have thorough training in the chemical products and methods for using the application equipment, as well as on natural enemies;
⇒ interventions are is based on threshold levels, and therefore increased research into loss assessments and economic thresholds is required.
• Drawbacks: harmful effects on the environment

General recommendation

In view of the possibilities offered by each of these methods, their advantages and drawbacks, and the resources available, lasting protection from locusts and grasshoppers necessarily requires integrated management of the ecosystem, giving priority to preventive methods aimed at avoiding a significant increase in locust populations and their detrimental effects on crops and pastures.

Control agents

Control agents	Most used or usable agents	Target groups — Stage	Target groups — Target	Control strategy	Formulation	Toxicity	Cost	Availability	Shelf-life	Remarks
Synthetic chemical products										
pyrethroids	deltamethrin cyhalothrine	adults	locusts grasshoppers	curative	ULV EC	significant / aquatic environment	high	yes	no particular problem	Avoid use in wetland.
organophosphates	fenitrothion malathion chlorpyriphos-ethyl	hoppers & adults	locusts grasshoppers	preventive and curative	ULV EC	high in case of fenitrothion	low	yes	—	Given the persistence of malathion and the toxicity of fenitrothion, prefer the first against hoppers and the second against adults.
carbamates	propoxur	hoppers	locusts grasshoppers	preventive	dusting powder	moderate	moderate	yes	—	Carbaryl, bendiocarb and carbosulfan can be found during locust campaigns.
insect growth regulators	diflubenzuron triflumuron teflubenzuron	hoppers	locusts grasshoppers	preventive	dust EC ULV	low	very high	yes	—	In view of cost, persistence and mode of action, these products are recommended for barrier treatment.
Natural products										
plant extracts	Meliacea extracts	hoppers	locusts grasshoppers	preventive	liquid	very low for humans, unknown for other animals	low	yes	—	Use on a small-scale. Otherwise need for increased knowledge and industrial-level production.
pheromones			Aggregation pheromone for *Z. variegatus* / Dispersion pheromone for locusts							Further research needed.
Biological agents										
fungi	*M. flavoviride* *B. bassiana*	larvae/adults larvae	locusts/grasshoppers	preventive	ULV	?	moderate	laboratory	spores: 3 months ULV: 2–3 weeks	Need to increase knowledge of toxicity and storage conditions. Possibility for local production.
other pathogenic agents	nematodes protozoa bacteria viruses					Need for greater knowledge				
parasitoids and predators	*Blaesoxipha filipjevi* meloid larvae *Trox* spp. birds					Need for greater knowledge				

EC = emulsifiable concentrate; ULV = ultra low volume

New Strategies in Locust Control
S. Krall, R. Peveling and D. Ba Diallo (eds)
© 1997 Birkhäuser Verlag Basel/Switzerland

Results and recommendations of the working group *Control agents and methods*

Working group 2

W. Meinzingen (Chairman) and C. Kooyman (Secretary)

Objective of the meeting

⇒ Identify (an) effective alternative method(s) of locust control and environmentally acceptable products or types of products.

Each class of control agent (IGRs, pathogens, botanicals, JHAs, semiochemicals) has been discussed according to the following points:

⇒ Type of target (bands, swarms)
⇒ Stage of development (operational, experimental)
⇒ Strategies (outbreak prevention, upsurge elimination, plague termination)
⇒ Formulation
⇒ Delivery systems (sprayers etc.)
⇒ Method of application (barrier, direct band, air/air)
⇒ Toxicology
⇒ Production/storage (shelf-life)
⇒ Cost of production
⇒ Registration
⇒ Areas of research needed
⇒ Training needs
⇒ Time frame (until operational use)
⇒ Disadvantages

The meeting agreed that, at the present time, conventional chemicals offer the only available and reliable option for locust control. However, we believe that they can be used even more effectively with better training and techniques. We also concluded that more ecotoxicological locust control work should enable sensitive areas to be defined and hence avoided. We believe that in some cases, dose rates may be reduced without loss of effectiveness. Among the newer classes of products and control techniques IGRs were identified as promising candidates for outbreak prevention and in particular for barrier spraying of hopper bands. In accordance with the FAO list of promising new products, the group agreed that the following two control agents are the most developed candidates:

⇒ *Metarhizium.* Although the group recognized that a lot of good work has been done, registration of practical commercial products is likely to be some time away. Several problems will need to be resolved, including commercial production, formulation (shelf-life etc.) and effects on swarms. We feel that they are unlikely to be available until the end of the century.

⇒ **Botanicals** (we considered extracts of *Melia volkensii* and neem). These are still at the experimental stage as far as locust control is concerned. Production on a large-scale is still problematic and problems with the registration of a variable product will limit adoption, but the group felt that development should continue.

The following two categories are still at the experimental stage:

⇒ **Semiochemicals** are scientifically interesting and may be useful as population monitoring tools in the longer term. It is not clear what role they would have in locust control.

⇒ **JHAs (juvenile hormone analogues)**. Manufacturers do not seem to be interested in marketing JHAs for locust control, nor is it clear what their role in locust control would be.

In summary, none of the new products will radically change control methods in the short to medium term. However, their eventual use in locust control where possible will reduce undesirable environmental side effects. All available methods and products should be used in an IPM context.

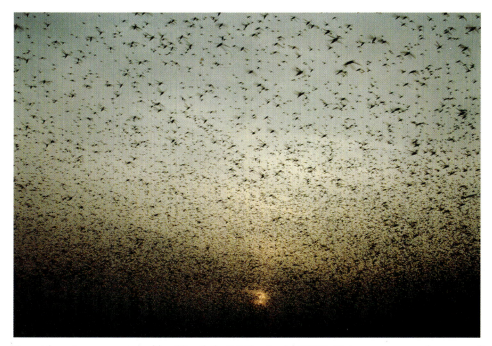

Desert locust swarm approaching Nouakchott (Mauritania, 1993). The swarm covered an area of 14 km^2 when settled and contained 12–14 billion insects.

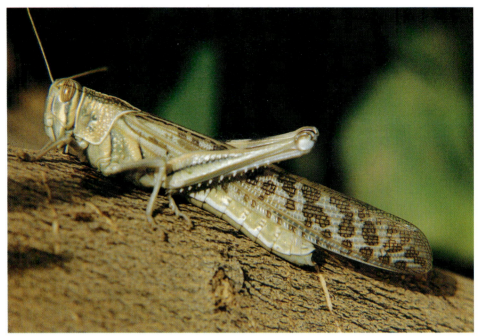

Solitary female desert locust (Agadez, Niger, 1992). During the first weeks after the adult moult the colour changes from light red to grey-brown and finally to beige-brown. The time course and the intensity of the various colours depend on climatic and intrinsic factors.

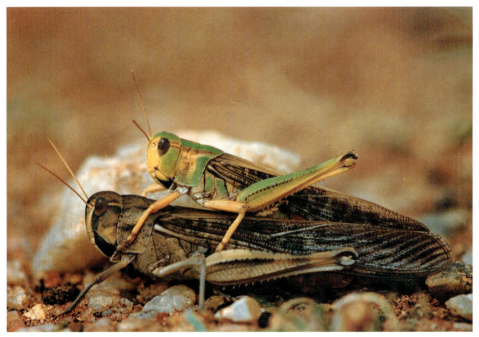

A solitary female and a transient male migratory locust in copula (South-West Madagascar, 1993).

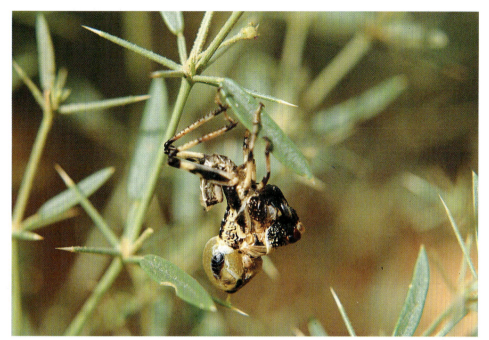

Sphecid wasps hunt for acridids and crickets, which serve as food for their offspring. A female wasp (cf. *Prionyx* sp.) drags a paralysed fifth instar desert locust nymph to its burrow. A single nymph is buried in each burrow (Inchiri, Mauritania, 1995).

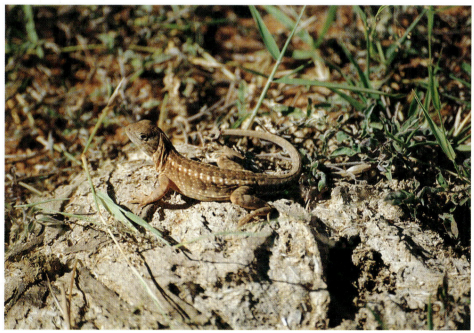

Reptiles make up an important part of the vertebrate fauna in locust habitats. *Chalarodon madagascariensis* (Iguanidae) feeds on small arthropods, including nymphs of migratory locust (Plateau d'Itamboina, South-West Madagascar, 1995).

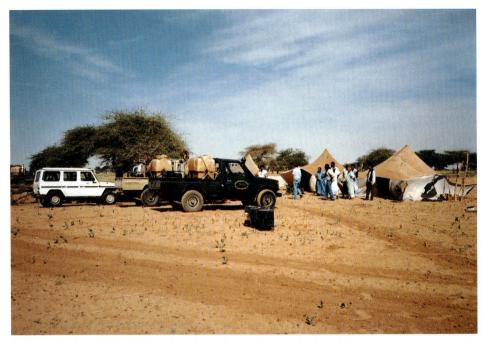

Survey camp in a breeding zone of the desert locust. The monitoring of locusts in remote areas relies on well-trained staff and logistics such as four-wheel drive vehicles or even helicopters and fixed-wing aircraft (Inchiri, Mauritania, 1995).

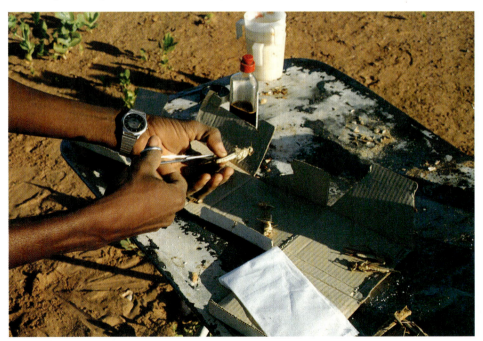

Gregarious, transient and solitary desert locusts differ in colour and morphology, but these features are not always reliable. The examination of fat body and ovaries provides additional information about the physiological state and the actual phase (Tamesna, Niger, 1989).

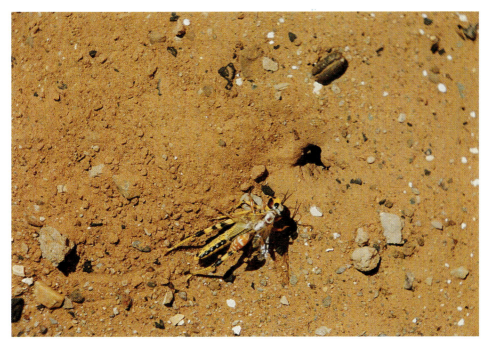

Malformation of a fourth instar desert locust nymph treated with neem oil containing azadirachtin (400 ppm/l) as active ingredient. During moult into the fifth instar the cuticle between pronotum and thorax disrupted, causing a drain of haemolymph, as indicated by the bubble (Inchiri, Mauritania, 1993).

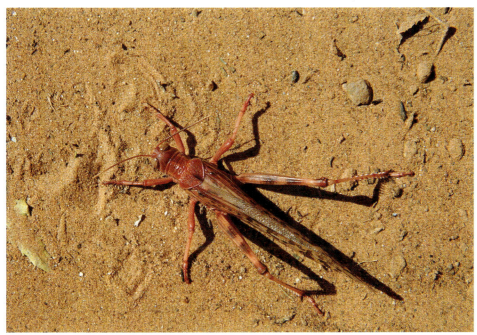

An adult desert locust killed by the entomopathogenic fungus *Metarhizium flavoviride*. The coloration turns dark red prior to death, providing clear evidence of fungal disease. The locust shown had been treated in its nymphal stage and only died after having successfully moulted into the adult stage (Inchiri, Mauritania).

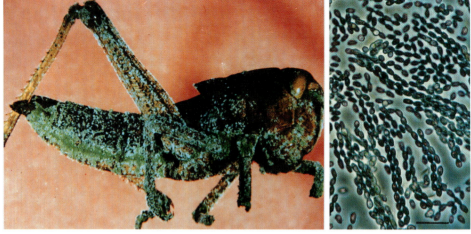

Metarhizium flavoviride: Infected larva of *Locusta migratoria* after sporulation of the fungus (left) and conidia (right; bar = 20 μm).

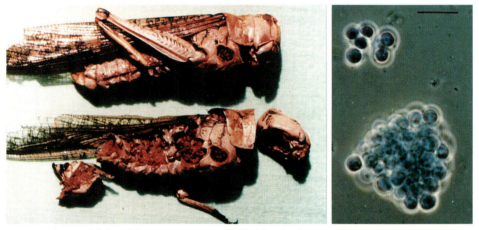

Sorosporella sp: Adults of *Locusta migratoria* killed by the fungus. The cadavers are fragile and entirely filled with resting spores (left). Agglutinated resting spores (right; bar = 20 μm)

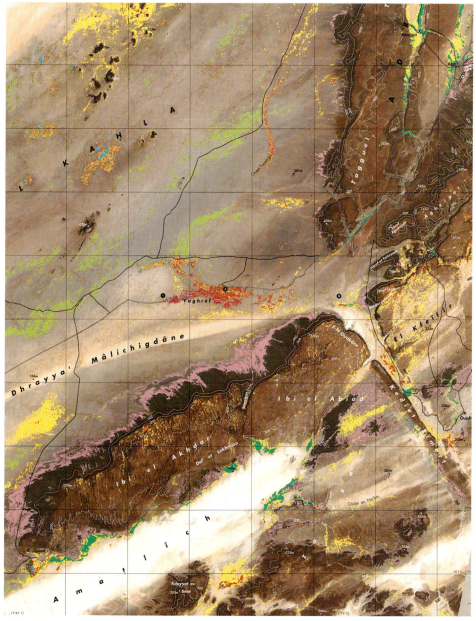

Remote-sensing techniques are a useful tool in habitat mapping. The detail from a habitat map of desert locust in Mauritania published by the Technical University of Berlin and GTZ shows the area to the North-East of Akjoujt. The red colour signifies annual *Schouwia thebaica* vegetation, one of the preferred breeding and feeding habitats of desert locusts.

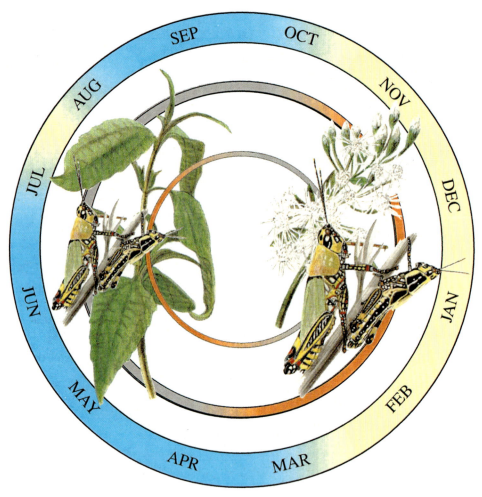

Zonocerus variegatus (L.) (Pyrgomorphidae) is a polyphagous African grasshopper. In parts of West Africa its dryseason population has reached pest status, apparently in coincidence with the spread of the introduced weed *Chromolaena odorata* (L.) K. & R. (Asteraceae: Eupatoriae), which, however, is not a food plant for *Zonocerus*.

Zonocerus sp. sequester pyrrolizidine alkaloids (PAs) not only from certain nutritional host plants but also independent of dietary requirements. Storage of PAs serves to protect the insects from antagonists, and thus aquisition of these secondary plant chemicals modulates the grasshopper's fitness. Flowers of *Chromolaena odorata* represent a novel and inexhaustible resource of PAs, but only for populations in the flowering season, and there is evidence that better performance related to the presence of *Chromolaena* is a reason that dry-season populations became a serious pest in coincidence with the spread of the weed.

The figure illustrates the two distinct and alternating populations of the univoltine *Zonocerus variegatus* in southern Benin. Outer circle: seasons (yellow: dry; blue: wet). Central circle: high abundance of dry-season *Zonocerus*; inner circle: low abundance of wet-season *Zonocerus*; orange: occurrence of larvae/adults; grey: eggs. Flowers of *Chromolaena* bloom in December and January only.

The chemoecological knowledge of *Zonocerus* and *Chromolaena* demonstrates the risk of introduction of foreign plants in (agro-)ecosystems by providing an example of the hidden and unpredictable effects secondary plant chemicals – even those which are not required for nutrition – may have on the population dynamics of insects. It also permits the development of selective baits as a new means for management, and with environmentally sound and cost-efficient application of insecticides, the species can be lured to its doom. (See Fischer and Boppré 1996, this volume).

Chemoecology and semiochemicals

New Strategies in Locust Control
S. Krall, R. Peveling and D. Ba Diallo (eds)
© 1997 Birkhäuser Verlag Basel/Switzerland

Chemoecological studies reveal causes for increased population densities of *Zonocerus* (Orth.: Pyrgomorphidae) and offer new means for management[*]

O.W. Fischer and M. Boppré

Forstzoologisches Institut der Albert-Ludwigs-Universität, D-79085 Freiburg i.Br., Germany

Summary. Grasshoppers of the genus *Zonocerus* sequester pyrrolizidine alkaloids (PAs) not only from certain nutritional host plants but also independent of dietary requirements. Storage of PAs serves protection of the insects from antagonists, and thus acquisition of these secondary plant chemicals modulates the grasshopper's population dynamics. Flowers of the introduced weed *Chromolaena odorata* (Asteraceae) represent a novel and inexhaustible resource of PAs – but only for populations in the dry-season. Evidence is provided that better performance related to the presence of *Chromolaena* is a reason that dry-season populations became a serious pest in coincidence with the spread of the weed. The chemoecological knowledge on the *Zonocerus*-PA relationship permits the development of selective baits, and with environmentally sound and cost-efficient application of insecticides the species can be lured to its doom. Multiple means of employing PA-baits within integrated pest management (IPM) concepts are possible, i.e., strategies of population management can be tailored according to actual demands and conditions. Apart from fighting the grasshopper in individual farms, a general reduction of *Zonocerus* populations is suggested to lower mean levels of abundance in areas with frequent upsurges; this could be done by combining PA-baits with mycoinsecticide technology.

Résumé. Les sauteriaux du type *Zonocerus* séquestrent les alcaloïdes de pyrrolicidine (AP) de certaines plantes hôtes non seulement à des fins nutritionnelles, mais également pour des raisons d'un tout autre ordre, les AP emmagasinés par les insectes leur servant à se protéger de leurs ennemis. Ces composants chimiques végétaux secondaires influent ainsi sur la dynamique des populations de sauteriaux. Les fleurs de la plante introduite dite Herbe du Laos, *Chromolaena odorata* (astéracées) constituent une source de AP renouvelable et inépuisable – toutefois uniquement pour ce qui est des populations de la saison sèche. Etant donné que les performances des insectes s'améliorent grâce à la présence de *Chromolaena*, il existe une corrélation certaine entre la pullulation de *Zonocerus* durant la saison sèche et la propagation de *Chromolaena odorata*. La connaissance du rapport chimio-écologique entre *Zonocerus* et les AP permet la mise au point d'appâts sélectifs attirant les sauteriaux vers des insecticides non destructeurs de l'environnement et rentables économiquement. Il existe de multiples moyens d'employer des appâts à base de AP selon les concepts de la lutte intégrée, c'est-à-dire qu'il est possible d'adapter les stratégies de contrôle des populations aux besoins et conditions existants. A part la lutte contre les sauteriaux menée au niveau des exploitations agricoles, il sera utile de réduire de façon générale les populations de *Zonocerus* afin d'abaisser les taux moyens d'abondance dans les zones fréquemment infestées. Ceci pourra être réalisé en associant les appâts à base de AP à la technologie des mycoinsecticides.

Introduction

The variegated grasshopper, *Zonocerus variegatus*, is extremely polyphagous and more than 60 arable crops, including cassava, maize and cotton, as well as plantation trees such as teak and *Citrus*, have been reported to be vulnerable to damage by this species. (For synoptic accounts on

---

[*] Dedicated with many thanks for stimulating discussions – not only on grasshoppers – and manifold support to Professor Dr. Wolfgang Wickler, Seewiesen, on the occasion of his 65th birthday.

Zonocerus see, e.g. Chapman et al. 1986 and Chiffaud and Mestre 1990.) *Z. variegatus* occurs all over West Africa, and in this large and diverse region its pest status varies considerably according to different climatic conditions, to plants cultivated and to land use systems. To date, no reliable data on economic losses caused by *Zonocerus* are available (see below), but locally and temporarily serious damage certainly occurs, necessitating management.

Due to an apparent linkage between the population dynamics of *Zonocerus* and the introduction and continuing spread of *Chromolaena odorata* in Africa (see below), an increase of problems with *Zonocerus* in both agriculture and silviculture is foreseeable (cf. FAO 1990).

Here, we report on ecological characters of *Zonocerus variegatus*, in particular on the influence of plant secondary chemistry on its population dynamics, and in consequence we suggest management means to be implemented in IPM concepts tailored to specific demands and conditions.

The information conveyed is principally also valid for *Z. elegans*, which inhabits South and East Africa; it is much less studied, but with respect to its biology and ecology it is most similar to *Z. variegatus* (Wickler and Seibt 1985).

Factors affecting population dynamics of *Zonocerus variegatus*

Seasonality

Generally, the variegated grasshopper is univoltine (egg diapause: six to eight months; six larval instars of approx. one to three weeks each; adult life-span approx. two months), but under certain climatic conditions it may occur in two distinct and alternating population peaks (e.g. in Benin). Interestingly, dry-season populations seem to achieve much higher densities than wet-season ones, and serious damage happens in dry seasons only (Anonymous 1977; Page 1978).

Antagonists

Conclusive studies on the role of antagonists on population dynamics as well as on influences of abiotic factors are missing. *Zonocerus* appears well protected, and comparatively few predators are known (Chapman and Page 1979). Upon disturbance, older larvae and adults eject large amounts of repulsive secretion (pyrazines; W. Francke, personal communication); also, secondary compounds from certain plants are stored for protection (see below). Reported predation by lizards, mantids, spiders, solifuges and tettigonids (e.g. Page 1978; Chapman 1962) apparently has little impact on *Zonocerus* populations, as does the nematode *Mermis* (Matanmi 1979) and the phorid fly *Megaselia* (Gregorio and Leonide 1980).

The pathogenic fungus *Entomophaga grylli* is considered to be an important mortality factor under wet conditions (Toye 1982; Chapman and Page 1979), and the parasitic fly *Blaesoxipha filipjevi* (Sarcophagidae) sporadically affects adults at oviposition sites and causes female *Zonocerus* to lay only one egg pod (Taylor 1964; Chapman et al. 1986).

Zonocerus-plant relationships

Zonocerus not only feeds on a wide variety of plants (refs in Chiffaud and Mestre 1990) but appears to require a mixed diet for proper development; therefore considerable movement between plants occurs: *Zonocerus* may leave a plant and change to another species even though there is still plenty of food. Our own observations support those of McCaffery and Harris (unpublished, quoted by Chapman et al. 1986): "A consequence of nymphal mobility is a continual turnover of the insects in any one area such as a field of cassava; e.g. a complete turnover of the population in a 100 m^2 cassava field may occur within 10 days."

Feeding experiments have revealed that very few plants – in particular cassava (*Manihot esculenta*) – fulfil the nutritional requirements of the grasshopper. Insects reared on cassava develop most quickly, gain most weight and produce most eggs (Bernays et al. 1975; Iheagwam 1979; McCaffery et al. 1978). Although many cassava varieties produce noxious cyanogens (Bernays et al. 1977a; McCaffery 1982), *Zonocerus* can utilize this plant through group attack, which circumvents the plant's defences by exhausting its protective devices (Chapman 1985).

Intensified cultivation of cassava and the use of non-cyanogenic varieties apparently is one factor responsible for increasing densities of dry-season populations. A number of native herbs and creepers which mediate good performance are annuals which are not available in the dry season; cassava, however, remains in full foliage deep into the dry season when most other potential host plants have dried up (Bernays et al. 1975; cf. Chapman et al. 1986).

Although he could not provide evidence of a possible link, Toye (1974) has suggested that the increased dry-season populations of *Zonocerus* might be related to the spread of the introduced weed *C. odorata*. Because *Chromolaena* is nutritionally inadequate for *Zonocerus* (see below), it has long been a puzzle as to how this plant influences this grasshopper's population dynamics.

Zonocerus' relationship to pyrrolizidine alkaloids (PAs)

Zonocerus sequesters pyrrolizidine alkaloids from plants and stores them for its defence (Bernays et al. 1977b; Biller et al. 1994; O.W. Fischer, A. Biller, M. Boppré and T. Hartmann, unpublished data). To non-adapted animals, vertebrates as well as invertebrates, PAs act as a taste deterrent, and PAs protect not only the plants producing these secondary chemicals from being eaten but also adapted insects which gather them from plants and store them (refs. in Boppré 1986, 1995).

Sources of PAs are found among the many host plants of the grasshopper: *Crotalaria* (Fabaceae), *Heliotropium* (Boraginaceae), *Emilia, Ageratum* (Asteraceae) and others. (For occurrence of PAs see, e.g. Smith and Culvenor 1980; Rizk 1991; Hartmann and Witte 1995.) Thus, as with many insects, for *Zonocerus* plants may represent much more than food sources because they not only utilize the plants' nutrients but also their noxious secondary compounds.

Although sequestration of secondary plant chemicals by insects is usually linked with feeding, there are so-called "pharmacophagous" insects that search for specific secondary compounds directly, consume them independently of food uptake and use them to increase their fitness (Boppré 1984, 1995). For example, pharmacophagy with respect to PAs is known for numerous butterflies and moths (Danainae, Arctiidae and others), some flea beetles (*Gabonia*) and chloropid flies which are attracted to dry parts of PA-plants, and also to the pure compounds. The Lepidoptera, for example, gather PAs for use as precursors for the biosynthesis of male pheromones and/or store these plant metabolites for their own defence; *Creatonotos* spp. (Arctiidae) even make use of them as morphogens which specifically regulate the growth of the male scent organs (for reviews on PA-pharmacophagy see Boppré 1986, 1990, 1995).

For *Zonocerus*, dry parts of various PA-plants, extracts of these plants as well as certain pure PAs provide very effective lures for all stages of both sexes; the insects take up PAs and store them (Boppré and Fischer 1993, 1994; Boppré et al. 1984; O.W. Fischer and M. Boppré, unpublished data). Therefore, *Zonocerus* is PA-pharmacophagous; it utilizes a variety of plants for obtaining nutrients ('grocer's shops'; e.g. *Manihot*), others for obtaining nutrients plus PAs ('supermarkets'; e.g. *Heliotropium*), and yet others solely to accumulate these secondary compounds ('pharmacies'/'drug stores'; dry parts of PA-plants); the latter case can only be recognized experimentally. The pharmacophagous behaviour not only affects the insects' population dynamics and provides an explanation for the puzzling role of *Chromolaena*, but it also enables the development of a bait to lure and concentrate *Zonocerus* (see below).

The special role of Siam weed, Chromolaena odorata, *for* Zonocerus

C. odorata K. & R. (*Eupatorium odoratum* L.) (Asteraceae: Eupatoriae) is a perennial shrub native to the tropical Americas. Following its introduction into India, *C. odorata* invaded South-East Asia from whence it subsequently reached Africa in the late 1930s and became a dominant weed in the 1970s. In its new habitats it spreads quickly, forming dense thickets of up to two meters in height which flower once a year during the dry season. It has become a major weed which seriously interferes not only with forestry, pastures and plantation crops but also with natural vegetation (e.g. Ambika and Jayachandra 1990; Goodall 1995). In favour of its invasive traits is its apparent chemical protection: vertebrate herbivores avoid it entirely, and there seem to be only a few adapted insect phytophages. (For synoptic accounts on *C. odorata* see, e.g. Audru et al. (1988), Cruttwell McFadyen (1989), Ambika and Jayachandra (1990) and M. Boppré, U. Ladenburger and O.W. Fischer (unpublished data).)

Although young hoppers of *Zonocerus* frequently aggregate overnight on the tips of *Chromolaena* plants and feed sporadically in small amounts, this plant is not adequate for normal development (Bernays et al. 1975; McCaffery et al. 1978). However, the flowers are consumed on a large-scale (Modder 1984), but they alone do not suffice as food (see Chapman et al. 1986).

Why then does the insect become a pest preferentially where the foreign weed occurs?

Modder (1984, 1986) reported that flowers of *Chromolaena* are attractive for all instars of *Zonocerus*; the attractive power of these inflorescences is highest when florets mature and show stigmata, which are preferred organs for starting consumption (Modder 1984, 1986). Interestingly, such flowers are not consumed entirely, as one might expect and as the grasshoppers do with flowers of other plants; rather *Zonocerus* is quite choosy; young hoppers select the stigmata, older ones and adults ingest the entire set of florets of a *Chromolaena* flower but leave the bracts alone as much as possible (Boppré and Fischer 1994, and Fig. 1 therein), i.e. in order to get access to the ovaries within these small capitulae.

Flowers of *Chromolaena* can be used to lure *Zonocerus* (Modder 1984, 1986), but its foliage does not elicit any response. However, roots of Siam weed exhibit strong attractive power, particularly if chopped into pieces, dried and re-moistened (see below and Boppré and Fischer 1994; O.W. Fischer and M. Boppré, unpublished data).

Biller et al. (1994) provide detailed chemical analyses showing that *C. odorata* produces a mixture of PAs with rinderine and intermedine as major components plus [7]O-angeloyl-retronecine, [9]O-angeloyl-retronecine and acetyl-rinderine, all occurring exclusively as N-oxides. In the ecological context, the distribution of PAs in *Chromolaena* is particularly interesting: highest concentrations occur in the roots and in the mature inflorescences with a maximum in the unripe ovaries. The foliage is devoid of PAs. (Non-PA secondary chemicals represent the anti-herbivorous mechanism of the foliage.) Moreover, as the florets mature and stigmata and style arms appear, the PA-content increases.

These chemical data precisely match the results of the behavioural studies mentioned above. Also, the insects have been shown to store PAs from *Chromolaena* and transfer them into the eggs (Biller et al. 1994; O.W. Fischer, A. Biller, M. Boppré and T. Hartmann, unpublished data; cf. Boppré 1991; Boppré et al. 1992). Thus, for dry-season populations of *Zonocerus* flowers of *Chromolaena* provide a novel, rich and most readily available – although temporally restricted – source of PAs.

In conclusion, the puzzle of the coincidence of the spread of *Chromolaena* and the increased abundance of *Zonocerus* seems to be explicable by the following hypothesis (cf. Boppré 1991): *Zonocerus* enjoys a non-nutritional association with *Chromolaena* which provides PAs; these secondary plant compounds are stored and chemically protect the grasshoppers and particularly their diapausing eggs from antagonists, thus giving rise to the increased fitness and higher densities of certain (e.g. dry-season) populations of *Zonocerus*. Without *Chromolaena*, i.e., either before its introduction or in areas where it is absent or in the wet season when *Chromolaena* does not bloom, PAs often seem to be a limited resource restricting the grasshoppers' reproductive success.

This explains why *Zonocerus* appears as a pest preferably where *Chromolaena* occurs, also why we have to envisage increasing problems with this grasshopper for the future. However, it does not imply that the novel source of PAs – flowers of *Chromolaena* – is the sole reason for increased and harmful dry-season populations, and it does not rule out that the increased cultivation of cassava, deforestation and/or lack of antagonists are additional factors favouring an increase in dry-season *Zonocerus* populations. In any case, *Chromolaena* appears to influence population dynamics to a greater extent than the indigenous PA-plants which are usually quite rare or contain small amounts of PAs. However, particularly high population densities can of course also be triggered by indigenous PA-plants. For example, an outbreak of *Zonocerus elegans* in 1987/88 in Tanzania where no *Chromolaena* occurs seems to be correlated to preferred feeding on *Ageratum* (Nyambo 1991). *Ageratum* is a common weed containing PAs similar to those in *Chromolaena* (Wiedenfeld and Röder 1991), but it is less competitive and much less persistent in comparison with *C. odorata*.

On the pest status of *Zonocerus variegatus*

Z. variegatus is a polyphagous species, and high population densities potentially may become harmful to a large number of cultures. In the literature, this insect is generally regarded as a serious pest. To date, hardly any data on damage to crops are available (see, e.g. Baumgart 1994), although the need for proper evaluation of its pest status as a basis for developing economically appropriate control strategies has often been recommended (e.g. Toye 1982). A recent questionnaire inquiry by J.A. Timbilla et al. (unpublished) at institutions in 36 African countries has provided only little data on damage and costs for control, respectively. However, the great attention this grasshopper receives is reflected in the publication of more than 250 papers within the past 60 years; for sure, this is not based on academic interests but underscores its economic importance. "There is a consensus among entomologists that, at least in some countries, the insect has changed in the last 15–20 years from a spasmodic, generally minor pest to a more regular and relatively major problem" (Chapman et al. 1986).

Obtaining reliable data – not only on quantitative but also on qualitative economic losses as well as on additional injuries such as transmission of bacterial (CBB) and viral (OMV) diseases by *Zonocerus* (Terry 1978; Givord and Den Boer 1980; Nkouka et al. 1981) – is probably difficult because of the many crops affected differently, the peculiar habits and bionomics of the grasshopper and the different agricultural systems involved. Dispersal of *Zonocerus* obstructs both assessment of damage and control: *Zonocerus* is not only polyphagous but usually requires changes in its diet for proper performance (cf. above); in consequence, high population densities may be found on a field, but damage does not become serious because this grasshopper leaves a host although it still provides plenty of food. We do not know of any other pest insect with such a trait. Movements related to changes of host plants has also been reported by Nwana (1984), who found that the insect stays longer in unweeded fields than in weeded ones, which is likely due to diversity of hosts.

Although the question is open under which circumstances control actions are justified and at which expenditure, there are many situations necessitating management of *Zonocerus*. Also, it is beyond doubt that there is great spaciotemporal variation. Thus, the goal must be a pest management concept permitting tailoring of means according to local conditions with respect to population density and also to availability of control means. In particular, prophylactic actions are required which have to be conducted at a community level (see below).

Current means and concepts for controlling *Zonocerus*

Various conventional control methods, i.e., use of insecticides, pathogens and mechanical means, are applicable to *Zonocerus*. Costly and environmentally hazardous spraying of synthetic chemicals are mainly applied, although IPM approaches have been advocated repeatedly (Anonymous 1977; Page 1978; Toye 1982). The most recent one by Modder (1986) consists of mechanical exposure of egg pods, spraying of insecticide on roosting nymphs and trapping nymphs and adults with flowers of *Chromolaena* (hoping to eventually find "the volatile chemical substance from the inflorescenses" and use this with insecticide after the flowering season and before egg laying).

Modder's (1986) concept is quite acceptable, but we disagree with his idea of protecting *Chromolaena*. Assuming that *Chromolaena* has no relevance to populations of *Zonocerus*, he believes it would be better to preserve *Chromolaena* in order to distract nymphs away from economically important plants. This opinion provokes contradiction apart from the erratic assessment of Siam weed on the fitness of *Zonocerus*: on the one hand, because the grasshoppers require nutrients not provided by *Chromolaena*, they cannot be confined to the weed; on the other hand, *C. odorata* is ecologically and economically harmful in many ways, e.g. through suppression of succession of natural vegetation and in being a fire hazard (e.g. Ambika and Jayachandra 1990; Crutwell McFadyen 1989; M. Boppré, U. Ladenburger and O.W. Fischer, unpublished data).

Management of pest populations of *Zonocerus* in view of PA pharmacophagy

The chemoecological knowledge on the relationship of *Zonocerus* to plants containing pyrrolizidine alkaloids, in particular the attractive and phagostimulatory power of PAs, can be utilized for developing a bait for IPM purposes (cf. Boppré et al. 1984; Boppré 1991; Boppré and Fischer 1993, 1994). Of course, as with other cases employing lures (e.g. pheromone baits used in the control of moth pests), there is competition between man-made lures and natural ones. A major peculiarity has to be observed in addition: PAs are not required to maintain the life of *Zonocerus*, rather these secondary plant compounds are utilized supplementarily. Thus, the motivation of the insect to search for PAs is secondary compared with ordinary feeding behaviour or any sexual activities, and *Zonocerus* responds to sources of PAs less 'automatically' than does a male moth to female sex attractants and an *instant* response cannot necessarily be expected.

Stimuli involved in locating sources of PAs

Although *Zonocerus* is pharmacophagous with respect to PAs and attracted by dry plants of various species and also by pure PAs (which proves that indeed only PAs and not any other secondary plant chemicals lure the insect), it is unable to discriminate between intact, living PA-containing plants and plants devoid of PAs over a distance. This is because in living plant tissue PAs are confined to cell vacuoles which prevents detection without physical contact; also, PAs are large molecules with insufficient volatility for olfactory perception. However, *Zonocerus* is capable of perceiving PAs with its gustatory (contact-chemo)receptors on the mouthparts and can thus only detect intact PA-plants upon contact; PAs then act as phagostimulants. (It is interesting to note that in combination with the 'good taste' of PAs, *Zonocerus* accepts higher doses of insecticides; i.e., repelling properties of pesticides are reduced.) However, when plants are mechanically damaged (e.g. by phytophages) or if they wither and wilt, PAs get exposed to the outside environment, and – as with pure PAs – the atmospheric conditions trigger their disintegration into a variety of derivatives, some of which are volatile and perceivable by olfactory receptors located on the insects' antennae. A major initial step in derivatisation is hydrolysis, and therefore the attractive power of dry plant material can be increased by chopping and re-moistening it with water. Also, the identical response of *Zonocerus* to a variety of PA-sources containing different PAs can be explained by the existence of a common volatile derivative (for details on the "PA-odour" see M. Boppré, unpublished data).

PA-baits – versatile tools

Attraction with flowers of *Chromolaena* is the simplest way of baiting *Zonocerus*; however, their attractivity quickly fades, and inflorescences are only available once a year for a few weeks (moreover at a time when there is heaviest competition with flowering stands of *Chromolaena*). PA-baits made up from roots (or foliage, in case) of PA-plants provide a year-round alternative. Other PA-pharmacophagous insects are usually rare or absent in areas where *Zonocerus* is present and can if necessary be kept off PA-baits by simple mechanical means. Thus, such simple baits represent versatile tools with high specificity to concentrate *Zonocerus* for killing and for monitoring purposes, respectively. (Monitoring of later instars and adults is otherwise difficult, because they do not congregate at the tips of foliage as do early hoppers.)

For control with PA-baits, insects can be lured to the poison instead of the poison being brought to the insects; this permits environmentally safe reduction of populations with a minimum of insecticide. Apart from spraying insecticides on insects gathering at baits, combinations of PA-bait and insecticide (attracticides) can be produced which work maintenance-free for more or less long times. Depending on the demand, attracticides employing PAs offer a menu of options which permit tailoring of the most appropriate control strategy:

Types of PA-baits/attracticides to lure Zonocerus

There are two general types of attracticide applications (O.W. Fischer and M. Boppré, unpublished data):

- Baits for mechanical trapping and for use in combination either with pathogens or stomach-acting pesticides, utilizing both the attractive and the phagostimulatory power of PAs; require regular re-moistening (necessary for emission of the volatile derivatives).

type of PA-source	comments
• mechanically damaged leaves of PA-plants (spp. of *Heliotropium*, *Crotalaria* and others)	easily obtainable; available all year; attractivity fades after a few days but can be regained by moistening
• dried, chopped and re-moistened roots of PA-plants (spp. of *Heliotropium*, *Chromolaena* and others)	easily obtainable; available all year; attractive for weeks if stored dry; attractivity can be regained after years by re-moistening

- Baits for mechanical trapping and for use in combination either with pathogens or pesticides which act upon contact. The attractive material is confined in polyethylene bags which act as dispensers for slow and continuous release of "PA-odour"; regular re-moistening in this case is not necessary, but the dispenser needs to be protected from being eaten by the insects.

type of PA-source	comments
• dried and chopped parts of PA-plants (spp. of *Heliotropium*, *Crotalaria*, *Chromolaena* (roots only))	easily obtainable; available all year; attractive for weeks if stored dry; attractivity can be regained after years by re-moistening
• methanolic raw extracts of PA-plants[1,2] (including spp. not occurring in the habitats of *Zonocerus*!)	easy to produce with simple laboratory equipment; can be standardized; shelf-life of many years
• purified extracts of PA-plants [1,2] (including spp. not occurring in the habitats of *Zonocerus*!)	easy to produce with laboratory equipment; can be standardized; shelf-life of many years
• pure PAs[1,2,3] (e.g. heliotrine, monocrotaline, axillarine, retrorsine) extracted from plant material	best for standardizing; requires professional production; shelf-life of many years

[1] Applied on substrates such as cardboard, filter paper, glass fibre filters, sponge clothes or any other material.
[2] Combination with stomach-acting insecticides is possible but would be a waste.
[3] Although in plants PAs usually occur as N-oxides, the respective free bases are attractive.

At present, neither PA-baits nor attracticides employing PAs are commercially available, but it is hoped that these will eventually be manufactured locally in a standardized way.

As indicated above, the attractive power of the various kinds of baits differs, varying and fading more or less quickly; therefore, absolute amounts of material needed for a good bait cannot be given. However, 5 – 10 g of dry PA-plant material and 200 mg of pure PAs, respectively, have given good results (O.W. Fischer and M. Boppré, unpublished data).

Zonocerus is susceptible to numerous insecticides including, BHC and fenitrothion (Anonymous 1977; Oyidi 1984), but also to various chitin synthesis inhibitors as well as to natural products such as dennetia oil (Iwuala et al. 1981) and neem (e.g. Olaifa and Adenuga 1988; Baumgart 1994); with respect to fungal pathogens, recently good success with *Zonocerus* has been obtained with *Metarhizium flavoviride* (Douro-Kpindou et al. 1995) but other mycoinsecticides are worthwhile testing, too.

As with other activities of *Zonocerus* (cf. Kaufmann 1965), responses to PA-baits are best when the temperature is above 23 °C and when there is full sunshine (see also Boppré et al. 1984; Modder 1984, 1986). The chemically mediated congregation of *Zonocerus* at PA-baits can be facilitated by visual cues. The grasshoppers are attractable by linear vertical patterns (cf. Kaufmann 1965), and hanging PA-baits are more attractive than ones placed on the ground. When we combined a lure on the ground with a stick in its vicinity, the majority of grasshoppers attracted jumped onto the stick and climbed it.

There is no indication that attraction to PAs is restricted in such a way that the 'hunger for PAs' terminates after ingestion of a certain amount of these plant substances; i.e., *Zonocerus* is attracted to PAs during its entire life independent of the amount of PAs already ingested. In laboratory tests where pure PAs had been offered ad libitum, no consistent pattern in PA-uptake could be recognized, except that on the average females took up larger amounts than did males (O.W. Fischer, A. Biller, M. Boppré and T. Hartmann, unpublished data).

Further prospects for future IPM of *Zonocerus*

The two *Zonocerus* species are peculiar grasshoppers with respect to their biology and their appearance as pests in agriculture and forestry, and there cannot be the 'one and only' recipe to combat high population densities. Rather, it is necessary to have an IPM concept which provides toolkits for selection and combination of the most appropriate control strategy in a given situation, considering population densities and instars occurring, and also availability of technical equipment, labour, pesticides etc. To date, this requirement is met to a great extent.

For implementing the most environmentally sound and cost-efficient means, farmers must be trained by plant protection services to properly assess the potential threat and take preventive measures against *Zonocerus* upsurges before they cause damage. The uncommon traits of this insect require action many months in advance, e.g. survey and marking of egg-laying sites and combatting early instar hoppers weeks before late instars and adults can cause damage. Because of the tendency to host-switching and the dispersal behaviour of *Zonocerus*, it is difficult in most cases to predict areas which might eventually be affected; in consequence, pest management should therefore be conducted at a community level.

Baiting Zonocerus *for infection with pathogens*

An appealing concept to *Zonocerus* control has its goal in a general reduction of population sizes in areas where the risk for damage is high for one reason or another; i.e., the objective should be to lower the mean level of abundance so that fluctuations above the economic threshold are reduced or eliminated. We are working on the development of a simple and cheap device which attracts the grasshoppers with a persistent PA-source and infects them with specific fungal spores while they are (unsuccessfully) trying to gather PAs. Due to the movements of hoppers (see above) over weeks, part of the population will be infected and disseminate the pathogen to conspecifics (cf. Thomas et al. 1995). Such a device with which control is self-perpetuating would have to be given to communities and co-operatives for distribution in their areas at low density and at times when young hoppers appear.

General conclusions

A plant – cassava – introduced to Africa as a crop with high resistance to grasshoppers (Schaefers 1978) nowadays contributes to increased population densities of dry-season *Zonocerus*, and these populations are, in turn, supported by another introduced plant – *Chromolaena*. This case nicely illustrates the uncertainties of establishing foreign plants in (agro-)ecosystems. Moreover, it provides an example of the effect secondary chemicals of plants not required for nutrition and in any case gathered independent of food may have on the population dynamics of insects. Similar non-nutritional phenomena might exist in many other insect-plant relationships but have not yet been recognized. Also, the relations of *Zonocerus* to plants exemplify that detailed basic knowledge on chemoecological interactions may lead to environmentally sound ways of pest management by employing secondary plant metabolites in simple formulations – just as in traditional medicine – or in a more 'high-tech style'.

Finally, the knowledge on storage of PAs by *Zonocerus* makes us to note that it is not advisable to use these grasshoppers as food items for humans or domestic animals. According to the literature, it is not rare that *Zonocerus* are eaten and even sold on local markets in West Africa (see, e.g. Page and Richards 1977; Koman 1983). To vertebrates, including humans, many PAs are toxic; usually they do not cause instant harm but have hepatotoxic, carcenogenic and other effects (e.g. Huxtable 1990).

Acknowledgements
Our studies are part of the project Integrated Biological Control of Grasshoppers and Locusts of the Deutsche Gesellschaft für Technische Zusammenarbeit (GTZ) and are largely funded by it. We are not only grateful to the GTZ for their financial support but also greatly indebted to the Projet GTZ de la Protection des Végétaux and the Service de la Protection des Végétaux (SPV), Porto-Novo, as well as to the Office National du Bois (O.NA.B.), Cotonou, for logistic support of our field work in Benin. Reinhold Loch and Niels Behn have contributed with their field studies in the cause of preparing their Diplomarbeiten, which is thankfully acknowledged. Our thanks are also due to Kodjo Nathegan and Hyacinth Ango for their effective field assistance.

References

Ambika SR, Jayachandra (1990) The problem of *Chromolaena* weed. *Chromolaena odorata* Newsletter 3: 1–6
Anonymous (1977) Control of *Zonocerus variegatus* (L.) in Nigeria. Final report and recommendations. (ODM Res Scheme R 2727) GB-London: Centre for Overseas Pest Research
Audru J, Berekoutou M, Deat M, Wispelaere G de, Dufour F, Kintz D, Masson A le, Menozzi PH (1988) L′Herbe du Laos. Etude et Synthèse de l'I.E.M.V.T. 28. F-Maisons-Alfort: I.E.M.V.T
Baumgart M (1994) Untersuchungen zur Wirkung von Öl und anderen Produkten aus den Samen des Niembaumes (*Azadirachta indica* A. Juss.) auf die Stinkheuschrecke *Zonocerus variegatus* L. (Orthoptera: Pyrgomorphidae) in Benin. D-Aachen: Verlag Shaker
Bernays EA, Chapman RF, Cook AG, McVeigh LJ, Page WW (1975) Food plants in the survival and development of *Zonocerus variegatus* (L.). Acrida 4: 33–45
Bernays EA, Chapman RF, Leather EM, McCaffery AR (1977a) The relationship of *Zonocerus variegatus* (L.) (Acridoidea: Pyrgomorphidae) with cassava (*Manihot esculenta*). Bull Ent Res 67: 391–404
Bernays EA, Edgar JA, Rothschild M (1977b) Pyrrolizidine alkaloids sequestered and stored by the aposematic grasshopper, *Zonocerus variegatus*. J Zool (Lond) 182: 85–87
Biller A, Boppré M, Witte L, Hartmann T (1994) Pyrrolizidine alkaloids in *Chromolaena odorata*.: chemical and chemoecological aspects. Phytochemistry 35: 615–619
Boppré M (1984) Redefining "pharmacophagy". J Chem Ecol 10: 1151–1154
Boppré M (1986) Insects pharmacophagously utilising secondary plant substances (pyrrolizidine alkaloids). Naturwissenschaften 73: 17–26
Boppré M (1990) Lepidoptera and pyrrolizidine alkaloids: exemplification of complexity in chemical ecology. J Chem Ecol 16: 165–185
Boppré M (1991) A non-nutritional relationship of *Zonocerus* (Orthoptera) to *Chromolaena* (Asteraceae) and general implications for weed management. Pages 153–157 in Muniappan R, Ferrar R (eds) Ecology and Management of *Chromolaena odorata*. Proc 2nd Int Workshop on Biol Control of *Chromolaena odorata*. (BIOTROP Special Publ no 44.) Bogor, Indonesia: ORSTOM and SEAMEO BIOTROP

Boppré M (1996) The diverse chemoecology of pyrrolizidine alkaloids: facts, fiction and prospects. Chemoecology: in press

Boppré M, Seibt U, Wickler W (1984) Pharmacophagy in grasshoppers? *Zonocerus* being attracted to and ingesting pure pyrrolizidine alkaloids. Entomol Exp Appl 35: 713–714

Boppré M, Fischer OWF (1993) *Zonocerus* et *Chromolaena* en Afrique de l´Quest: une approche chimioecologique de lutte biologique. Sahel PV Info (Bamako, Mali) 56: 7–21

Boppré M, Fischer OWF (1994) *Zonocerus* and *Chromolaena* in West Africa: a chemoecological approach towards pest management. Pages 107–126 in Krall S, Wilps H (eds) New trends in locust control. D-Eschborn: GTZ

Boppré M, Biller A, Fischer OW, Hartmann T (1992) The non-nutritional relationship of *Zonocerus* (Orthoptera) to *Chromolaena* (Asteraceae). Pages 89–90 in Menken SBJ, Visser JH, Harrewijn P (eds) Proc 8th Intern Symp Insect-Plant Relationships. NL-Dordrecht: Kluwer Acad Publ

Chapman RF (1962) The ecology and distribution of grasshoppers in Ghana. Proc Zool Soc Lond 139: 1–66

Chapman RF (1985) The paradoxical biology of a West African grasshopper. Proc R Entomol Soc Queensland 13: 51–54

Chapman RF, Page WW (1979) Factors affecting mortality of the grasshopper, *Zonocerus variegatus*, in southern Nigeria. J Anim Ecol 48: 271–288

Chapman RF, Page WW, McCaffery AR (1986) Bionomics of the variegated grasshopper (*Zonocerus variegatus*) in West and Central Africa. Annu Rev Entomol 31: 479–505

Chiffaud J, Mestre J (1990) Le criquet puant *Zonocerus variegatus* (Linné, 1758). F-Paris: CIRAD

Crutwell McFadyen RE (1989) Siam weed: a new threat to Australia's north. Plant Prot Quart 4: 3–7

Douro-Kpindou O-K, Godonou I, Houssou A, Lomer CJ, Shah PA (1995) Control of *Zonocerus variegatus* by ultra-low volume application of an oil formulation of *Metarhizium flavoviride* conidia. Biocontrol Sci Technol 5: 131–139

FAO (1990) Groupe de travail sur le *Zonocerus*. Compte rendu de la Réunion, Rome, 31 May–1 June 1990

Givord L, Den Boer L (1980) Insect transmission of okra mosaic virus in the Ivory Coast. Ann appl Biol 94: 235–241

Goodall J (1995) *Chromolaena*: what hope for Southern Africa? Plant Prot News 39: 2–5

Gregorio R, Leonide JC (1980) Un nouveau cas de phoride parasite d'orthoptères adultes. Bull Soc Entomol France 85: 103–105

Hartmann T, Witte L (1995) Chemistry, biology and chemoecology of the pyrrolizidine alkaloids. Pages 155–233 in Pelletier SW (ed) Alkaloids: chemical and biological perspectives. Vol 9. GB-Oxford: Pergamon Press

Huxtable RJ (1990) Human health implications of pyrrolizidine alkaloids and herbs containing them. Pages 41–86 in Cheeke RR (ed) Toxicants of plant origin. Vol 1: Alkaloids. Boca Raton/FL: CRC Press

Iheagwam EU (1979) Host plant effects on fecundity and adult survival of *Zonocerus variegatus* L. Rev Zool Afr 93: 760–765

Iwuala MOE, Osisiogu IUW, Agbakwuru EOP (1981) Dennettia oil, a potential new insecticide: tests with adults and nymphs of *Periplaneta americana* and *Zonocerus variegatus*. J Econ Entomol 74: 249–252

Kaufmann T (1965) Observations on aggregation, migration and feeding habits of *Zonocerus variegatus* in Ghana (Orthoptera: Acrididae). Ann Entomol Soc Am 58: 426–436

Koman J (1983) Notes sur le régime alimentaire de *Zonocerus variegatus* (L.) (Orthoptera, Pyrgomorphidae) en République de Guinée. Bull Inst Fond Afrique Noire 45: 118–125

Matanmi BA (1979) *Mermis* sp. (Nematoda: Mermithidae) as a parasite of *Zonocerus variegatus* Linnaeus (Orthoptera: Pyrgomorphidae). Ife J Agric 1: 150–161

McCaffery AR, Cook AG, Page WW, Perfect TJ (1978) Utilisation of food by *Zonocerus variegatus* (L.) (Orthoptera: Pyrgomorphidae). Bull Entomol Res 68: 589–606

McCaffery AR (1982) A difference in the acceptability of excised and growing cassava leaves to *Zonocerus variegatus*. Ent Exp Appl 32: 111–115

Modder WWD (1984) The attraction of *Zonocerus variegatus* (L.) (Orthoptera: Pyrgomorphidae) to the weed *Chromolaena odorata* and associated feeding behaviour. Bull Entomol Res 74: 239–247

Modder WWD (1986) An integrated pest management strategy for the African grasshopper *Zonocerus variegatus*. Nigerian Field 51: 41–52

Nkouka N, Onore G, Fabres G (1981) Eléments d'un inventaire de l'entomofaune phytophage du manioc en vue de l'identification des insectes vecteurs de la bactériose vasculaire. Cah O.R.S.T.O.M. sér Biol 44: 9–10

Nwana IE (1984) The dispersal of the variegated grasshopper, *Zonocerus variegatus* (Linnaeus)(Orthoptera, Acridoidea, Pyrgomorphidae), in open fields and cultivated farms. Insect Sci Appl 5: 273–278

Nyambo BT (1991) The pest status of *Zonocerus elegans* (Thunberg) (Orthoptera: Acridoidea) in Kilosa District in Tanzania with some suggestion on control strategies. Insect Sci Appl 12: 231–236

Olaifa JI, Adenuga AO (1988) Neem products for protecting field cassava from grasshopper damage. Insect Sci Appl 9: 267–270

Oyidi O (1984) A preliminary note on laboratory and field tests of some insecticides against *Zonocerus variegatus* in northern Nigeria. Sumaru J Agric Res 2: 75–85

Page WW (1978) The biology and control of the grasshopper *Zonocerus variegatus*. PANS 24: 270–277

Page WW, Richards P (1977) Agricultural pest control by community action: the case of the variegated grasshopper in southern Nigeria. Afr Environm 2: 127–141

Rizk A-FM (ed) (1991) Naturally occurring pyrrolizidine alkaloids. Boca Raton/CA: CRC Press

Schaefers GA (1978) Grasshoppers (*Zonocerus* spp.) on cassava in Africa. Pages 221–226 in Brekelbaum T, Bellotti A, Lozano JC (eds) Proc Cassava Protection Workshop. Cali, Colombia: Centro Internacional de Agricultura Tropical

Smith LW, Culvenor CCJ (1980) Plant sources of hepatotoxic pyrrolizidine alkaloids. J Nat Prod 44: 129–152

Taylor TA (1964) *Blaesoxipha filipjevi* Rohd. (Diptera, Sarcophagidae) parasitising *Zonocerus variegatus* (L.) (Orthoptera, Acridoidea) in Nigeria. Bull ent Res 55: 83–86

Terry ER (1978) Cassava bacterial diseases. Pages 75–84 in Brekelbaum T, Bellotti A, Lozano JC (eds) Proc Cassava Protection Workshop. Cali, Colombia: Centro Internacional de Agricultura Tropical

Thomas MB, Wood SN, Lomer CJ (1995) Biological control of locusts and grasshoppers using a fungal pathogen: the importance of secondary cycling. Proc R Soc Lond B 259: 265–270

Toye SA (1974) Feeding and locomotory activities of *Zonocerus variegatus* (L.) (Orthoptera, Acridoidea). Rev Zool Afr 88: 205–212

Toye SA (1982) Studies on the biology of the grasshopper pest *Zonocerus variegatus* (L.) (Orthoptera: Pyrgomorphidae) in Nigeria: 1911–1981. Insect Sci Appl 3: 1–7

Wickler W, Seibt U (1985) Reproductive behaviour in *Zonocerus elegans* (Orthoptera: Pyrgomorphidae) with special reference to nuptial gift guarding. Z Tierpsychol 69: 203–223

Wiedenfeld H, Röder H (1991) Pyrrolizidine alkaloids from *Ageratum conyzoides*. Planta Med 57: 578–579

New Strategies in Locust Control
S. Krall, R. Peveling and D. Ba Diallo (eds)
© 1997 Birkhäuser Verlag Basel/Switzerland

Attraction and diurnal behaviour of the African pest grasshopper, *Zonocerus variegatus* (L.), at oviposition sites

W.W.D. Modder

Plant Health Management Division, International Institute of Tropical Agriculture, BP 08-0932, Cotonou, Benin

Summary. Zonocerus variegatus oviposition sites (OSs) of different types were studied in southern Benin, as a first step in characterising OS attractants for bait traps. OSs have more males (70–85%; ca. 50% outside). Two to three times more males than females were attracted to males used as lures. Females were not as attractive, even to other females. Supernumerary single males in foliage above OSs suggest that they attract each other and initiate OSs. Almost all the females were copulating; extra, competing males probably enhance the reproductive success of the species. During one week, the females arriving at an OS increased, suggesting that females are attracted as they become ready to oviposit. Most in copula pairs were in the foliage, but many descended to the ground at ca. midday to oviposit. The highest number of ovipositions occurred after rain. Many single males were on the ground during the heat of the day, probably seeking moisture. Numbers peaked at night, suggesting that OSs also serve for roosting. More adults approached a recently emptied OS upwind than downwind, indicating olfactory attraction, perhaps to buried egg pods or residual male odour.

Résumé. Différents types de champs de ponte (CP) établis par *Zonocerus variegatus* dans le sud du Bénin ont fait l'objet d'études qui constituaient une première étape vers la mise au point de substances attirant les insectes vers les CP. Les mâles sont en surnombre dans les champs de ponte (70 à 85%; environ 50% à l'extérieur). Deux à trois fois plus de mâles ont été attirés par d'autres mâles utilisés comme leurres. Les femelles ont exercé une attraction moindre, même sur d'autres femelles. Les mâles seuls en surnombre dans les feuillages au-dessus des CP suggèrent une inter-attractivité entre mâles et la détermination des CP par les mâles. La plupart des femelles étaient en copulation; les mâles concurrents en surnombre permettent probablement d'améliorer la reproductibilité de l'espèce. Pendant une semaine, le nombre de femelles arrivant dans un CP a augmenté. On pourrait en déduire que les femelles sont attirées lorsqu'elles sont sur le point de pondre. La plupart des femelles en copulation se trouvaient dans les feuillages, mais beaucoup sont descendues vers le sol vers le milieu de la journée pour déposer leurs oeufs. La majorité des ovipositions a eu lieu après la pluie. De nombreux mâles seuls s'étaient rassemblés sur le sol pendant la chaleur du jour, recherchant probablement l'humidité. Les rassemblements maxima au sol ayant lieu durant la nuit, il semble que les CP servent également de perchoirs. Plus d'adultes se dirigeaient vers un CP récemment vidé contre le vent que sous le vent, ce qui indique une attraction olfactive, peut-être vers des oothèques enterrées ou des résidus d'odeur mâle.

Introduction

Zonocerus variegatus (L.) is the main grasshopper pest of crops in the extensive forest and savannah areas of West and Central Africa. The adults aggregate at oviposition sites (OSs) in thickets and bush, in the shade of trees or shrubs which may have ground cover such as fallen leaves, or under heaps of stalks or withered vegetation resulting from harvesting or weeding. OSs are usually <30 m from farmers' fields with soil soft for ovipositor insertion (Page and McCaffery 1979) and moist for stages of egg development (Chapman and Page 1978; Modder

1978). They are relatively small (<20 m^2, Page 1978) and closely packed with egg pods <10 cm below the surface. Both sexes are attracted olfactorily, not to the egg pods, but to the males already present (Chapman et al. 1986). However, both sexes were attracted to an OS recently cleared of grasshoppers. The present study is a first step in characterising OS attractants such as pheromones which could be useful in devising bait traps for control, and perhaps in disrupting oviposition.

Materials and methods

Observations at OSs

Z. variegatus singles and copulating pairs at eight OSs in five varied locations in southern Benin were observed (Tab. 1). At OS 7, daily observations were made at 07.00, 11.00, 15.00 and 19.00 h (Tab. 2).

Attraction experiments at a cleared OS

All the adults at OS 1 (the shade of a banana mat) were collected. Around midday the same day, 709 were marked white with enamel paint on the pronota and released 10 m south, or upwind, of the OS. The remaining 775 were marked red and released 10 m north, or downwind, of it. Two concentric circles of 12- and 10-m radius, with the OS as centre, were staked out to form sectors A and B (Fig. 1), and 24 h later marked adults were recovered from A, B and the OS.

Attraction experiments with live lures

A. Five wood and wire-mesh cages (30 × 30 × 38 cm) containing reproductive adults as lures (Tab. 3A) were arranged 2.5 m apart in a straight line, in a bare field, 10 m from and parallel to a large bank of *Chromolaena odorata* (L.) King and Robinson containing other reproductives. Adults at the outside of the cages 24 h later were counted.

B and C. OS 6 was cleared of adults but not egg pods. Adults were brought from elsewhere and placed as lures in bottomless cages (70 × 70 × 40 cm). Adult males and females just collected from the surroundings were released as indicated below. Those at the outside of the cages 3−4 days later were counted.

Table 1. The numbers and distribution of *Z. variegatus* adults at and near oviposition sites (OSs) in southern Benin

A. Onigbolo, Ouémé Province; 6.5.93; OSs at bases of oil palm trees

	OS 2		OS 3	
	Males	Females	Males	Females
Singles	51 (53.7%)	2 (2.1%)	196 (62%)	16 (5.1%)
In copula	21 (22.1%)	X 21 (22.1%)	52 (16.5%)	X 52 (16.5%)
Total	72	23	248	68
Total males + females		95 (100%)		316 (100%)
% Males	75.8		78.5	

B. Ilou Olofin, Ouémé Province; 8.4.94; OSs at bases of mango trees

	OS 4		OS 5		<50m from OSs	
	Males	Females	Males	Females	Males	Females
Singles	80 (46.8%)	7 (4.1%)	64 (71.9%)	9 (10.1%)	36 (33.6%)	59 (55.1%)
In copula	40 (23.4%) X 40 (23.4%)		7 (7.9%)	X 7 (7.9%)	6 (5.6%)	X 6 (5.6%)
Males "in copula"	2 X 2		1 X 1			
Total:	124	47	73	16	42	65
Total males + females:		171 (100%)		89 (100%)		107 (100%)
% Males:	72.5		82.0		39.2	

C. Niaouli, Atlantique Province; 3.9.93; OS 6, in overgrown cassava

	In foliage and on ground		In foliage		On ground		<50m from OS	
	Males	Females	Males	Females	Males	Females	Males	Females
Singles	21 (67.7%)	4 (12.9%)	19	0	2	4		
In copula	3 (9.7%)	X 3 (9.7%)	0	0	3	X 3		
Total:	24	7	19	0	5	7	55	81
Total males + females:	31 (100%)						136 (100%)	
% Males:	77.4						40.4	

D. IITA, Abomey-Calavi, Atlantique Province; 20.4.94; OS 7, in *Chromolaena odorata*

	In foliage and on ground		In foliage		On ground	
	Males	Females	Males	Females	Males	Females
Singles	170 (75.9%)	8 (3.6%)	139	8	31	0
In copula	22 (9.8%)	X 22 (9.8%)	18	X 18	4	X 4
Males "in copula"	1 X 1		1 X 1		0	
Total:	194	30	159	26	35	4
Total males + females:	224 (100%)					
% Males:	86.6					

B. Males and females as lures together in one cage (Tab. 3B).

(a) Lure cage at the OS. 109 males released at N (5 m north of the OS) and 126 females at S (5 m south of it).

(b) Lure cage at the OS. 122 males released at S and 118 females at N.

(c) Lure cage at S, empty cage at N. 72 males and 48 females released together at the OS.

C. Males and females as lures in separate cages (Tab. 3 C). Lure cage 1 at S, lure cage 2 at N.

(a) 104 males and 102 females released together 10 m to the west of the OS.

(b) 81 males and 83 females released together, as in replicate 1.

(c) 95 males and 85 females released together at the OS.

Results and discussion

Distribution of Z. variegatus at oviposition sites

The preponderance of males at OSs (ca. 70–85%; Tab. 1), mostly as singles in the foliage, suggests that males may initiate OSs, probably before they begin to copulate. Single females were much fewer than single males, most of the females being in copula (Tab. 1, 2). The total

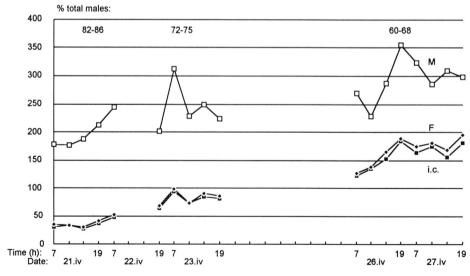

Figure 1. Variations in percentages of total males, and numbers of single males (M), single females (F) and in copula pairs (i.c.), with time at a *Chromolaena odorata* oviposition site (OS 7) in southern Benin.

number of females is only a little higher than that of the in copula pairs (Fig. 1). The few single females at OSs are probably newly arrived, or have just finished copulation or oviposition, because single females occur (on ground or in foliage) mostly where copulation is taking place (Tab. 1C, D; Tab. 2). The presence of supernumerary, "waiting" males, and mostly only paired females, indicates that the OS is an adaptation for ensuring insemination by the most competitive males and enhancing the reproductive success of the species.

Less than 50 m from OSs 4–6, the percentage of males was ca. 40 (Tab. 1B, C), but in the general population (80–200 m from OS 6), it was ca. 52. These facts suggest that males, unlike females, are particularly attracted to OSs over distances of <50 m, and remain there for longer periods. McCaffery and Page (1982) made a similar finding.

During a week of observation, the total numbers at OS 7 more than doubled (Tab. 2). More females than males arrived, the percentage of males declining from 86 to 60 (Fig. 1). As females

Table 2. The numbers and diurnal distribution of *Z. variegatus* adults in a *Chromolaena odorata* oviposition site (OS 7) in southern Benin. M - males; F - females

Date:		20.4.	21.4.				22.4.		23.4.			
Time (h):		15	7	11	15	19	7	19	7	11	15	19
Total M + F:		224	213	210	220	254	299	267	411	302	341	310
Singles M:	In foliage	139	138	111	151	163	196	136	211	122	151	137
	On ground	31	9	31	9	13	0	1	7	32	15	5
Singles F:	In foliage	8	3	0	4	4	5	4	4	0	5	2
	On ground	0	1	0	0	0	0	0	1	0	2	2
In copula M, F:	In foliage	18+18	29+29	27+27	26+26	37+37	48+48	60+60	88+88	51+51	83+83	78+78
	On ground	4+4	2+2	_7+7_	1+1	0+0	0+0	4+4	6+6	_23+23_	1+1	4+4
In copula F ovipositing:				7				1	3	10		

Date:		26.4.				27.4.				29.4.
Time (h):		7	11	15	19	7	11	15	19	11
Total M + F:		398	368	453	544	498	468	479	494	410
Singles M:	In foliage	146	55	84	167	160	82	145	108	102
	On ground	2	39	52	3	0	28	10	9	35
Singles F:	In foliage	6	4	11	4	12	6	12	15	9
	On ground	0	0	2	0	0	0	2	0	8
In copula M, F:	In foliage	121+121	107+107	146+146	185+185	163+163	148+148	142+142	181+181	43+43
	On ground	1+1	_28+28_	6+6	0+0	0+0	_27+27_	13+13	0+0	_85+85_
In copula F ovipositing:			15			12	6			80

in the general population become ready to oviposit, they probably become attracted to OSs (McCaffery and Page 1982).

Table 3. The numbers of reproductive adults of *Z. variegatus* attracted to others used as lures

A. Males and females used together, and separately, as lures

Cage No.	Adults used as lures, 6.5.93			Adults attracted, 7.5.93			
	Males	Males + Females	Females	Males		Females	
1	100			6		2	
2			37		0		0
3		51 + 51		1		1	
4	147			3		1	
5		52 + 52		3		0	
Total attracted to:	Male			9		3	
	Males + Females			4		1	
	Females				0		0

B. Males and females used together as lures

Expt	Adults used as lures			Adults attracted		
	Date	Males	Females	Date	Males	Females
(a)	28.9.93	208	187	1.10.93	18	14
(b)	1.10.93	199	176	5.10.93	34	15
(c)	15.10.93	60	72	19.10.93	7	3
Total attracted:					59	32

C. Males and females used separately as lures

Expt	Cage No	Adults used as lures			Adults attracted			
		Date	Males	Females	Date	Males		Females
(a)	1	5.10.93	187		8.10.93	24		6
	2			162			0	2
(b)	2	8.10.93	150		12.10.93	7		7
	1			143			2	3
(c)	2	12.10.93	110		15.10.93	15		2
	1			97			2	0
Total attracted to males:						46	15	
Total attracted to females:						4		5

Diurnal behaviour at an oviposition site

Total numbers at OS 7 peaked at either 07.00 or 19.00 h (Fig. 1), suggesting that OSs are also roosting sites. There were more singles in the foliage than on the ground, but a higher proportion of the single males descended at 11.00 and 15.00 h (Tab. 2). They are probably seeking moist conditions during the heat of the day, because many more males descended to OS patches that were experimentally watered than to patches that were not.

At 11.00 h, the number of in copula pairs on the ground increased considerably, with many of the females ovipositing (Tab. 2). McCaffery and Page (1982) also found maximal oviposition at 11.00–12.00 h. In addition, they found peak oviposition after rain. Here too the highest number of in copula pairs and ovipositing females on the ground occurred on 29.iv, after the only rain during the observations, on 28.iv (27.5 mm).

Attraction to a cleared OS

More of the adults released downwind than upwind of the empty OS arrived there, or were en route to it, after 24 h (Fig. 2). Conversely, more upwind than downwind releases moved away from the OS. McCaffery and Page (1982) also found that more *Z. variegatus* approached an

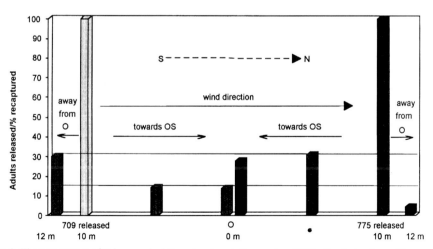

Figure 2. The percentages of colour-marked *Z. variegatus* adults recaptured 24 h after their release 10 m up- and downwind of their experimentally cleared oviposition site (OS).

OS from downwind. The attraction is therefore olfactory and acts over 10 m at least. The sexes do not respond differently: the sex ratios in the recoveries from all the sectors were similar.

Attraction between reproductive adults

More males and females were attracted to males than to females; females were only slightly attractive, even to other females (Tab. 3A, C). Also, ca. 2–3 times more males than females were attracted to males, or to males and females (Tab. 3A, B, C). These facts suggest that mutual attraction, mediated probably by pheromones, brings mature males together as the first step in OS establishment. Obeng-Ofori et al. (1994) found with *Schistocerca gregaria* (Forskål) that mature adult males, but not females, produce volatiles that cause aggregation in both sexes.

Conclusion

The olfactory attraction to an OS recently cleared of grasshoppers suggests an odour source other than the males, although it is possible that concentrated male odour may take time to dissipate. A plant odour is unlikely because OSs are not uniform in plant composition. Egg pods in the soil probably exert some attraction. Although released adults did not move to an OS (OS 6), recently cleared of adults but containing egg pods, when there were male lures a similar distance (5 m) away, a small proportion (comprising more males than females) released at OS 6 itself remained there and continued reproductive behaviour.

    Z. variegatus OSs are probably initiated when mature males aggregate by mutual attraction, at locations that supply shade and moisture. More males and females are then attracted to the aggregations. The sequence and numbers of arrivals, male and female responses, and the timing of mating and oviposition require study. Nothing is known also about the departure of females after oviposition and their subsequent behaviour leading to second and more cycles of oviposition. These are being investigated.

Acknowledgements
I thank Dr C.J. Lomer for useful comments on the manuscript, and Messrs Yacinthe Bocco, Firmin Obognon and Comlan Gbongboui for field assistance.

References

Chapman RF, Page WW (1978) Embryonic development and water relations of the eggs of *Zonocerus variegatus* (L.) (Acridoidea: Pyrgomorphidae). Acrida 7: 243–252

Chapman RF, Page WW, McCaffery AR (1986) Bionomics of the variegated grasshopper (*Zonocerus variegatus*) in west and central Africa. Ann Rev Entomol 31: 479–505

McCaffery AR, Page WW (1982) Oviposition behaviour of the grasshopper *Zonocerus variegatus*. Ecol Entomol 7: 85–90

Modder WWD (1978) Respiratory and weight changes, and water uptake, during embryonic development and diapause in the African grasshopper *Zonocerus variegatus* (L.) (Acridoidea: Pyrgomorphidae). Acrida 7: 253–265

Obeng-Ofori D, Njagi PGN, Torto B, Hassanali A, Amiani H (1994) Sex differentiation studies relating to releaser aggregation pheromones of the desert locust, *Schistocerca gregaria*. Entomol Exp Appl 73: 85–91

Page WW (1978) Destruction of eggs as an alternative to chemical control of the grasshopper pest *Zonocerus variegatus* (L.) (Orthoptera: Pyrgomorphidae) in Nigeria. Bull Entomol Res 68: 575–581

Page WW, McCaffery AR (1979) Characteristics and distribution of oviposition sites of the grasshopper *Zonocerus variegatus* (L.). Ecol Entomol 4: 277–288

New Strategies in Locust Control
S. Krall, R. Peveling and D. Ba Diallo (eds)
© 1997 Birkhäuser Verlag Basel/Switzerland

Potential for the use of semiochemicals against *Locusta migratoria migratorioides* (R. & F.)

M. Rosa Paiva

Universidade Nova de Lisboa, FCT/DCEA, Q.da Torre, P-2825 Monte de Caparica, Portugal

Summary. Pheromones, both of the primer and releaser type, have been detected in *Locusta migratoria*. Research is in progress aiming at the identification and future synthesis of semiochemicals that might find application in programmes of integrated management for this pest. In laboratory experiments, the oviposition rhythm and fecundity of virgin females were to some extent stimulated by the proximity of males. Chromatographic and mass spectrometric (MS) analysis of the semiochemicals of *L. migratoria migratorioides* were performed, and important variations in the composition of the bouquet of odours emitted by different stages, and sexes, were detected. Thus benzyl cyanide was only produced by sexually mature males, while by contrast, guaiacol was detected in nymphs and adults of both sexes, although females contained larger amounts. Different strategies, based on the use of semiochemicals, can be devised, aiming at the control and particularly the monitoring of populations of the migratory locust. Among them, the application of aggregation/arrestant pheromones to concentrate egg laying in pre-selected sites, where the eggs would afterwards be destroyed, preferably by bio-pesticides, should be considered. The use of maturation synchronisers could also be taken into account, to time adult development with unfavourable climatic periods. However, the implementation of methods resorting to the application of pheromones must be contemplated in combination with other techniques, such as cultural practices, within the scope of an encompassing Integrated Pest Management (IPM) programme.

Résumé. Des phéromones, tant du type phéromones modificatrices que du type phéromones de déclenchement, ont été décelées chez *Locusta migratoria*. Des recherches sont en cours en vue d'identifier et de synthétiser des substances sémio-chimiques pouvant être utilisées dans des programmes de lutte intégrée. Au cours d'essais conduits en laboratoire, le rythme des pontes et la fécondité de femelles vierges ont été dans une certaine mesure stimulés par la proximité des mâles. Des analyses chromatographiques et la spectrométrie de masse des substances sémio-chimiques de *L. migratoria migratorioides* ont permis la détection d'importantes variations dans la composition du bouquet d'odeurs émises à différents stades et par chacun des sexes. Ainsi, le cyanure de benzyle était produit uniquement par les mâles sexuellement mûrs, tandis que le guaïacol a été détecté sur les larves et les individus adultes des deux sexes, les femelles en sécrétant toutefois de plus grandes quantités. Différentes stratégies basées sur l'emploi de substances sémio-chimiques peuvent être élaborées pour lutter contre et surtout contrôler les populations de criquets migrateurs. Parmi ces stratégies, il conviendra de considérer l'utilisation de phéromones d'agrégation/de blocage afin de concentrer l'oviposition dans des sites préalablement sélectionnés et dans lesquels les oeufs seront ensuite détruits, préférablement par des bio-insecticides. On pourra également envisager l'emploi de synchroniseurs de maturation pour programmer le développement de l'adulte durant des périodes climatiques qui lui sont défavorables. Toutefois, l'application de méthodes basées sur l'emploi de phéromones devra s'effectuer en association avec d'autres techniques, telles que certaines pratiques culturales, dans le cadre d'un programme de lutte intégrée.

Introduction

Control of the migratory locust: brief summary

Similarly to other locusts, the economic and social impact caused by *Locusta migratoria migratorioides* (R. & F.) is difficult to quantify, its assessment depending largely on the spatial and temporal scales considered. Thus, at the world level economic damage is sometimes estimated as negligible, while on a regional basis, like in the Sahel, up to 90% of crop losses can occur (e.g. Wewetzer et al. 1993). In spite of an intensive search for alternative methods of control conducted over the last decades, insecticide spraying, mainly with organophosphates and carbamates, is still the primary weapon used against locusts (e.g. Onyeocha and Fuzeau-Braesch 1990).

Among the alternative methods tested, entomopathogenic fungi and bacteria achieved variable degrees of success (e.g. Krall and Knausenberger 1992). Botanicals, and particularly extracts of *Melia volkensii*, showed a high efficiency against the migratory locust (Rembold 1994) and appear as promising control agents, in particular due to their low environmental persistence (Peveling et al. 1994). Insect growth regulators (IGRs), including juvenile hormone analogues (JHAs) and benzoylphenyl ureas (BPUs), yielded positive results under laboratory conditions (Dorn et al. 1994; Peveling et al. 1994), but complete field data regarding their efficacy against *L. migratoria* and environmental impact studies are still lacking. Complementary to all other methods, remote sensing now offers a valuable contribution to the implementation of forecast systems and management options for locust populations (e.g. Voss and Dreiser 1994).

Research on behavioural chemicals of *L. m. migratorioides* has been initiated (Francke and Schmidt 1994; Martinho et al. 1995), but field tests have not yet been conducted. An analysis of the potential of semiochemicals, as monitoring and control agents of the migratory locust, is presented.

Semiochemical terminology

Karlson and Lüscher (1959) proposed the term *pheromone* to describe a volatile released by an organism that elicits a response from a receiver of the same species. Wilson (1963) further differentiated between pheromones of the releaser type, which trigger an immediate and reversible behavioural response in the receiver, and primers, which elicit either a physiological or behavioural alteration, occurring after a time-lag. On the other hand, the word *allomone* is used to describe a message aimed at an organism of a species different from that of the emitter.

Under the general designation of semiochemicals, both types of olfactory messages, pheromones plus allomones, are included. Another term, *infochemicals*, has been proposed (e.g. Dicke and Sabelis 1989) to express a concept identical to that of semiochemicals.

Pheromones of Locusta migratoria migratorioides

In addition to visual, acoustical and tactile stimuli, olfactory communication plays a key role in the bioecology of the Acrididae, pheromones being involved in the regulation of the gregarization, maturation and oviposition processes (e.g. Norris 1970; Schmidt and Osman 1988; Loher 1990).

The semiochemicals so far detected in *L. m. migratorioides* can be placed in two broad categories: pheromones influencing the pattern of oviposition, and/or fecundity parameters, and pheromones promoting gregarisation and/or synchronising development. However, the same substance may sometimes be involved in multiple functions, for example aggregation and oviposition regulation.

Oviposition and/or fecundity primers and releasers
Norris (1950), hinted at the existence of a female pheromone that would influence the egg-laying behaviour of neighbouring females. Highnam and Haskell (1964) reported a slower oocyte growth in crowded females of *L. m. migratorioides* in comparison to isolated ones, which was correlated with an accumulation of neurosecretory material in the pars intercerebralis. An inhibitory agent emitted by the other females prevented its release. Such findings agree with the fact that the duration of the pre-oviposition period is longer in crowded females of *L. migratoria* than in solitary ones (e.g. Pener 1990).

Lauga and Hatte (1977, 1978) observed that solitary females were attracted to oviposit on sand previously used by gregarious females; furthermore, their egg-laying rhythm was also modified. Laboratory observations of *L. m. migratorioides* detected a clear tendency for oviposition-prone females to become immobilised around the first one initiating egg laying, sometimes even grasping or partially mounting her (pers. observ.). Some field observations confirm this tendency (e.g. Ferenz et al. 1994). The probable existence of an oviposition-mediating pheromone of the arrestant type is now widely accepted, although its isolation has not yet been achieved. Lange and Laughton (1985) showed that an oviposition-stimulating factor was produced in the male accessory reproductive gland of the migratory locust. Investigations of the possible effects of male stimulation, upon female fecundity are in progress (Martinho et al. 1995).

Gregarisation pheromones and developmental synchronisers
Uvarov (1937) first pointed out that phase transformation in *L. migratoria* "does not depend on increase in numbers alone, but also on the sensory reactions of individuals to one another". Nolte (1963) detected the production of an olfactory stimulus by crowded locusts of *S. gregaria*

which affected the coloration of locusts reared in isolation. It is now believed that a gregarisation pheromone similarly exists in other species of Acrididae. In *L. migratoria*, this pheromone should influence phase transformation and induce aggregation (e.g. Loher 1990; Byers 1991).

Reported effects of a hypothetical gregarisation pheromone include colour and morphometric changes (e.g. Rowell 1971; Byers 1991), variations in the chiasmata formation rate during meiosis (Nolte 1976), shortening of developmental time for the 5th nymphal stage (Nolte 1976) and, in general, gregarisation powers. However, information about such indicators is contradictory (e.g. Nolte et al. 1970; Dearn 1974; Nolte 1976), thus rendering most conclusions questionable. Greenwood and Chapman (1984) further observed that solitarious 5th instar nymphs and adults of *L. migratoria* possess a larger number of olfactory sensillae in the antennae than gregarious forms, an evolutive trace that could present an adaptive value.

Guaiacol was one of two main components extracted from the faeces of nymphs of both sexes of *L. m. migratorioides* by Nolte et al. (1973). The second one was locustol (2-methoxy-5-ethylphenol, also called 5-ethyl-guaiacol), a substance indigitated to be a moulting synchroniser (Nolte et al. 1973; Nolte 1976). Nevertheless, the action as a primer of this nymphal pheromone could not be confirmed (e.g. Gillett 1983; Ferenz et al. 1994). Phenol, guaiacol and veratrol were identified from the air surrounding *L. m. migratorioides* (Fuzeau-Braesch et al. 1988), and a mixture of the three alcohols was shown to act as a "cohesion" pheromone for males and females alike. However, several authors criticised the bioassays performed (e.g. Byers 1991), so that final conclusions about the potential of these chemicals to mimic the effect of a gregarisation pheromone cannot be drawn.

Effect of male-female stimulation in *Locusta migratoria migratorioides*

Antecedents

For *Aiolopus thalassinus* and *S. gregaria* it has been shown that the presence of males, or even their proximity, can influence female longevity and fecundity (Schmidt and Albütz 1994; Schmidt and Othman 1994). Comparable experiments were carried out with *L. m. migratorioides* to determine the possible influence of primer pheromones emitted by sexually mature males upon the females, particularly their effect on patterns of oviposition and fecundity. A parallel aim was to detect and identify semiochemicals emitted by males or by females that could play a role in the process of olfactory communication.

Experimental procedure

The locusts used in all experiments originated from a culture of *L. m. migratorioides* maintained under controlled conditions (Schmidt and Osman 1988) at the University of Hannover, Germany. For each experiment, treatments consisted of 6 to 10 females kept in cages under the following conditions: Females mated with an equal number of males (A); virgin females kept in isolation from males (B); virgin females separated from an equal number of males by either a single or double net panel (mesh = 2 mm), through which visual, acoustical, olfactory and to some extent tactile contact was possible (C). Previous experiments conducted at the New University of Lisbon, Portugal (Martinho et al. 1995), compared treatments A and B with another treatment, where virgin females were kept separated from males by a perforated transparent acrylic wall, thus receiving visual, acoustical and some olfactory stimulation from them. The parameters quantified were the number of egg pods deposited, the number of viable larvae/egg pod produced per female per week, longevity and the duration of the periods of pre-oviposition, oviposition and post-oviposition.

A comparative analysis of the semiochemicals emitted by nymphs and adults of both sexes of *L. m. migratorioides* was also carried out. The volatiles were collected by freeze-drying the locusts, followed by washing with pentane. Alternatively, the air surrounding the insects was suctioned and concentrated over poropak, which was afterwards extracted with a solvent. The volatiles were analysed by gas chromatography and mass spectrometry (Mateus et al., in preparation).

Results and discussion

Table 1 and Figure 1 show some of the results obtained, referring to treatments A–C. Experiments are still in progress, and a complete analysis will be presented elsewhere (Paiva et al., in

Table 1. *L. migratoria migratorioides*. Mean ± SD for the number of egg pods and nymphs produced per female per week by females kept under different experimental conditions: mated ($n = 12$), virgin isolated from males ($n = 12$), virgin stimulated by males through a net ($n = 24$). a, b, c – differences encountered for all pairs, $p < 0.01$, non-parametric Wilcoxon rank sum test.

Fecundity parameters	Female condition		
	Mated $\bar{x} \pm s$	Virgin isolated $\bar{x} \pm s$	Virgin stimulated $\bar{x} \pm s$
Egg pods per female per week	1.2±0.6	0.7±0.2	1.1±0.6
Nymphs per female per week	31.6[a]±16.5	1.8[c]±2.4	6.5[b]±4.2

preparation). Table 1 expresses the mean number of egg pods and of nymphs produced per week per female over a period of nine weeks, under three experimental conditions. Using the non-parametric Wilcoxon rank sum test (Sokal and Rohlf 1981), a difference significant at $p <$ 0.01 was detected between the three groups of females regarding the number of nymphs produced. Figure 1a shows that the pattern of oviposition of virgin females, which were stimulated by males through a net, follows an intermediate trend between that of the mated and of the virgin isolated females. A similar tendency can be seen for the number of nymphs produced (Fig. 1b).

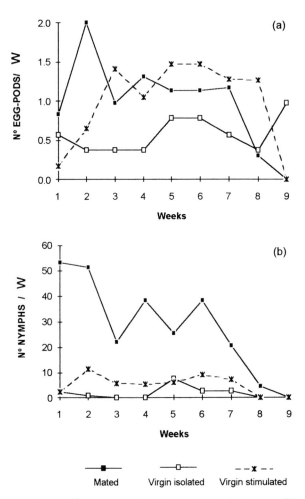

Figure 1. *L. migratoria migratorioides*: mean number of egg pods (a) and of nymphs (b) produced per week per female, under different experimental conditions. Mated females ($n = 12$), virgin females isolated from males ($n = 12$), virgin females separated from males by a net ($n = 24$).

Martinho et al. (1995) found a significant difference between the number of eggs/egg pods and the number of nymphs produced by mated females in comparison with virgin females whether isolated from males or stimulated by them, but without tactile contact.

Results of the analysis of the semiochemicals emitted by *L. m. migratorioides* indicate that certain substances are mainly produced by one of the sexes or by certain stages. Thus, sexually mature males produce benzyl cyanide, which was neither detected in the immature stages nor in the females (Mateus et al., in preparation). It is interesting to note that the same substance was also detected in mature males of *S. gregaria* (Francke and Schmidt 1994). Guaiacol was detected in nymphs and adults of both sexes of *L. m. migratorioides*, but females seem to produce larger amounts. The biological activity of these substances will be investigated next. It is probable that the substances detected in sexually mature stages only might have pheromonal action, influencing the life cycle of females. However, contact pheromones also appear to be involved in the process of chemical communication for this species.

Prospects for the use of semiochemicals in IPM strategies

From a purely economic perspective, it has been demonstrated that pesticide application can only be recommended under specific circumstances, such as the protection of high-value crops (e.g. Krall 1994). Regrettably few data exist regarding the assessment of environmental hazards resulting from large-scale insecticide spraying against locusts. Storage for up to several decades and final disposal of unused toxic products pose additional problems to developing countries (pers. observation). Given the non-periodic character of locust outbreaks, and the widely disparate ecological and social characteristics of the affected areas, flexible and diversified strategies of monitoring and control are clearly needed.

The role played by ecological factors in the development of outbreaks of *L. m. migratorioides* should be considered when delineating IPM strategies. Environmental disturbances, mostly anthropogenic, can be responsible for upsurges of the migratory locust (e.g. Farrow 1987). To diminish the risk of outbreaks, cultural practices such as preventing further destruction of secondary forest cover and scrub patches, avoiding burning and overgrazing of perennial grasslands and planting of soils that become exposed after flood recession must be considered. In general, densities of specialist herbivorous insects, such as *L. migratoria*, are higher in areas supporting monocultures than in diversified agro-habitats. The benefits of modifying the vegetation through diversification, rotation, inter cropping or trap cropping should be implemented, whenever possible.

Extensive field work was conducted by Farrow (1975) between 1963 and 1969 in Mali on *L. m. migratorioides,* while Price (1991) studied its the oviposition behaviour in South Africa. However, further behavioural and ecological investigations must be undertaken in nature before a field campaign is designed. Among other points, learning behaviour has been documented in the Acrididae (Szentesi and Jermy 1990), a feature which might compromise the long-term effectiveness of an initially successful IPM scheme in a way similar to the evolution of pest resistance to insecticides (e.g. Prokopy and Lewis 1993).

In spite of the ecological constraints that to a large extent shape the distribution and growth of this pest, it is believed that semiochemicals could in the future play a valuable role in locust monitoring and control (e.g. Byers 1991; Ferenz et al. 1994). Figure 2 summarises the sequential application of different control methods in population management schemes of *L. m. migratorioides.*

A possible strategy would consist in the application of female pheromones of the aggregation/arrestant type used to concentrate ovipositing females in pre-selected areas. Price (1991)

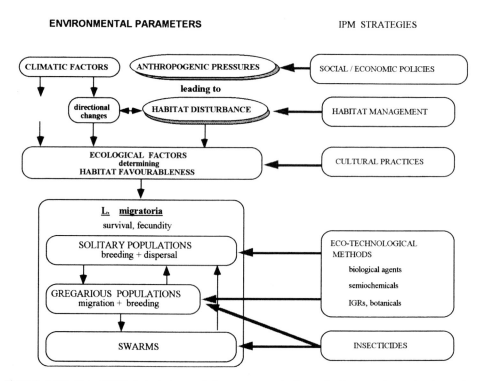

Figure 2. Application of IPM strategies in population management schemes for *Locusta migratoria migratorioides.*

noticed an aggregation of egg pods of the migratory locust in maize field areas where planting had failed or soil erosion had occurred, even if no arrestant effect of the females was observed. A higher concentration of egg pods could thus be achieved by maintaining ecologically suitable oviposition spots, such as cleared patches within crops and field edges, and reinforcing its attractiveness with pheromone dispensers. The egg pods would afterwards be destroyed, preferably by pathogenic organisms. Alternatively, an opposite strategy could aim at the dispersion of egg-laying sites to prevent swarm forming. Yet the range of attraction of these semiochemicals must be previously established, and further research is needed.

Phase change follows and does not precede variations in locust density, but the mechanisms underlying this process are not yet clearly understood. Corpora allata activity and the production of juvenile hormone are certainly important contributors, but they might not constitute the precursors of the physiological chain of events leading to phase change (e.g. Pener 1990). In the desert locust the production of a maturation accelerating pheromone is apparently controlled by the juvenile hormone (JH) titers (Loher 1961). Should the male specific semiochemicals detected in *L. m. migratorioides* act as development synchronisers, its application coupled with the use of JH analogues could be envisaged to time adult development with the occurrence of unfavourable climatic periods. Nevertheless, when attempting to manipulate phase changes caution must be excised, and experiments should first be conducted under strictly controlled seminatural conditions.

Acknowledgements
Warm thanks are due to Ms. R. Albütz and Ms. A. Martinho for technical assistance, respectively at the University of Hannover and at the New University of Lisbon. The research in progress is financed by the EU, contract no. TS 2*-CT90-0295. I thank the Deutsche Gesellschaft für Technische Zusammenarbeit (GTZ), Eschborn, for a travel grant to attend the meeting where this paper was presented, and the Alexander von Humboldt Stiftung, Bonn, for a fellowship that enabled my research stay at the University of Hannover.

References

Byers JA (1991) Pheromones and chemical ecology of locusts. Biol Rev 66: 347–378
Dearn JM (1974) Phase transformation and chiasma frequency variation in locusts. II. *Locusta migratoria*. Chromosoma 45: 339–352
Dicke M, Sabellis MW (1989) Does it pay to advertise for bodyguards? Pages 341–358 in Lambers H. et al. (eds) Causes and consequences of variation in growth rate and productivity of higher plants. The Hague, The Netherlands: SPB Acad. Publishing
Dorn A, Wiesel G, Schneider M (1994) Juvenile hormone analogues in locust control. Pages 91–106 in Krall S, Wilps H (eds) New trends in locust control. Schriftenreihe no 245. Eschborn: GTZ
Farrow R (1975) The african migratory locust in its main outbreak area of the middle Niger: quantitative studies of solitary populations in relation to environmental factors. Locusta 11: 197 pp
Farrow R (1987) Effects of changing land use on outbreaks of tropical migratory locust, *Locusta migratoria migratorioides* (R. & F.). Insect Sci Applic 8: 969–975

Ferenz HJ, Luber K, Wieting J (1994) Pheromones as a means of controlling migratory locusts. Pages 81–89 in Krall S, Wilps H (eds) New trends in locust control. Schriftenreihe no 245. Eschborn: GTZ

Francke W, Schmidt G (1994) Potential of semiochemicals for locust control. Pages 48–52 in Rembold H et al. (eds) New strategies for locust control in natural product and receptor research. ATSAF: Bonn

Fuzeau-Braesch S, Genin E, Jullien R, Knowles E, Papin C (1988) Composition and role of volatile substances in atmosphere surrounding two gregarious locusts, *Locusta migratoria* and *Schistocerca gregaria*. J Chem Ecol 14(3): 1023–1033

Gillett SD (1983) Primer pheromones and polymorphism in the desert locust. Animal Behaviour 31: 221–230

Greenwood M, Chapman RF (1984) Differences in numbers of sensilla on the antennae of solitarious and gregarious *Locusta migratoria* L. (Orthoptera, Acrididae). Internat J Insect Morphol Embryol13: 295–301

Highnam KC, Haskell PT (1964) The endocrine systems of isolated and crowded *Locusta* and *Schistocerca* in relation to oocyte growth, and the effects of flying upon maturation. J Ins Physiol 10: 849–864

Karlson P, Lüscher M (1959) Pheromones: a new term for a class of biologically active substances. Nature 183: 55–56

Krall, S. 1994. Importance of locusts and grasshoppers for African agriculture and methods for determining crop losses. Pages 7–22 in Krall S, Wilps H (eds) New trends in locust control. Schriftenreihe no 245. Eschborn: GTZ

Krall S, Knausenberger W (1992) Efficacy and environmental impact for biological control of *Nosema locustae* on locusts in Cape Verde: a synthesis report. Eschborn: GTZ

Lange AB, Laughton BG (1985) An oviposition-stimulating factor in the male accessory reproductive gland of locust, *Locusta migratoria*. Gen Comp Endocrin 57: 208–215

Lauga J, Hatte M (1977) Propriétés grégarisantes acquises par le sable dans lequel ont pondu à de nombreuses reprises des femelles grégaires de *Locusta migratoria migratorioides* R. & F. (Orthoptere, Acrididae) Acrida 6(4): 307–311

Lauga J, Hatte M (1978) L'activité grégarisante du sable de ponte chez *Locusta migratoria*: action sur le comportement et la réproduction des individus. Ann Sci Naturelles Zool Paris 20: 37–52

Loher W (1961) The chemical acceleration of the maturation process and its hormonal control in the male of the desert locust. Proc Royal Soc B 153: 380–397

Loher W (1990) Pheromones and their role in phase transformation in locusts. Pages 45–53 in Chapman RF, Joern A (eds) The biology of grasshoppers. New York: Wiley

Martinho AP, Santos T, Paiva MR (1995) Role of male-female stimulation in the bio-ecology of *Locusta migratoria migratotioides* (R. & F.). Avances en Entomología Ibérica, pp 421–430

Nolte D J (1963) A pheromone for melanization of locusts. Nature 200: 660–661

Nolte DJ (1976) Locustol and its analogues. J Insect Physiol 22: 833–838

Nolte DJ, Eggers SH, May IR (1973) A locust pheromone: Locustol. J Insect Physiol. 19: 1547–1554

Nolte DJ, May IR, Thomas BM (1970) The gregarization pheromone of locusts. Chromosoma 29: 462–473

Norris MJ (1950) Reproduction in the migratory locust (*Locusta migratoria migratorioides* R. & F.) in relation to density and phase. Anti-locust Bull no. 6: 1–48

Norris MJ (1970) Aggregation response in ovipositing females of the desert locust, with special reference to the chemical factor. J Insect Physiol 16: 1493–1515

Onyeocha FA, Fuzeau-Braesch S (1990) Comparative toxicity of some synthtic insecticides, and a growth inhibitor, in the migratory locust, *Locusta mirgratoria*. Comp Biochem Physiol 100(3): 361–363

Pener MP (1990) Endocrine effects on locust phase change: basic and applied aspects. Bol San Veg Plagas 20: 39–55

Peveling R, Weyrich J, Müller P (1994) Side effects of botanicals, insect growth regulators and entomopathogenic fungi on epigeal non-target arthropods in locust control. Pages 147–176 in Krall S, Wilps H (eds) New trends in locust control. Schriftenreihe no 245. Eschborn: GTZ

Price RE (1991) Oviposition by the African migratory locust, *Locusta migratoria migratorioides*, in a crop environment in South Africa. Entomol Exp Appl 61: 169–177

Prokopy RJ, Lewis WJ (1993) Application of learning to pest management. Pages 308–342 in Papaj DR, Lewis AC (eds) Insect learning – ecological and evolutionary perspectives. New York: Chapman & Hall

Rembold H (1994) Controlling locusts with plant chemicals. Pages 41–49 in Krall S, Wilps H (eds) New trends in locust control. Schriftenreihe no 245. Eschborn: GTZ

Rowell CHF (1971) The variable coloration of the acridoid grasshoppers. Adv Insect Physiol 8: 145–198

Schmidt G, Albütz R (1994) Laboratory studies and reproduction in the desert locust *Schistocerca gregaria* (Forsk.). J Appl Ent 118: 378–391

Schmidt G, Othman KSA (1988) Male pheromones and egg production in Acrididae. Pages 701–706 in Sehnal F, Zabza A, Denlinger D (eds) Endocrinological frontiers in physiological insect ecology. Wroclav. Tech. Univ. Press Wroclav

Schmidt G, Othman KSA (1994) Studies on the influence of pheromones on the reproduction of virgin and mated females of the Acridid *Aiolopus thalasinus* (Fabr.) (Insecta, Orthoptera, Acrididae). Zool Anz 233 (3/4): 75–116

Sokal RR, Rohlf F (1981) Biometry. San Francisco: Freeman

Szentesi A, Jermy T (1990) The role of experience in host plant choice by phytophagous insects. Pages 39–74 in Bernays EA (ed) Insect/plant interactions. Vol 2. Boca Raton: CRC Press

Uvarov BP (1937) Biological and ecological basis of locusts phases and their practical application. Fourth Intern. Locust Conference, Cairo, Egypt, 1936. Appendix 7: 16 pp

Voss F, Dreiser U (1994) Mapping of desert locust and other migratory pests habitats using remote sensing techniques. Pages 23–39 in Krall S, Wilps H (eds) New trends in locust control. Schriftenreihe no 245. Eschborn: GTZ

Wewetzer A, Krall S, Schulz FA (1993) Methods for the assessment of crop losses due to grasshoppers and locusts. Roßdorf: TZ-Verl.-Ges, 54pp

Wilson EO (1963) Pheromones. Sci Amer 208: 100–114

New Strategies in Locust Control
S. Krall, R. Peveling and D. Ba Diallo (eds)
© 1997 Birkhäuser Verlag Basel/Switzerland

Alternative strategy and tactics for the management of the desert locust, *Schistocerca gregaria* (Forsk.)

S. El Bashir

The International Center of Insect Physiology and Ecology, P.O. Box 30772, Nairobi, Kenya

Summary. The current locust control strategy has been modified from what was originally a preventive strategy to a crisis management strategy. This is because instead of pre-empting swarm development through surveillance and timely control, locust management efforts are withheld until a plague becomes imminent. For this reason the current strategy has become heavily dependent on the use of quick-acting, broad spectrum and environmentally hostile pesticides. An alternative strategy which focuses on pregregarious locusts and whose objective is to keep locusts permanently solitarious through environmentally benign tactics is discussed. This strategy and these tactics would be based on a good understanding of locust biology, behaviour and ecology, as well as on the application of the integrated pest management (IPM) concept. Locust semiochemicals will be used either to attract nymphs and adults to contaminated sites or to disperse an already gregarising population, thus preventing development of swarms.

Résumé. La stratégie de lutte contre le Criquet pèlerin est aujourd'hui une stratégie de gestion de crise alors qu'elle était auparavant une stratégie de lutte préventive. La raison en est qu'au lieu de prévenir le développement des essaims par une surveillance et un contrôle en temps opportun, les opérations de lutte sont retenues jusqu'au moment où le fléau acridien devient imminent. La réussite de la stratégie actuellement employée est donc devenue très fortement tributaire de la rapidité des opérations entreprises et est basée sur l'emploi de pesticides à large spectre d'action et déprédateurs de l'environnement. Cette étude analyse une stratégie alternative centrée sur les locustes en phase pré-grégaire et dont l'objectif est de maintenir constamment les criquets en phase solitaire par des techniques n'ayant qu'un impact faible sur l'environnement. Cette stratégie et ces techniques reposeront sur une bonne connaissance de la biologie, du comportement et de l'écologie des locustes, ainsi que sur l'application des principes de la lutte intégrée (integrated pest management - IPM). Des substances sémio-chimiques seront utilisées soit pour attirer des larves ou des ailés vers des sites contaminés soit pour disperser une population déjà en phase de grégarisation afin d'éviter la formation d'essaims.

Introduction

Desert locust upsurges usually develop in remote and thinly populated desert and semi-desert environs, hence their threat to rural farming communities is detected at very late stages. Because of their ability to migrate long distances, swarms of locusts may invade large areas within a short time, overwhelm pest control units in the affected countries and jeopardise community participation. As there is no reliable preventive control measure against gregarising populations, the fire-fighting approach is the most widely accepted practice. Preventive control strategies require heavy investment in human and material resources, even at times when there is no eminent threat of locust resurgence, an effort so far much less supported by donors and governments. On the other hand, the costs of current locust control practices are also prohibitive, as they depend on aerial and ground application of large quantities of insecticides to widely scattered infested sites. However, because of the emergency nature of the locust invasions and the accompanying political pressures, generous donations are provided by various donors to locust-affected countries. More often than not, a large proportion of the donated pesticides become a liability to recipients, especially after the end of a plague, because of inadequate storage and disposal facilities.

The high costs of the current strategy, and the potential environmental risks involved, prompted a vigorous search for more effective and environmentally acceptable alternatives. The development of an alternative strategy requires thorough understanding of factors mediating phase change, and better knowledge of the dynamics of locust populations in recession and breeding habitats.

The current strategy and tactics of locust control

The current locust control strategy is claimed to be a preventive one which, during upsurges, changes into a plague containment and eventually to a crop protection or plague elimination effort (Symmons 1992). Effective surveillance is essential for a successful preventive control strategy. Information on the state of locust development, population density and degree of gregarisation can be obtained only by active ground survey teams, as faster methods are not yet available. Ground surveys require well-trained and motivated field staff in all countries within the recession zone, in addition to reliable transport facilities and efficient means of communication. Only a few locust-affected countries provide funds for surveys during recession periods, because locust control is not a priority at such times. Most of the donors also find it difficult to support locust-affected countries during recession periods for fear of mismanagement of donated funds and materials. As a result, almost a total breakdown of locust control units is witnessed in plagued countries, especially during prolonged recession periods, as was the case preceding the 1986–1989 desert locust plague. On the other hand, governments of locust-affected countries and donor agencies become extremely supportive for any locust control activities during plague upsurges. This was very well illustrated in the 1986–1989 desert locust plague control effort (Skaf et al. 1990). The political environment during plague periods is very favourable for government spending, especially in donor countries in which the electronic media focus on the ravages of locust swarms. However, in view of the ever-increasing costs of locust control campaigns, the high environmental risk involved and the fact that the insecticide-based strategy has never succeeded in ending a plague, future support of the current approach is likely to diminish.

The choice of the currently used chemical control methods and tactics depends very much on the developmental stage of the insect, and the size and location of the target; but in general, aerial spraying of ultra low volume (ULV) formulations of insecticides is the most preferred method; this is because water is a rare commodity in many of the infested areas. Aerial spraying is only feasible where large areas are involved; thus in the case of scattered hopper bands and swarm-lets, knapsack and vehicle-mounted sprayers as well as dusting equipment are commonly used. Sometimes emulsifiable insecticide concentrates (EC) are also sprayed in very restricted areas.

Alternative strategy and tactics of locust control

The proposed alternative strategy is a preventive, environmentally friendly and sustainable one; its focus is on pregregarious locusts, and its goal is to keep locusts permanently solitarious, through the implementation of integrated pest management tactics.

Locusts occur in distinct gregarious and solitarious phases, as well as in transitional forms. In the solitarious phase, locusts are found in low numbers, but as soon as they transform into the gregarious phase and develop hopper bands and swarms, they pose a serious threat to agriculture and natural resources. The goal of the alternative strategy is to keep locusts permanently solitarious. This formidable task may be attained through the manipulation of solitary populations so that numbers are kept constantly at low levels. Alternatively, the process of gregarisation can be disrupted so that rapid population build-up is prevented. Successful interventions at these two levels should virtually contain the locust menace and decrease dependence on environmentally hostile chemical pesticides.

The development of viable interventions at the pre-swarming phase requires research on the elements of an integrated desert locust management strategy, embracing the use of semiochemicals (chemical signals produced by one organism which initiate behavioural or physiological responses in another organism), in conjunction with biological and other control agents, within a proven knowledge of locust behaviour, ecology and population dynamics. Our emphasis has been on the study of the fundamental biological processes responsible for the control and modification of locust behaviour. In this respect, much attention has been focused on the role of the semiochemicals mediating the processes of gregarisation, synchronisation and acceleration of sexual maturation. Investigations of the chemical identity of the pheromones which mediate sex attraction in solitary locusts and oviposition behaviour of gravid females were also conducted.

Aggregation pheromone complex

The pheromone system of the gregarious phase of the desert locust is a complex one, derived both from live insects and their faeces (Obeng-Ofori et al. 1994). Behavioural bioassays showed two distinct sets of releaser pheromones which affect the aggregation behaviour of the desert locust: a juvenile aggregation pheromone specific to nymphs and an adult aggregation phero-mone specific to the adult stage. The nymphal pheromone system is produced by and stimulates individuals of both sexes, while that of the adults is produced only by males, but it is equally responded to by both sexes. Sexually immature adults of either sex do not produce a stimulus with a significant activity (Obeng-Ofori et al. 1993). The adult pheromone system consists of major and minor components, while the nymphal pheromone system consists of a number of components of which the following have so far been identified: phenol, guaiacol, benzaldehyde, acetophenone and phenylethanol. Phenol and guaiacol are the most common electrophysiolo-gically active components of the nymphal and young adult faeces, while phenylacetonitrile, phe-nol and guaiacol are the most predominant compounds in the older adult faecal volatiles. It is interesting to note that phenylacetonitrile, which is only found in the adult faecal volatiles, has been shown to have a significant solitarising stimulus on nymphs (D. Obeng-Ofori, ICIPE, per-sonal communication). This finding supports the conclusions of Gillett and Phillips (1977) that adult faeces had the effect of making nymphs less gregarious. This finding may have an impor-tant practical implication, since an effective dispersant could prevent or delay gregarisation of nymphs, thus help keep locusts in a solitary state.

Maturation pheromones

Maturation synchrony and group oviposition help to sustain critical locust population densities necessary for maintaining the gregarious phase. Pheromones have been implicated in regulating maturation in the gregarious desert locust, thus a maturation-accelerating pheromone associated with mature males was suggested (Norris 1954) and a maturation-retarding pheromone associa-ted with the immature stages of locust was also proposed. The two pheromonal systems operate in a manner that retards and accelerates maturation according to population structure and the prevailing ecological conditions, hence ensuring cohesiveness and sustaining the gregarious phase. Analysis of mature male volatiles shows that there are at least five compounds implicated in the process of maturation-acceleration, and that these compounds are also known to induce aggregation in adults (Mahamat et al. 1993). This suggests that the same pheromone blend is implicated in a parsimonious role as an adult aggregation signal and as an accelerant of maturation, and indicates a similar dual role for volatile pheromone emissions of the nymphs (Mahamat et al. 1993). Volatiles from fifth instar nymphs have been found to retard maturation of immature adults. These findings confirm earlier observations and provide evidence of pheromonal mediation in the process of maturation synchrony in the desert locust. However, it is not clear how these pheromones can be effectively used as components of a practical locust management strategy.

Oviposition aggregation pheromones

Under field conditions gravid females were observed to lay eggs in close proximity to one another. Although this group oviposition behaviour could be stimulated by visual, tactile and chemical cues, emphasis was more on the chemical stimulus. Behavioural experiments clearly indicate that females are attracted to a common egg-laying site by a chemical signal associated with the froth of the egg pods and that females preferred to oviposit in moist sand contaminated with froth. Electroantennogram recordings confirmed the presence of olfactory receptors on the antennae that were responsive to compounds in the extracts and the volatile collections of the froth. The results implicate froth-derived chemicals in the communal oviposition behaviour of gregarious desert locust females, but it is also possible that this behaviour is modulated by both the froth-derived oviposition pheromone system and the adult aggregation pheromone. The components of the oviposition pheromone system are not yet fully identified.

Sex pheromones

Mate finding in gregarious locusts is relatively easy because of the high densities at which these insects occur however, solitarious phase locusts, which usually occur in thinly scattered populations, must have a mechanism that brings the opposite sexes together for mating, and it should preferably be of a long-range type so as to minimise the search effort. Visual and acoustic cues do not seem to play a major role in mate finding in the desert locust, because solitarious males are attracted toward virgin unmated females in a wind tunnel, in the absence of visual and acoustic cues, which affirms the presence of a female-produced volatile sex pheromone (Inayatullah et al. 1993). Complimentary gas chromatograph electroantenn-ographic detector (GC-EAD) studies also indicate that the volatile collections from solitarious females elicit response in olfactory receptors of male antennae. Investigations to determine the chemical identity of the sex pheromone components are now nearly complete.

Tactics

Pheromones have been used in the field for mating disruption in the cotton bollworm (Baker et al. 1990) and for mass trapping of the spruce bark beetle (Bakke and Lie 1989), but it is unlikely that they can be employed for mating disruption or mass trapping of the desert locust. However, sex pheromones may be incorporated in colour or light traps for monitoring locust populations in a recession and breeding habitat. The trap may also be treated with spores of a virulent pathogen which infects escaping males that can spread the disease among the locust population in the vicinity. Similarly, the oviposition-aggregating pheromone can be used for attracting gravid females to a contaminated common egg-laying site. On the other hand, the aggregation pheromones could be employed to concentrate hoppers at certain focal points where they form easy targets for treatment with a suitable control agent, provided that the pheromones are perceived from a reasonably long distance.

Another tactic embraces the application of dispersants or anti-aggregants on hopper bands to break up the cohesive groupings and force individuals into a solitarious state. However, these pheromones have to be sufficiently stable so that they may remain active for a long time in the field, because repeated treatment of remote sites with unstable pheromones in order to suppress gregarising behaviour of hoppers may prove to be a highly unsustainable effort. There is also a need to select suitable sites within the extensive recession and breeding zone where these pheromones can be dispensed. The proper location of these sites requires new technologies such as remote sensing, Geographic Information System (GIS) and simulation modelling in which the information generated from the extensive field testing of semiochemicals is incorporated. Accurate forecasting of population movements and of locust breeding and development conditions are of paramount importance for the success of this approach.

Discussion and conclusions

Although semiochemicals have been successfully used in the field for the management of some pests, they are not generally considered to be sufficiently robust or reliable in their action to be used alone (Smart et al. 1994). They are less persistent than most pest control chemicals, hence, they have to be repeatedly applied to achieve satisfactory pest control (Griffiths 1990). These non-toxic, behaviour-modifying compounds are not known to have significant negative environmental impact. However, they are only effective when used as part of integrated control strategies, for monitoring or for direct manipulation of pest populations. Not all the discovered locust semiochemicals can be used in the development of an alternative control strategy, but there are a few which hold reasonable promise. Of these the aggregation/solitarisation, oviposition-aggregating and sex pheromones offer possibilities for use mainly against gregarising and pregregarious solitary living individuals. The use of semiochemicals for the manipulation of gregarious locusts is not envisaged, because there is hardly a better alternative to quick-acting pest control agents against swarms and hopper bands.

At present we can only speculate about possible uses of locust semiochemicals for the management of this pest, because only laboratory data and very limited field experience are at hand. Nonetheless, the aggregation/solitarisation pheromone complex appears to operate under field conditions. This complex and the oviposition-aggregating pheromones could be used for suppressing locust populations at the early stages of gregarisation, while the sex pheromone is mainly for monitoring. Yet the problem is how to detect those early stages in time, how to apply the material and for how long the semiochemicals and the incorporated locust control agents would remain active. There is no answer yet to any of these questions, hence research must continue to resolve these and other important issues. It is also necessary to take note of the logistics required to cover all the complementary breeding areas within the locust recession zone, which is vast, sparsely populated and has poor infrastructure.

In this connection, the role of locust-affected countries, regional and international organisations and the donor community should be emphasised. Rural communities in countries affected by locust plagues should be motivated by their respective governments to participate in monitoring and control activities. Regional and international organisations should provide technical and material support to affected countries, and donors should not wait until the last moment before pledging their support. The success of the proposed alternative strategy very much depends on improved forecasting, efficient surveillance of recession areas, effective community participation, good information exchange, continuous training of locust control personnel and adequate funding.

References

Baker TC, Staten RT, Flint HM (1990) Use of pink bollworm pheromone in the Southwestern United States. Pages 417–436 in Ridgway RL, Silverstein RM, Inscoc MN (eds) Behaviour modifying chemicals for insect management. New York, Basel: Marcel Dekker

Bakke A, Lie R (1989) Mass trapping. Pages 67–87 in Jutsum AR, Gordon RFS (eds) Insect pheromones in plant protection. Chichester: Wiley

Gillett SD, Phillips M (1977) Faeces as a source of a locust gregarisation stimulus. Effects on social aggregation and on cuticular colour of nymphs of the desert locust, Schistocerca gregaria (Forskål). Acrida 6: 279–286

Griffiths DC (1990) Opportunities for control of insects in arable crops using semiochemicals and other unconventional methods. Proc 1990 Br Crop Prot Confr Pests Diseases, Brighton: 487–496

Inayatullah C, El Bashir S, Hassanali A (1993) Sexual communication in the desert locust (Orthoptera: Acrididae): an evidence of a sex pheromone. Environmental Entomology 23: 1544–1551

Mahamat H, Hassanali A, Odongo H, Torto B, El Bashir ES (1993) Studies on the maturation-accelerating pheromone of the desert locust Schistocerca gregaria (Orthoptera:Acrididae). Chemoecology 4: 159–164

Norris MJ (1954) Sexual maturation in the desert locust, Schistocerca gregaria (Forskål), with special reference to the effects of grouping. Anti-Locust Bull 18: 1–4

Obeng-Ofori D, Torto B, Hassanali A (1993) Evidence for mediation of two releaser pheromones in the aggregation behaviour of gregarious desert locust, Schistocerca gregaria (Forskål) (Orthoptera: Acrididae). J Chem Ecol 19: 1665–11676

Obeng-Ofori D, Torto B, Njagi PGN, Hassanali A, Amiani H (1994) Faecal volatiles as part of the aggregation pheromone complex of the desert locust, Schistocerca gregaria (Forskål) (Orthoptera: Acrididae). J Chem Ecol 20: 2077–2087

Skaf R, Popov GB, Roffey J (1990) The desert locust: an international challenge. Phil Trans R Soc Lond B 328: 525–538

Smart LE, Blight MM, Pickett JA, Pye BJ (1994) Development of field strategies incorporating semiochemicals for the control of the pea and bean weevil, Sitona lineatus L. Crop Protection 13: 127–135

Symmons P (1992) Strategies to combat the desert locust. Crop Protection 11: 206–212

New Strategies in Locust Control
S. Krall, R. Peveling and D. Ba Diallo (eds)
© 1997 Birkhäuser Verlag Basel/Switzerland

Pheromones in *Schistocerca gregaria* (Forsk.): the present situation

G.H. Schmidt

Lehrgebiet Zoologie-Entomologie, FB Biologie, Universität Hannover, Herrenhäuser Straße 2, D-30419 Hannover, Germany

Summary. Chemical signals play an important role in species-specific communication of Acrididae, and the following were observed in *Schistocerca gregaria*: accelerated maturation among grouped immature adults in the presence of a single mature (yellow) male; stimulation of egg pod deposition among virgin females separated from males by a perforated foil; reduction of melanisation among nymphs reared in isolation; acceleration of chiasma formation during meiosis; a positive reaction to releaser pheromones in nymphs and adults; mass deposition of egg pods mediated by strips of paper contaminated by female locusts. Head-space chromatographic analysis identified 13 volatile compounds in mature males and six in mature females. The chromatograms obtained for 5th instar nymphs were similar to those of the females. The main compounds identified were guaiacol, veratrole, phenol and benzylnitrile, the latter being found only in mature males and their faeces. All substances *"per se"* elicited an antennal reaction. A specific strong response was observed in immature adults when a mixture, corresponding to that in the head space of sexually mature males, was used.

Résumé. Chez les locustes et les sauteriaux (Acrididae), les signaux chimiques jouent un rôle important dans la communication entre individus co-spécifiques. Chez *S. gregaria,* les signaux chimiques suivants ont pu être observés: Accélération de la maturation chez des insectes adultes immatures groupés en présence d'un seul mâle mature (jaune); stimulation du dépôt d'oothèques dans les groupes de femelles vierges séparées des mâles par une feuille d'aluminium finement perforée; réduction du mélanisme parmi les larves élevées dans l'isolation; accélération de la formation de chiasmata durant la méiose; réaction positive à des phéromones de déclenchement tant chez les larves que chez les individus adultes; dépôt en masse d'oothèques provoqué par des bandelettes de papier contaminées préalablement par des locustes femelles. L'analyse chromatographique de l'espace de tête a permis l'identification de 13 composés volatiles chez les mâles matures et de 6 chez les femelles matures. Les chromatogrammes obtenus pour les larves de 5ème stade étaient similaires à ceux des femelles. Les principaux composants identifiés étaient le guaïacol, le vératrol, le phénol et le cyanure de benzyle, ce dernier composant n'ayant été trouvé que chez les mâles matures et dans leurs fèces. Chacune des substances «per se» a déclenché une réaction des antennes. Toutefois, une réaction spécifique très nette a pu être observée chez les adultes immatures lorsque nous avons utilisé un mélange de composants correspondant à celui que l'on trouve dans l'espace de tête de mâles sexuellement mûrs.

Introduction

There is no doubt that apart from optical, tactile and acoustic signals, pheromones have an influence on behavioural and physiological processes of locusts and grasshoppers. These pheromones (Karlson and Lüscher 1959) are produced in glands and transferred to individuals of the same species at close range or by contact. Primer pheromones effect long-term morphometric, behavioural and genetic changes, while releaser pheromones cause an immediate behavioural response. These chemical compounds are species specific with varying responses in different species. Often the response is to a mixture (bouquet) of chemical compounds varying between species.

Pheromones are perceived at extremely low concentrations through the antennae (Slyfer et al. 1959) and affect the sexual, aggregation and oviposition behaviour and physiology. These three pheromone effects combine to cause gregarisation in desert and migratory locusts. The aim is to control locusts with the least impact on the environment by applying pheromones and antipheromones to manipulate aggregation behaviour. In *Schistocerca gregaria* six pheromones have been reported.

Maturation-acceleration pheromone

Norris (1954) suggested that pheromones stimulate sexual maturation in the desert locust, affecting behaviour, body coloration in aggregated locusts, especially males (from brown to yellow), and maturation of the gonads. Paired adults copulated about four weeks after emergence and after 17 days (though with a wide range) if a single mature male was added. The change of colour was enhanced, and oviposition occurred earlier. This chemical acceleration factor is more significant in locusts reared in groups than singly or in pairs.

Loher (1960, 1961) demonstrated that yellow males produce an oily aromatic substance in vacuolised epidermal cells of the abdominal tergites. The pheromonal effect was not identified. Thomas (1972) found these epidermal cells in smaller numbers also in mature females. Kendall (1972) found that a glandular epidermis is also present in the dorsal part of the first segments of the tarsi and that vacuoles appear only at the onset of sexual maturation.

It is unknown whether the gland product is the maturation-acceleration pheromone. However, Norris (1954, 1962, 1963, 1964, 1968) showed that males matured faster if treated with cotton wool impregnated with extracts. Sexual maturation, yellow coloration and pheromone production are influenced through the corpora allata stimulated by an airborne factor through the antennae. Allatectomy and antennal cutting stopped these physiological processes in *Aiolopus thalassinus* (Fabr.) (Schmidt and Othman 1994). However, males reared singly and not yellow also accelerated the maturation process of conspecific adults (Amerasinghe 1978).

Recently Mahamat et al. (1993) confirmed the acceleration effect of mature *S. gregaria* males on immature males and females by placing mature male head-space volatiles in the upper chamber and the recipients in the lower chamber of a two-chamber bioassay system. The volatiles were a mixture of anisole, veratrole, benzaldehyde, benzylnitrile and 4-vinylveratrole, roughly in the ratio of 4.8 : 3.3 : 7.0 : 79.8 : 5.0.

Egg pod-forming stimulation pheromone

In *S. gregaria* grouped virgin females kept far away from males produce significantly fewer egg pods, and the interval between two ovipositions is more than twice as long as for those paired with males (30.1 and 14.3 days, respectively). The egg-laying interval can be shortened, if virgin females are separated from males by a wirenet or perforated aluminium foil, indicating that males produce an airborne stimulus (pheromone). While the number of egg pods produced increased, the total number of eggs per female was slightly lower compared with paired females. On the other hand, if males were kept separated, females were disorientated in finding the moist spots, resulting in an increase in mislaid egg pods (Schmidt and Albütz 1994).

Melanisation pheromone

All nymphal stages of locusts reared in groups have more black spots than ones reared singly. Melanisation resulted in totally black 1st instar nymphs being produced. Melanin appears partly in the exuviae of grouped nymphal stages, and is lost in the next moult in singly reared ones. In grouped nymphs, the melanin lost is resynthesised, but in isolated nymphs the body coloration becomes lighter, and the next exuviae contains no pigment (Schmidt, 1996).

Nolte (1963) observed that melanin is lost only in part, and more slowly in isolated nymphs, if reared with aggregated locusts in the same room. If *S. gregaria* is reared in isolation, the pigment is lost faster and is almost totally reduced. Results from translocation experiments indicate that a pheromone surrounding aggregated *S. gregaria* nymphs is responsible for the melanisation and also for morphometric changes.

Gillett (1968) experienced difficulties in attempting to reverse the gregarious behaviour of locusts to that of isolated individuals in a mass-rearing room. If the locusts were reared far from the breeding room, the grouping behaviour was lost, indicating an airborne factor not only influenced the nymphs but also intensified the grouping behaviour and melanisation of adults. Nolte et al. (1970) introduced, prematurely, the term "gregarisation pheromone".

Fuzeau-Braesch et al. (1988) analysed the volatile compounds present in cages with 5th instar nymphs, immature adults or copulating and ovipositing adults of various locust species by gas chromatography and mass spectroscopy. Four aromatic substances were found, and phenol, guaiacol and veratrole were identified. The four compounds were produced by *S. gregaria* and *Locusta migratoria* (L.), but in different ratios, and various factors may be operating. In all cases, guaiacol was the main compound which alone, or in combination with the other substances, induced aggregation effects.

Chiasma induction factor

Nolte (1968) found a volatile factor trapped using one or two solvents in rearing rooms of *S. gregaria*. It increases chiasma formation in chromosomes of the spermatocytes during meiosis, which facilitates genetic recombination. A pad of cotton wool, impregnated with the extract, was placed under a wire mesh at the bottom of one-litre jar containing a solitarious 4th instar hopper which had been isolated during the 3rd instar. This exposure caused a high chiasma frequency also with 4th and 5th nymphal instars in the three long and five medium chromosomes of testes cells, during the mid-diplotene stage of meiosis, counted during the first week of adult life. Individuals retained the remaining dark coloration during their nymphal life, but no significant morphometric changes towards the gregarious phase were found in the adult stage (Nolte et al. 1970).

Oil extracts from different body parts of crowded hoppers showed that the highest values of chiasma frequency (up to 30%) were obtained from the foregut, particularly from the crop. Treatment with crop extracts also caused retention of 65% of the initial 3rd instar black coloration; the elytron/femur length (E/F) and femur length/head (caput) (F/C) ratios tended to change towards the gregarious form. The compound is probably synthesised in the crop and excreted with the faeces. This could be demonstrated by exposing solitarious, single hoppers to faecal material from solitarious hoppers, but also from gregarious ones of either sex. Autostimulation did not occur probably because concentrations would be too low. The compound also acted to some extent on at least three other locust species. This means that no "pheromone" exists which induces chiasmata; the substance may be present in all faeces of grass-feeding hoppers and locusts. Faeces from adults had no effect on transformation towards the gregarious phase.

The gregarisation effect of faeces from crowded nymphs, reflected in the retention of black pigmentation in solitary hoppers, has been confirmed for 2nd instar nymphs of *S. gregaria*. The pink/beige background coloration persisted as well (Gillett and Phillips 1977). In addition, the hoppers exhibited strong social behaviour by grouping closely together under the influence of the faeces, in contrast to the controls. According to the authors mentioned above, gregarisation criteria of black colour retention and grouping behaviour were linked to the same factor. In spite of these observations, it remains unclear whether a factor from the faeces increases gregarisation or not, since Dearn (1974) could not find any difference in the chiasma frequency of the chromosomes in testes between isolated and grouped locusts.

Nolte (1976) used steam to distil two kilograms of faeces of grouped hoppers, and extracted the distillate with pentane. After purification a brownish oil was obtained, and thin-layer chromatography yielded two major and several minor compounds. Guaiacol and 5-ethyl-guaiacol were identified by gas chromatography and mass spectrometry, and both showed considerable activity in increasing chiasma frequency. After exposure to guaiacol, only 20% of the black hopper colour was retained (10% in the controls), whereas 5-ethylguaiacol preserved 80% of the pigmentation. Guaiacol had no effect on the F/C ratio, but 5-ethyl-guaiacol significantly lowered it approaching the gregarious state. Finally, guaiacol had no effect on nymphal marching behaviour, whereas 5-ethyl-guaiacol enhanced it. For these reasons, 5-ethyl-guaiacol was considered to posses all the properties exhibited by the pheromone from the hopper faeces. The substance, named locustol (Nolte et al. 1973), was considered to gregarise isolated solitarious hoppers. In our studies, it was found neither in faeces nor in volatiles obtained by head space of various developing stages of *S. gregaria* and *L. migratoria* (Francke and Schmidt 1994).

Nymphal and adult releaser pheromones

Using an olfactometer constructed specifically for this purpose, Obeng-Ofori et al. (1993) found a positive reaction to air columns coming from grouped nymphs and adults of *S. gregaria*. Nymphs tested singly or in groups preferred the part of the air column with volatile head space of nymphs, and were indifferent to that of the adults. In contrast, older adults reacted only to their own volatiles, and not to those of nymphs or young adults, whereas the latter were lured only by volatiles from older adults. Volatile compounds from nymphs and young adults absorbed on charcoal filters, produced the same effect as living locusts. Torto et al. (1994) showed by different synthetic blends that the volatile extract of older adult locusts consists of benzylnitrile, guaiacol, phenol and benzaldehyde, which belong to the aggregation pheromone system of the adult gregarious locust. Locust nymphs reacted neither to the volatile extract nor to the adult pheromone blend. The results showed that in *S. gregaria* there are two different aggregation pheromones: a juvenile attracting pheromone produced by nymphs, and an adult attracting one, acting specifically on the imagoes. A sexual specificity was not found.

Oviposition-mediating pheromone

Field observations and laboratory experiments have shown that mature females of various acridid species aggregate near an ovipositing female to lay eggs, and Norris (1963) observed that conspecific females even remained near a site less favourable for egg laying.

In experiments with *S. gregaria* live males and nymphs of the last instar were used as decoys. In the dark, touching of decoys, dead or alive, was necessary for an egg-laying locust to oviposite near them. Using paper strips, across which female locusts had crawled previously, has shown that a chemical factor was involved.

Females without antennae still found live decoys but were much less responsive if separated by gauze or to dead ones, suggesting that chemotactile stimuli must be involved. According to Norris (1970) the pheromone which is involved in aggregating egg-laying females is not only present in the 5th nymphal instar but also in the freshly produced exuviae. Interestingly, sand into which *S. gregaria* had formerly laid many egg pods was not attractive to females ready for egg laying in spite of relicts of oviposition ducts, faeces or pieces of froth plugs (Norris 1970). To a lesser extent isolated desert locusts also produce such a substance, but its chemical structure and how it is perceived are unknown.

Chemical compounds with possible pheromonal action

Some years ago a collaboration with Prof. W. Francke, Hamburg University, was begun to isolate and identify the volatile substances produced by the nymphal instars and adults of *S. gregaria*. We extracted the volatiles using the head-space technique and by washing the cuticle with pentane (Francke and Schmidt 1994).

Head-space volatiles

In a closed-loop-system the volatiles emitted by locusts were trapped by means of micro-charcoal filters and extracted with CS_2 for GC-MIS-analysis. Several aromatic compounds were identified, of which phenol, guaiacol and veratrole had already been described by Fuzeau-Braesch et al. (1988). Benzylnitrile was always found to be a main sex-specific component in adult males, the amount increasing with maturation. 2-Methoxy-5-ethylphenol (locustol), which Nolte et al. (1973) had described as a locust pheromone, was never found, instead we identified 4-vinylveratrole, the structure of which is closely related to locustol.

Less volatile compounds

These compounds, soluble in pentane, may be transported through the air, absorbed on scales upon release and act as pheromones over short distances or by direct contact. Extracts obtained by washing adult males with pentane contained a number of straight-chain hydrocarbons dominated by nonacosane. The co-eluting compounds could be identified by mass spectrometry and retention indices.

Oxygen-containing compounds are present as *cis-trans* mixtures of tetrahydrofuranes, and the compounds with the molecular formulas $C_{29}H_{58}O$ and $C_{30}H_{60}O$, respectively, were identified as 3,7-dimethylheptacosan-2-one, while the homologue shows an additional methyl-branching. Their biological function is under investigation.

Proof of perceiving volatile compounds with electroantennography

Some substances identified from the head space of the desert locust were phenol, veratrole, guaiacol, 1,2,3-trimethoxybenzol and benzylnitrile. Each substance, and a mixture of these (found in sexually mature males), was tested electroantennographically on sexually mature and immature males and females.

All compounds had a significant reaction on the antenna indicating that receptors are located on the antenna. The strong reaction observed to the mixture of these substances in immature males and females could not be attributed to a single substance. Therefore, we assume that these are additive or synergistic effects (Klause-de-Pupka et al., in press).

Discussion and conclusion

Work has been done on the pheromones of African locusts and grasshoppers over the last 40 years. Reference has been made to a pheromone accelerating the maturation of adult males and females of the desert locust and synchronising oviposition. This effect seems to be caused by a volatile chemical. However, touch produced a greater response than did airborne response received by the antennae. The production of volatile compounds is controlled by the corpora allata. Electroantennographic investigations have shown that immature males and females are very sensitive to a mixture of benzylnitrile, guaiacol, veratrole, phenol and 1,2,3-trimethoxybenzol contained in the head space of mature males. This has been partly confirmed by olfactometer measurements at ICIPE/Nairobi. Experiments have shown that older adults react to their own volatiles not to those of nymphs and immature adults, while the latter are attracted by volatile compounds from the head space of mature adults. Thus we are dealing with a nymphal and adult releaser pheromone.

An airborne male factor, possibly from the head space of males, found in *S. gregaria* and *A. thalassinus*, stimulates egg laying and egg pod formation in virgin females but is connected with disorientation in females in finding moist substrate for egg laying. The mechanism that induces melanisation during nymphal development is still unclear. Whether guaiacol is responsible for the physiological process in aggregation behaviour and whether there is a chemical factor besides the reaction to substrate moisture influences aggregated oviposition needs to be established.

Locustol is considered responsible for the gregarisation of isolated solitarious hoppers by chiasma induction, but so far has not been isolated recently by any research group. However, the chiasma-inducing factor has been found in the faeces of several locust species. If confirmed, the active substance is not a pheromone. An increase in chiasma frequency of chromosomes in spermatocytes can facilitate genetic recombination, which may be of adaptive value. Furthermore, if the active substance is found in all faeces of grass-feeding acridids, it may signal to the insects that the site is overcrowded, stimulating them to migrate and reducing the risk of food shortage.

In summary, locust pheromones are various volatile compounds that act as bouquet. Their most efficient composition and effect on physiological and behavioural processes still needs to be researched through special rearing experiments, electroantennography and olfaction measurements.

The action of the low volatile pentane extracts seems to be different. These are compounds with straight and branched hydrocarbon chains of different lengths and configurations. Analysis and synthesis are needed to test the biological activity of these compounds.

References

Amerasinghe FP (1978) Pheromonal effects on sexual maturation, yellowing and the vibration in immature male desert locust (*Schistocerca gregaria*). J Insect Physiol 24: 309–314

Dearn, JM (1974) Phase transformation and chiasma frequence variation in locusts. I. *Schistocerca gregaria*. Chromosoma 45: 321–338

Francke W, Schmidt GH (1994) Potential of semiochemicals of locust control. Pages 48–52, in New strategies for locust control in natural product and receptor research. ATSAF, Proceedings of the CEC-Workshop, Hamburg, Germany, 10–11 June 1993

Fuzeau-Braesch S, Genin E, Jullien R, Knowles E, Papin R (1988) Composition and role of volatile substances in atmosphere surrounding two gregarious locusts: *Locusta migratoria* and *Schistocerca gregaria*. J Chem Ecol 14: 1023–1033

Gillett SD (1968) Airborne factor affecting the grouping behaviour of locusts. Nature 214: 782–783

Gillett SD, Phillips M (1977) Faeces as a source of a locust gregarization stimulus: effects on social aggregation and on cuticular colour of nymphs of the desert locust, *Schistocerca gregaria* (Forsk.). Acrida 6: 279–286

Karlson P, Lüscher M (1959) Pheromone – Ein Nomenklaturvorschlag für eine Wirkstoffklasse. Naturwissenschaften 46: 63–64

Kendall MP (1972) Glandular epidermis on the tarsi of the desert locust, *Schistocerca gregaria* (Forskål). Acrida 1: 121–147

Klause-de-Pupka A, Schmidt GH, Brunnemann U, Francke W (in press) Nachweis der Perception von arteigenen volatilen Substanzen bei der Wüstenheuschrecke *Schistocerca gregaria* (Forsk.) mittels Elektroantennographie. Entomologia generalis

Loher W (1960) The chemical acceleration of the maturation process and its hormonal control in the male of the desert locust. Proc R Soc Lond B 153: 380–397

Loher W (1961) Die Beschleunigung der Reife durch ein Pheromon des Männchens der Wüstenheuschrecke und die Funktion der Corpora allata. Naturwissenschaften 48: 657–661

Mahamat H, Hassanali A, Odongo H, Torto B, El-Bashir El-S (1993) Studies on the maturation-accelerating pheromone of the desert locust *Schistocerca gregaria* (Orthoptera: Acrididae). Chemoecology 4: 159–164

Nolte DJ (1963) A pheromone for melanization of locusts. Nature 200: 660–661

Nolte DJ (1968) The chiasma-inducing pheromone in locusts. Chromosoma 23: 346–358

Nolte DJ (1976) Locustol and its analogues. J Insect Physiol 22: 833–838

Nolte DJ, May IR, Thomas BM (1970) The gregarization of locusts. Chromosoma 29: 462–473

Nolte DJ, Eggers SJ, May IR (1973) A locust pheromone: locustol. J Insect Physiol 19: 1517–1554

Norris MJ (1954) Sexual maturation in the desert locust (*Schistocerca gregaria* Forskål) with special reference to the effect of grouping. Anti-Locust Bull 7: 1–44

Norris MJ (1962) Group effects on the activity and behaviour of adult males of the desert locust (*Schistocerca gregaria* Forsk.) in relation to sexual maturation. Anim Behav 10: 275–291

Norris MJ (1963) Laboratory experiments on gregarious behaviour in ovipositing females of the desert locust (*Schistocerca gregaria* Forsk.). Entomol Exp Appl 6: 279–303

Norris MJ (1964) Accelerating and inhibiting effects of crowding on sexual maturation in two species of locusts. Nature 203: 784–785

Norris MJ (1968) Some group effects on reproduction in locusts. Colloq Int CNRS173: 147–161

Norris MJ (1970) Aggregation response in ovipositing females of the desert locust, with special reference to the chemical factor. J Insect Physiol 16: 1493–1515

Obeng-Ofori D, Torto B, Hassanali A (1993) Evidence for mediation of two releaser pheromones in the aggregation behaviour of the gregarious desert locust, *Schistocerca gregaria* (Forskål) (Orthoptera: Acrididae). J Chem Ecol 19(8): 1665–1676

Schmidt G, Othman KSA (1994) Studies on the influence of pheromones on the reproduction of virgin and mated females of the Acridid *Aiolopus thalassinus* (Fabr.) (Insecta, Orthoptera, Acrididae). Zool Anz 233 (3/4): 75–116

Schmidt GH (1996) Notes on the effect of population density and parthenogenesis in hopper colouration of the desert locust, *Schistocerca gregaria* (Forsk.) (Saltatoria, Acrididae). Fragm Entomol 27(2): 273–287

Schmidt GH, Albütz R (1994) Laboratory studies on pheromones and reproduction in the desert locust *Schistocerca gregaria* (Forskål). J Appl Ent 118: 378–391

Slyfer EH, Prestage JJ, Beams HW (1959) The chemoreceptors and other sense organs on the antennal flagellum of the grasshopper (Orthoptera: Acrididae). Journ Morphol, New York 105: 145–191

Thomas JG (1972) Epidermal glands in the abdomen of acridids. Acrida 1: 223–232

Torto B, Obeng-Ofori D, Niagi PGN, Hassanali A, Amiani H (1994) Aggregation pheromone system of adult gregarious desert locust *Schistocerca gregaria* (Forskål). J Chem Ecol 20(7): 1749–1762

Chemoecology and semiochemicals

Poster contribution

New Strategies in Locust Control
S. Krall, R. Peveling and D. Ba Diallo (eds)
© 1997 Birkhäuser Verlag Basel/Switzerland

Electrophysiological studies of *Schistocerca gregaria* (Forsk.) with volatile compounds

A. Klause-de-Pupka

Universität Hannover, Lehrgebiet Zoologie-Entomologie, Herrenhäuser Straße 2, D-30419 Hannover, Germany

Volatiles from *Schistocerca gregaria* (Forsk.) were collected with the "closed-loop-stripping" technique. After identification, 15 volatile compounds were found in the "head space" of mature males (Francke and Schmidt 1994). Five of these compounds (phenol, guaiacol, veratrole, 1,2,3-trimethoxybenzene and benzylcyanide) and a mixture of these five substances, which corresponds to the "head space" of mature males, were selected to be tested in an electroantennogram (EAG). The antennae from immature and mature females and males were exposed to streams of air containing the volatile substances in different concentrations.

The results of these experiments revealed a clear reaction to all single substances and to the mixture tested (Tab. 1). Figure 1 shows the different reactions to the mixture in immature and mature females and males.

Immature females (3.37 [mV]) and males (4.07 [mV]) showed significantly stronger reactions than mature females (1.5 [mV]) and males (1.69 [mV])($\alpha = 0.01$).

The experiments show clearly that these differences were not a result of reactions to any of the individual substances (Tab. 1) but can be attributed only to the exposure of the locusts to the

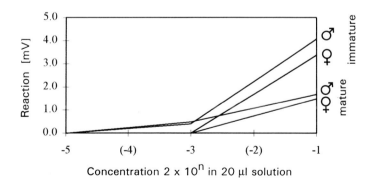

Figure 1. Diagram of the electrophysiological reactions from *S. gregaria* (Forsk.) to the mixture.

Table 1. Electrophysiological reactions in mV (from immature and mature females and males from S. gregaria (Forsk.) to the single substances

Phenol

mol/l	1×10^{-9}	1×10^{-8}	1×10^{-7}	1×10^{-6}	1×10^{-5}	1×10^{-4}	1×10^{-2}	1×10^{-1}
♀♀ mature				0		0	2.63±0.39	
♀♀ immature				0		0.54±0.22	3.09±0.43	
♂♂ mature				0		0.57±0.51	2.86±0.47	
♂♂ immature				0		0.27±0.32	3.57±0.59	

1,2,3-Trimethoxy-benzene

mol/l	1×10^{-9}	1×10^{-8}	1×10^{-7}	1×10^{-6}	1×10^{-5}	1×10^{-4}	1×10^{-2}	1×10^{-1}
♀♀ mature				0.42±0.04		0.49±0.10	1.54±0.15	1.44±0.17
♀♀ immature				0.44±0.005		0.58±0.15	1.23±0.43	1.19±0.33
♂♂ mature				0.66±0.52		0.66±0.19	1.40±0.30	1.09±0.18
♂♂ immature				0		0.36±0.35	1.21±0.15	1.62±0.24

Benzyl-cyanide

mol/l	1.74×10^{-9}	1.74×10^{-8}	1.74×10^{-7}	1.74×10^{-6}	1.74×10^{-5}	1.74×10^{-4}	1.74×10^{-2}	1.74×10^{-1}
♀♀ mature	0.13±0.19		0.63±0.14		3.41±0.28			
♀♀ immature	0.43±0.06		0.86±0.28		3.69±0.74			
♂♂ mature	0.38±0.39		1.61±0.40		3.05±0.27			
♂♂ immature	0.39±0.18		0.69±0.16		4.39±0.78			

Veratrole

mol/l	9.85×10^{-9}	9.85×10^{-8}	9.85×10^{-7}	9.85×10^{-6}	9.85×10^{-5}	9.85×10^{-4}	9.85×10^{-2}	9.85×10^{-1}
♀♀ mature	0.45±0.07	0,74±0.23	2.80±0.20	2.60±0.23	2.78±0.30			
♀♀ immature	0.45±0.05	0.76±0.15		2.38±0.23	2.37±0.47			
♂♂ mature	0.45±0.20	0.66±0.23	2.88±0.39	2.67±0.43	2.46±0.27			
♂♂ immature	0.47±0.38	0.60±0.23		2.74±0.35	2.66±0.56			

Guaiacol

mol/l	4.46×10^{-9}	4.46×10^{-8}	4.46×10^{-7}	4.46×10^{-6}	4.46×10^{-5}	4.46×10^{-4}	4.46×10^{-2}	4.46×10^{-1}
♀♀ mature		0.44±0.31		2.44±0.63	3.78±0.97	3.59±0.30		
♀♀ immature		0.54±0.22		0.88±0.21	3.12±0.56	3.38±0.39		
♂♂ mature		0.48±0.32		1.55±0.33	2.02±0.52	4.12±0.47		
♂♂ immature		0.47±0.42		0.95±0.36	3.16±0.76	3.65±0.97		

tested mixture. However, it remains to be clarified whether the observed reactions were the result of an additive or a synergistic effect among the compounds.

References

Francke W, Schmidt GH (1994) Potential of semiochemicals of locust control. New strategies for locust control in natural product – and receptor research. Proceedings of the CEC Workshop, Hamburg, Germany, 10–11 June 1993. ATSAF, 48–52

Environmental impact

Environmental effects of locust control: state of the art and perspectives[*]

J.W. Everts[1] and L. Ba[2]

[1]FAO, Project LOCUSTOX, B.P. 3300, Dakar/Senegal
[2]Direction de la Protection des Végétaux, B.P. 20054, Thiaroye/Senegal

Summary. Chemical pesticides applied for locust control represent a risk for humans, terrestrial non-target fauna and aquatic ecosystems. This paper reviews the field experience on side-effects. Humans most at risk are field operators themselves. Of the insecticides recommended by the Food and Agriculture Organisation of the United Nations (FAO) specifically, organophosphates and carbamates should be handled with the most care. These compounds also pose a risk to birds, either by direct poisoning or by food depletion. Among the terrestrial non-target invertebrates, there are beneficial species. They appear to be generally affected by treatments, in some cases causing upsurges of secondary pests. Long-term disturbances (over one year) were observed in terrestrial invertebrate communities. The risk of environmental damage can be mitigated considerably by proper selection and use of pesticides. An improvement in the information given decision makers and in the training of operators are essential tools to achieve these goals.

Résumé. Les pesticides chimiques qui sont utilisés dans la lutte antiacridienne représentent un risque pour l'homme, la faune non-cible terrestre et pour les écosystème aquatiques. Cette revue est une synthèse des effets néfastes observés sur le terrain. Parmi les humains, ceux qui manipulent les produits sont le plus en danger. Ce sont spécifiquement les organophosphorés et les carbamates qui méritent une haute vigilance. Les mêmes molécules représentent des risques pour les oiseaux, soit par intoxication directe, soit par privation de nourriture (insectivores). Parmi les invertébrés terrestres non-cibles on trouve beaucoup d'espèces utiles. En général, ils sont toujours touchés par les traitements, parfois résultant des résurgence de déprédateurs secondaires. Ce n'est que dans ce groupe d'invertébrés qu'on a pu constater des effets à long terme, c'est-à-dire se prolongeant sur plus d'une année. Le risque de dégâts environnementaux peut être limité considérablement par une sélection propre et une utilisation judicieuse des produits. A cet effet, il est essentiel que les décideurs soient mieux informés sur les méthodes les moins néfastes et que le personnel opérationnel soit mieux formé.

Introduction

Synthetic pesticides are still an essential weapon in the war against locusts. The combination of large-scale treatment and the relatively high dosage required for effective control results in large amounts of pesticides being used. These are applied to a wide variety of ecosystems. In recession areas it concerns primarily "green islands" in an otherwise barren environment, such as in wadis and oases. Plagues, on the other hand, spread into cultivated and inhabited areas as well as pasture zones, forests and wetlands. Because of infrastructural limitations, the use of less discriminate methods of spraying, e.g. by fixed-wing aircraft, is often unavoidable.

---

[*]Extended abstract of an article to be published in *Pesticide News for West Africa*, FAO Regional Office, Accra, Ghana.

Furthermore, in the emergency of plagues poorly trained personnel are employed and the choice of pesticides is often limited. In arid zones, the areas most at risk are those with high biological productivity, i.e., where agriculture is concentrated and where crop protection is important. There are, however, factors that mitigate the risk of environmental damage.

Most communities of organisms in arid zones, for instance, are adapted to highly variable physical conditions and therefore exhibit remarkable resilience to disturbance. The fact that locust interventions are rarely repeated at the same place over consecutive seasons enhances the chances of recovery from damage, provided unaffected reservoirs for recolonisation (refugia or non-affected dormant stages) are available. High UV radiation and elevated temperatures in locust areas also accelerate degradation of pesticides.

Despite the limited training possibilities in emergency situations, the more regular control in recession areas is nevertheless carried out by professionals who are well aware of the risks involved.

Environmental risk

The potential risk from pesticides used in locust control can be derived through various models. We combined toxicity data available from the literature. These data from laboratory-based studies clearly indicate a general potential hazard for aquatic invertebrates. Fenitrothion is particularly toxic to bees and may also present a hazard to birds, as is the case with bendiocarb. Chlorpyrifos and lambdacyhalothrin exhibit the highest fish toxicity. On the other hand, the low vertebrate toxicity of diflubenzuron is striking. Toxic effects as observed under field conditions in these risk groups are discussed below.

Human exposure

There are three principal human risk groups: persons handling pesticides, persons exposed to the treatments and consumers of contaminated food products. The first is the most important. In a recent study carried out in Senegal, toxic effects were monitored in operators of vehicle-mounted sprayers (ULVA mast and airblast canons). The latter was found the most hazardous device for operators, even those trained in the safe handling of pesticides. On the other hand, ground support teams for aerial operations appeared to work with utmost care whenever observed by us. For the second risk group, i.e., those directly exposed to the spray, the hazard is reduced. It concerns inhabitants or passers-by of areas that are treated by aircraft. In virtually all cases inhabitants are warned beforehand by radio by the local authorities. If they remain present in the spray zone, the pilots are often able to avoid direct overspray. Even when oversprayed by full dose, however, such exposure represents only a fraction of the highest, non-toxic dose. Contaminated crops are a risk to consumers. Although subject to rapid degradation, the residues may be unacceptably high shortly after spraying, with waiting periods of over two weeks after treatment.

Animal husbandry

There are two risk groups among domestic animals: those directly exposed to spray and those feeding on contaminated vegetation or fodder. Very often, herds are not removed from areas to be sprayed, even after extensive warning. However, dosages to which the animals may be exposed are too low to pose a serious problem (see: human exposure). Contamination of forage grass or fodder, on the other hand, may give rise to waiting periods of over two weeks. In the field, no proven cases of intoxication of grazing animals have been reported thus far.

Wildlife

Although most operators (both aerial sprayers and ground teams) avoid spraying of open water as much as possible, the risk of contamination is real, and is substantiated by reports of fish kills. These are likely to be observed. However, the aquatic invertebrate fauna (crustaceans and insects) is more sensitive. Experimental treatments have demonstrated devastating effects on these groups. The risk of unacceptable damage largely depends on the type of water involved. Three main types have to be considered: temporary pools, perennial standing water, streams and rivers. The fauna of temporary pools consists of organisms with a rapid life cycle in the active stage (mostly crustaceans), of immigrants (flying insects) and a few vertebrates which have a dormant stage in the dry season (toads, tortoises and (rarely) lungfish). Side-effects of locust treatments in these groups have been studied in experiments with fenitrothion, diflubenzuron, deltamethrin and bendiocarb. The primary concern for these waters is the risk of wiping out active stages of poorly migrating organisms, resulting in long-term perturbations. Despite some devastating acute effects, long-term effects (i.e., having consequences for the following season) have not been demonstrated thus far.

In perennial standing water the presence of fish often implicates an entirely different invertebrate community. Of the insecticides tested, i.e., fenitrothion, chlorpyrifos and diflubenzuron, only chlorpyrifos proved toxic to fish.

Running waters generally harbour large crustaceans, specifically shrimps, some of which may be of economic importance. Shrimps are known to be sensitive to insecticides, in particular to pyrethroids. FAO has demonstrated that two common Sahelian species (i.e., *Palaemonetes africanus* and *Caridina africana*) are at risk after treatments with fenitrothion and chlorpyrifos. Running water, however, is unlikely to become contaminated by locust treatments to such a degree that survival of populations is at risk. Locust treatments take place mostly in the wet season when water levels are high, thus avoiding the risk of wiping out relict communities in dry-season pools (an important reservoir for recolonisation of the lotic fauna).

The acute effects on birds are generally limited to individual cases of poisoning, and in many cases, no effects have been observed at all. The risk for birds includes both direct intoxication and deprivation of food supplies. Exposure to spray is supposed to be hazardous when toxic amounts of chemicals are ingested through preening. Uptake of contaminated food is another important risk factor: debilitated or dead insects provide easy prey. Although not quantitatively substantiated, this route of exposure is considered most important. Lasting effects on bird populations have yet to be proven. However, it has been suggested that the decline of stork populations in Western Europe since the 1950s is related to the success of locust control operations depriving migrant storks of an important source of food.

Although reptiles and amphibians play a key role in arid ecosystems, up to now the taxa have not been included in environmental impact surveys for locust control. Direct toxic effects are unlikely to occur. Occasionally, observed tadpoles exposed to experimental sprays did not appear to be sensitive. However, poisoning through uptake of contaminated food (the vast majority of species are either insectivorous and/or carrion eaters) is a risk which has yet to be studied. The lack of information on this group is a serious omission which will be addressed in the near future.

The insecticides used in locust control have been selected for low mammalian toxicity. Side-effects, if any, are to be expected among the insectivores. However, only in rodents have indications of toxicity been demonstrated thus far.

Terrestrial invertebrates

Insecticides are meant to kill insects. The dosage rates required for locust control, represent a high potential risk for non-target insects. This has been confirmed in all field studies carried out thus far. Nevertheless, there is a sharp differentiation between the various pesticides with respect to the taxa and, more important, the functional groups that are affected.

The functional groups we are primarily interested in are pollinators, natural enemies of locusts and other pests, and insects essential for maintaining soil functions. It has been demonstrated that bees can be seriously affected by malathion. Of the other recommended pesticides, fenitrothion is classified as "highly toxic" to bees, while bendiocarb and chlorpyrifos are classified as "dangerous". Of all side-effects, those on parasitoids and predators of crop pests have been most extensively studied. Serious effects have been observed in species which correlated with pest upsurges.

Ants and termites are essential for the productivity of tropical and semi-arid soils. In many places tree growth is directly related to termite activity, aiding root penetration and transport of organic material into the subsoil. Side-effects on ants have been observed by various authors, malathion and fenitrothion being especially harmful. The few observations made on termites indicate that the latter insecticide was toxic to this group as well.

Key soil processes

Studies on key soil processes such as respiration, nitrification and chlorophyll production showed only marginal disturbances, even at high dosages. The insecticides tested (i.e., fenitrothion, chlorpyrifos, diflubenzuron and deltamethrin) may be considered not harmful for key soil processes, under the given circumstances.

Evaluation

A number of conclusions can be drawn from the recorded side-effects of chemical control:
- All the current insecticides present a risk to non-target organisms.
- The groups of organisms at risk differ for each insecticide.
- Long-term effects are rare and, as far as known, limited to secondary disturbances within insect communities.
- Terrestrial vertebrates are primarily at risk at the individual level.
- Fish are at risk where chlorpyrifos is used near open water.
- Aquatic invertebrates are sensitive to all recommended locust pesticides.
- Terrestrial invertebrates are at risk in all cases, sometimes leading to undesirable effects (i.e., upsurges of secondary pests).

In order to appraise the risk posed by chemical locust control to the ecosystems in the invasion area, we should compare the scale and intensity of treatments to the surface area covered by the ecosystems or communities concerned. It is clear that the treatments may have a deleterious effect, specifically on invertebrates, sometimes resulting in long-lasting disturbances in numerical relationships. However serious these effects may be, they are always characterised by their limited scale when compared to the size of the ecosystem concerned. In some cases the majority of wadis within a certain area may be treated and, thus, damaged. However, not all wadis in the invasion area are likely to be sprayed. In an extremely serious upsurge probably not more than 10% of the (potentially) productive (green) area is infested. Recovery will always occur, albeit in some cases slowly. This holds for the terrestrial communities and for temporary aquatic communities. Perennial aquatic communities found in arid areas, on the other hand, may harbour entirely isolated relict populations (e.g. aquatic tortoises in oases). Local extinction in such cases could affect biodiversity in the desert locust area. Fortunately, this risk is limited. Locally appointed operators are generally very aware of the risk of contaminating open waters (= drinking water) in arid zones.

Although recent research has revealed some of the hazards related to chemical locust control, for the most part the potential risk is still largely unknown. We know, for instance, virtually nothing about the risk to reptiles and insectivorous mammals. The mechanisms of observed disturbed interspecies relationships in invertebrate communities are unknown, which hinders extrapolation to other situations. We know that ants are at risk. However, which species are affected and the ecological consequences of their temporary disappearance is not known. Furthermore, in describing the resilience of some of this fauna, we still refer to qualitative or phenomenological observations. Until the underlying processes have been studied, recovery rates cannot be predicted and the factor "recovery" cannot be used for risk assessments.

Wherever insecticides are used, humans are at risk. The most important risk group, the personnel handling the chemicals, can be easily trained and provided with protective material at low cost. Negligence, however, is a global problem and accidents will consequently occur.

The final solution to all ecotoxicological problems is to reduce the use of toxic chemicals for locust control. This can be achieved primarily by improving the selectivity and efficacy of the available chemical methods and also by further development of non-chemical methods of control.

Acknowledgements
The Locustox project is a joint research programme by the Food and Agriculture Organisation of the United Nations and the Senegalese Crop Protection Directorate. The studies mentioned in this paper as being part of a project were funded by the Government of the Netherlands under projects ECLO/SEN/003/NET, GCP/SEN/041/NET and by the Government of Senegal.

New Strategies in Locust Control
S. Krall, R. Peveling and D. Ba Diallo (eds)
© 1997 Birkhäuser Verlag Basel/Switzerland

Side-effects of locust control on beneficial arthropods: research approaches used by the Locustox project in Senegal

H. van der Valk[1] and A. Niassy[2]

[1]*Food and Agriculture Organisation of the United Nations (FAO). The Locustox Project. B.P. 3300, Dakar, Senegal*
[2]*Ministry of Agriculture, Plant Protection Directorate (DPV) B.P. 20054, Dakar-Thiaroye, Senegal. Present address: International Centre for Insect Physiology and Ecology (ICIPE), ARPIS Programme, PO Box 30772, Nairobi, Kenya*

Summary. A large variety of methods are used to study the side-effects of insecticides on non-target terrestrial invertebrates. These methods are most often organised in some sort of tiered system in which simple laboratory tests precede more complex field bioassays, full field tests and eventually monitoring schemes. The FAO Locustox project applies most of these techniques in its research on the impact of locust and grasshopper control on beneficial arthropods in the African Sahel. A number of weaker points in the types of field studies carried out to date are discussed. It is argued that ecological monitoring of side-effects of operational locust control on non-target invertebrates will be nearly impossible.

Résumé. Des méthodes très variées sont utilisées pour étudier les effets secondaires des insecticides sur les invertébrés terrestres non-cibles. L'expérimentation comporte généralement plusieurs stades : de simples essais en laboratoire précèdent des bio-essais plus complexes sur le terrain. Ils sont suivis de tests en plein champ et finalement de différents contrôles. Le projet FAO Locustox applique la plupart de ces techniques dans ses travaux de recherche concernant l'impact sur les arthropodes utiles dans le Sahel africain de la lutte contre les locustes et sauteriaux. Cet article présente quelques-unes des faiblesses des études menées à ce jour sur le terrain. Il est démontré que le contrôle écologique des effets secondaires de la lutte antiacridienne opérationnelle sur les invertébrés non-cibles sera quasiment impossible.

Introduction

Most, if not all, of the insecticides used in locust and grasshopper control have broad spectrum activity, and thus kill non-target terrestrial arthropods. Many of these arthropods perform important functions in (agro-)ecosystems: Some are responsible for organic matter cycling; others are predators and parasitoids of crop pests (including locusts and grasshoppers). Some assure pollination of crops and wild plants, while others again produce honey or silk. Apart from having specific ecological functions with direct benefit for humans, arthropods are also a key part of almost any terrestrial ecosystem in the world, at all trophic levels. Unintentional side-effects of insecticides on non-target arthropods should thus be avoided as much as possible.

Studying the negative impact of insecticides on beneficial arthropods is almost as old as the use of these compounds itself, and goes back to the late 1800s (Croft 1990). Not surprisingly, the earliest studies concerned natural enemies of crop pests, which had a direct agricultural importance. Over the last two decades ecotoxicological studies on terrestrial arthropods have become more important, especially within the framework of integrated pest management.

Different from aquatic, wildlife and human toxicology, no standard set of testing and hazard assessment methods has yet been developed for terrestrial invertebrates. Therefore, we will discuss hereafter in some detail the approaches chosen in the Locustox project.

Tiered testing

Insecticide hazard and risk assessment for beneficial arthropods is generally based on a tiered approach. One of the most detailed schemes developed so far is the one recently published by the European and Mediterranean Plant Protection Organisation (EPPO 1994). To start with, a limited number of simple laboratory toxicity tests is carried out on organisms which are relevant for the crop or ecosystem to be treated. Results of these tests allow the pesticides to be classified as probably harmless, in which case no further fieldwork is required, or as possibly harmful, with the suggestion to carry out further studies to clarify their real impact. Field or semi-field studies may follow, depending on the outcome of the laboratory screening as well as on the proposed use pattern of the insecticide. Post-registration monitoring of the operational use of the pesticide may be carried out if field studies have given rise for concern, albeit not enough to refuse registration. The Locustox project generally follows this tiered approach, although sometimes second- or third- tier studies have preceded the simple screening tests, for reasons which will be discussed below.

Laboratory toxicity tests

A number of standard laboratory testing methods have been compiled by the Working Group Pesticides and Beneficial Arthropods of the International Organisation for Biological and Integrated Control of Noxious Animals and Plants/West Palearctic Region Section (IOBC/WPRS) (Hassan et al. 1985; Hassan 1992). A hazard assessment procedure for bees, also part of the EPPO scheme but following a different approach, has already existed for some time (Felton et al. 1986). Data collected under such schemes, as well as other published studies, can be used in a first assessment of the potential risk of locust control to non-target arthropods (Murphy et al. 1994). A drawback of using existing toxicity data from the literature is that almost all of these studies have been executed in temperate or sub-tropical ecosystems or with organisms originating from such ecosystems. Relatively few studies have been carried out in tropical, hot arid or semi-arid environments (van der Valk and Koeman 1988; Bourdeau et al. 1989), despite differences in potential impact of insecticide use (Balk and Koeman 1984).

As part of its overall objectives, the Locustox project is developing laboratory toxicity tests with beneficial insects which are relevant for arid and semi-arid (agro-)ecosystems. Most of this work was done over the last two years, however, after a number of larger-scale field studies had been carried out. This disgression from the evaluation sequence described above was necessary to gather enough ecological and ecotoxicological data to be able to chose the appropriate organisms for which laboratory tests were to be developed.

A simple but reliable rearing method of *Bracon hebetor* (Hym., Braconidae) has been developed, as well as a toxicity test which evaluates both mortality and reproductive parameters of this parasitoid (van der Valk et al. 1994). *B. hebetor* is an ectoparasitoid of, among others, the larvae of *Heliocheilus albipunctella* (Lep., Noctuidae), a major millet pest in the western Sahel. Toxicity tests are also carried out on a regular basis on *Pimelia senegalensis* and *Trachyderma hispida* (Col., Tenebrionidae) (Danfa and van der Valk 1993; Danfa 1994). Tenebrionid beetles are a major component of arid ecosystems, both in biomass as well as in their ecological function. They often play a key role in the degradation of organic matter (Crawford 1991), and the larvae of some species have been reported to attack grasshopper egg pods (Greathead et al. 1994). The IOBC testing programme does not include tenebrionid beetles, while the only regularly used test with a braconid refers to an endoparasitoid. The laboratory tests developed in Senegal thus add to existing knowledge rather than duplicate it.

Semi-field tests and in situ bioassays

Field cage trials, tunnel tests, *in situ* bioassays and similar techniques combine the simplicity, limited scale and repeatability of laboratory tests with the environmental fate and behaviour of the insecticide under more or less natural conditions. As such they have an important function as a bridge between the laboratory and the field, providing information for the extrapolation of laboratory data to actual field circumstances (Sotherton et al. 1988). In some cases, e.g. insecticide effects on bees, these semi-field methods are widely used and highly standardised. Most often though, techniques are developed on an *ad hoc* basis, depending on the ecology of the organisms to be studied. An elegant approach, integrating *in situ* bioassays in the overall insecticide hazard assessment, is described by Wiles and Jepson (1992, 1994). Bioassays presently used by us include field arenas for Tenebrionidae and "micro-cages" to assess the toxicity of leaf residues on Coccinellidae and Braconidae.

Field experiments

A field experiment should be the final proof of the existence of a deleterious effect of an insecticide. However, ecotoxicological field studies, especially with terrestrial arthropods, are notoriously difficult to design, execute and interpret. Requirements for experimental design relevant for ecotoxicological field studies, as well as many of the classical pitfalls, have been described by Green (1979), Hurlbert (1984), Sotherton et al. (1988), Hairston (1989), Eberhardt and Thomas (1991) and Fairweather (1991), among others. FAO (1989) and Everts (1990a, b) specifically addressed field study methods for locust control.

Matteson (1992) evaluated a number of the studies on side-effects of locust control, and suggested that "few of the experiments followed the ideal experimental guidelines ... [described by FAO (1989)]. Results are thus of limited applicability". In an evaluation of some of the earlier studies, van der Valk (1990b) also argued that conclusions drawn following these studies were often not supported by the actual data.

Having learned from such experiences, we have chosen a more or less standard design for our entomological field experiments. It uses elements of the BACI approach described by Stewart-Oaten et al. (1986), which requires taking samples, replicated in time, "Before the insecticide treatment and Afterwards, at both a Control and an Impact site". Following a number of critical suggestions which followed publication of this approach (Smith et al. 1993; Underwood 1991, 1994), we have adapted our experimental set-up, blocking treatments in the form of a Randomised Complete Block design. As a rule the field studies cover at least one rainy season, i.e., 3–4 months. Data collected in such a way can be analysed by classical analysis of variance (ANOVA), and it allows differences in location of the treatments to be separated from the actual treatment effects (Dutilleul 1993). This has the additional practical advantage that the area in which the experiments are to be done does not have to be completely homogeneous, which facilitates setting up the study. This approach is a compromise, however, between analytical power to distinguish pesticide impact on the one side and logistical feasibility on the other. A consequence is that with the design one detects only large and acute effects. Both subtle changes in population sizes and longer-term effects will not be found. More powerful study designs exist (e.g. Underwood 1994) but would require a larger assessment and sampling effort than we could presently manage.

Fieldwork by the Locustox project concentrates on side-effects in the millet agro-ecosystem (van der Valk and Kamara 1993), especially with respect to natural enemies of millet pests (e.g. ichneumonoid and dipteran parasitoids). Additional work is being done in semi-arid savannah systems, both on natural enemies of grasshoppers (e.g. sphecid wasps, asilid flies and tenebrionid beetles) and on insects which are important for organic matter cycling in the soil (e.g. tene-brionid beetles, ants and termites) (van der Valk 1990a; Gueye and Everts 1990).

A limitation in these field studies is the absence of spatial scale as an explicit experimental parameter. Obviously, large-scale treatments have a higher probability of causing prolonged effects than smaller ones. With a few exceptions, most experimental treatments in the project have been carried out on plots of 1–4 hectares. This is considerably smaller than many pesticide applications against locusts. Apart from affecting the speed of population recovery (Jepson and Thacker 1990; Duffield and Aebischer 1994) changing the scale at which we study insecticide impact may require a "change of glasses" through which we try to observe such impacts. At different ecological hierarchical scales, both in space and in time, different types of processes dominate. Therefore, pesticide disturbance may need to be described in a different way as well (O'Neill et al. 1986; Levin 1989; Jepson 1989). One possibility to better integrate spatial aspects in ecotoxicological assessment may be the use of mathematical (simulation) models (Levin 1989; Thomas et al. 1990; Sherratt and Jepson 1993). We hope to become more "spatially conscious" in the research which has been planned for the next few years.

Monitoring

When insecticides are used on a large operational scale, it may be possible to monitor side-effects on non-target arthropods, i.e. to assess in one way or another if the treatments had any ecological impact under "real life" circumstances. Such ecological monitoring has as a common characteristic that the investigator does not control in any way the event being studied (Herricks et al. 1989), in this case the insecticide applications. Ecological monitoring tends to be quite successful when pollutants are either persistent or are being discharged continuously in the environment. Examples of such monitoring schemes include cases such as heavy metal pollution caused by smelters, bio-accumulating chemicals in mussels, lead in human hair or the impact of eutrophication on freshwater organisms.

Unfortunately, locust control does not have any of the required characteristics to allow for practical ecological monitoring of terrestrial invertebrates. The insecticides have low persistence, insect biomarkers which may be used to assess exposure tend to be transitory, arthropod populations are often extremely variable in arid ecosystems, and the location and timing of insecticide applications are rather unpredictable. The latter means that one will almost always be too late on site to use one of the few monitoring techniques which remain.

The project has field-tested one method, which assessed grasshopper egg pod density and natural mortality in blocks treated with insecticides by the Senegalese Crop Protection Directorate (Niassy et al. 1993; van der Valk et al. 1995). Power analysis revealed, however, that a fairly large number of independent cases would need to be monitored to be able to distinguish ecologically significant effects. Even though the work suggested that some intriguing effects might occur, an obvious explanation for the observed effects was difficult to provide, especially due to the high variability in the data.

If ecological monitoring of (migratory) locust control is going to be required in the future, extreme care will have to be taken with respect to the design of such a programme to avoid a complete waste of time and money. It is relatively easy to set up programmes which will collect a large number of data, but much more difficult to collect ecologically meaningful data. Too many examples exist of monitoring programmes which failed their objectives (Stout 1993). Unfortunately, monitoring of locust control seems to be an almost ideal candidate for what has been described as the "data-rich but information-poor" syndrome (Rose and Smith 1992).

Acknowledgements
The Locustox project is a joint research programme by the Food and Agriculture Organisation of the United Nations and the Senegalese Crop Protection Directorate. The studies mentioned in this paper as being part of the project were funded by the Government of the Netherlands under projects ECLO/SEN/003/NET and GCP/SEN/041/NET, and by the Government of Senegal.

References

Balk F, Koeman JH (1984) Future hazards from pesticide use: With special reference to West Africa and Southeast Asia. IUCN/Commission on Ecology Paper no 6. The Environmentalist 4 (suppl.6): 1–100

Bourdeau P, Haines J, Klein W, Krishna Murti CR (eds)(1989) Ecotoxicology and climate. With special reference to hot and cold climates. SCOPE 38. ICPS Joint Symposia 9. Chichester: John Wiley and Sons

Crawford CS (1991) The community ecology of macroarthropod detritivores. Pages 89–112 in Polis GA (ed) The ecology of desert communities. Tucson: The University of Arizona Press

Croft BA (1990) Arthropod biological control agents and pesticides. New York: John Wiley and Sons

Danfa A (1994) Tests de toxicité de *Metarhizium flavoviride* (Deuteromycetes-Moniliales) sur *Bracon hebetor* (Hymenoptera, Braconidae), *Pimelia senegalensis* et *Trachyderma hispida* (Coleoptera, Tenebrionidae). Rapport Locustox 94/1. Organisation des Nations Unies pour l'Alimentation et l'Agriculture projet ECLO/SEN/003/NET. FAO, Rome

Danfa A, van der Valk H (1993) Tests de toxicité du fénitrothion sur *Pimelia senegalensis* et *Trachyderma hispida* (Coleoptera, Tenebrionidae). Rapport Locustox 93/6. Organisation des Nations Unies pour l'Alimentation et l'Agriculture projet ECLO/SEN/003/NET. FAO, Rome

Duffield SJ, Aebischer NJ (1994) The effect of spatial scale of treatment with dimethoate on invertebrate population recovery in winter wheat. J Appl Ecol 31: 263–281

Dutilleul P (1993) Spatial heterogeneity and the design of ecological field experiments. Ecology 74(6): 1646–1658

Eberhardt LL, Thomas JM (1991) Designing environmental field studies. Ecological Monographs 61(1): 53–73

EPPO (1994) Decision making scheme for the environmental risk assessment of plant protection products. Chapter 9. Arthropod natural enemies. European and Mediterranean Plant Protection Organisation. Council of Europe. Bulletin OEPP/EPPO Bulletin 24: 17–35

Everts JW (1990a) Methods for monitoring the impact of chemical control of locusts and grasshoppers in Africa. Pages 45–54 in Proceedings of the workshop on health and environmental impact of alternative control agents for desert locust control. Oslo, 14–17 January, 1990. NORAGRIC occasional papers series C, no 5. NORAGRIC, Oslo

Everts JW (ed) (1990b) Environmental effects of chemical locust and grasshopper control. A pilot study. Project ECLO/SEN/003/NET. FAO, Rome

Fairweather PG (1991) Statistical power and design requirements for environmental monitoring. Australian J Marine Freshwater Res 42: 555–567

FAO (1989) Report of the working group on environmental side-effects of desert locust control. 14–16 February 1989. FAO, Rome

Felton JC, Oomen PA, Stevenson JH (1986) Toxicity and hazard of pesticides to honeybees: harmonization of test methods. Bee World 67(3): 114–124

Greathead DJ, Kooyman C, Launois-Luong MH, Popov GB (1994) Les ennemis naturels des criquets du Sahel. Collection Acridologie Opérationelle no.8. CILSS/DFPV/PRIFAS, Niamey

Green RH (1979) Sampling design and statistical methods for environmental biologists. New York: John Wiley and Sons

Gueye N, Everts JW (1990) Termites. Pages 231–235 in Everts JW (ed) Environmental effects of chemical locust and grasshopper control. A pilot study. Project ECLO/SEN/003/NET. Food and Agriculture Organisation of the United Nations (FAO), Rome

Hairston NG Sr (1989) Ecological experiments: purpose, design, and execution. Cambridge: Cambridge University Press

Hassan SA (ed) (1992) Guidelines for testing the effects of pesticides on beneficial organisms: description of test methods. Bulletin IOBC/WPRS, 1992/xv/3: 1–186

Hassan SA, Bigler F, Blaisinger P et al. (1985) Standard methods to test the side-effects of pesticides on natural enemies of insects and mites developed by the IOBC/WPRS Working Group "Pesticides and Beneficial Organisms". Bulletin OEPP/EPPO Bulletin 15: 214–255

Herricks EE, Schaeffer DJ, Perry JA (1989) Biomonitoring: closing the loop in environmental sciences. Pages 351–366 in Levin SA, Harwell MA, Kelly JR, Kimball KD (eds) Ecotoxicology: problems and approaches. New York: Springer

Hurlbert SH (1984) Pseudoreplication and the design of ecological field experiments. Ecological Monographs 54: 187–211

Jepson PC (1989) The temporal and spatial dynamics of pesticide side-effects on non-target invertebrates. Pages 95–127 in Jepson PC (ed) Pesticides and non-target invertebrates. Wimborne: Intercept

Jepson PC, Thacker JRM (1990) Analysis of the spatial component of pesticide side-effects on non-target invertebrate populations and its relevance to hazard analysis. Functional Ecology 4: 349–355

Levin SA (1989) Models in ecotoxicology: methodological aspects. Pages 211–220 in Levin SA, Harwell MA, Kelly JR, Kimball KD (eds) Ecotoxicology: problems and approaches. New York: Springer

Matteson PC (1992) A review of field studies of the environmental impacts of locust/grasshopper control programmes in Africa. Pages 347–355 in Lomer CJ, Prior C (eds) Biological control of locusts and grasshoppers. Wallingford: CAB International

Murphy CF, Jepson PC, Croft BA (1994) Database analysis of the toxicity of antilocust pesticides to non-target, beneficial invertebrates. Crop Prot 13(6)413–420

Niassy A, Beye A, van der Valk H (1993) Impact of fenitrothion applications on natural mortality of grasshopper eggpods in Senegal (1991 treatments). Locustox report 93/1. Food and Agriculture Organisation of the United Nations project ECLO/SEN/003/NET. FAO, Rome

O'Neill RV, DeAngelis DL, Waide JB, Allen TFH (1986) A hierarchical concept of ecosystems. Monographs in Population Biology no 23. Princeton: Princeton University Press

Rose KA, Smith EP (1992) Experimental design: the neglected aspect of environmental monitoring. Environ Manage 16(6): 691–700

Sherratt TN, Jepson PC (1993) A metapopulation approach to modelling the long-term impact of pesticides on invertebrates. J Appl Ecol 30: 696–705

Smith EP, Orvos DR, Cairns J jr (1993) Impact assessment using the Before-After-Control-Impact (BACI) model: concerns and comments. Canad J Fisheries Aquat Sci 50: 627–637

Sotherton NW, Jepson PC, Pullen AJ (1988) Criteria for the design, execution and analysis of terrestrial non-target invertebrate field tests. Pages 183–190 in Greaves MP et al. (eds) Field methods for the study of environmental effects of pesticides. BCPC Monograph no 40. Thornton Heath: British Crop Protection Council Publications

Stewart-Oaten A, Murdoch WW, Parker KR (1986) Environmental impact assessment: "pseudoreplication" in time? Ecology 67(4): 929–940

Stout BB (1993) The good, the bad and the ugly of monitoring programs: defining questions and establishing objectives. Environ Monit Assess 26: 91–98

Thomas CFG, Hol EHA, Everts JW (1990) Modelling the diffusion component of dispersal during reco-
    very of a population of linyphiid spiders from exposure to an insecticide. Funct Ecol 4: 357–368
Underwood AJ (1991) Beyond BACI: experimental designs for detecting human environmental
    impacts on temporal variations in natural populations. Australian J Marine Freshwater Res 42: 569–
    587
Underwood AJ (1994) On beyond BACI: sampling designs that might reliably detect environmental
    disturbances. Ecol Applic 4(1): 3–15
van der Valk HCHG (1990a) Beneficial arthropods. Pages 171–224 in Environmental effects of
    chemical locust and grasshopper control. A pilot study. Project ECLO/SEN/003/NET. FAO, Rome
van der Valk HCHG (1990b) Environmental impact studies of chemical locust and grasshopper control.
    A review. Report to the Scientific Advisory Committee of the Coordinating Group on Locust
    Research. FAO, Rome
van der Valk H, Kamara O (1993) The effect of fenitrothion and diflubenzuron on natural enemies of
    millet pests in Senegal (the 1991 study). Locustox report 93/2. Project ECLO/SEN/003/NET. FAO,
    Rome
van der Valk HCHG, Koeman JH (1988) Ecological impact of pesticide use in developing countries.
    Netherlands' IRPTC-IPCS Committee. Ministry of Housing, Physical Planning and Environment, The
    Hague
van der Valk H, Niassy A, Beye A (1995) Effects of grasshopper control with fenitrothion on natural
    mortality of eggpods in Senegal (1992 treatments). Locustox report 95/1. Project
    GCP/SEN/041/NET. FAO, Rome
van der Valk H, van der Stoep J, Fall B, Dieme E (1994) A laboratory toxicity test with *Bracon hebetor*
    (Say)(Hymenoptera, Braconidae) – first evaluation of rearing and testing methods. Locustox report
    94/1. Project GCP/SEN/041/NET. FAO, Rome
Wiles JA, Jepson PC (1992) In situ bioassay techniques to evaluate the toxicity of pesticides to bene-
    ficial invertebrates in cereals. Aspects of Applied Biology 31: 61–68
Wiles JA, Jepson PC (1994) Substrate-mediated toxicity of deltamethrin residues to beneficial inver-
    tebrates: estimation of toxicity factors to aid risk assessment. Arch Environ Contam Toxicol 27: 384–
    391

New Strategies in Locust Control
S. Krall, R. Peveling and D. Ba Diallo (eds)
© 1997 Birkhäuser Verlag Basel/Switzerland

Side-effects of the insect growth regulator triflumuron on spiders

R. Peveling[1], J. Hartl[2] and E. Köhne[2]

[1]*Deutsche Gesellschaft für Technische Zusammenarbeit (GTZ), Postfach 5180, 65726 Eschborn, Germany*
[2]*Institut für Biogeographie, Universität des Saarlandes, Postfach 151150, 66041 Saarbrücken, Germany*

Summary. Laboratory bioassays and small-scale field trials were conducted to study side-effects of the insect growth regulator triflumuron (TFM) on different spider species from Europe, Mauritania and Madagascar. Various formulations were tested, depending on the desired mode of exposure. Technical-grade TFM was used in long-term bioassays with sub-adult *Pisaura mirabilis* (Clerck) [Pisauridae], a European species. Alsystin 25 WP and 050 UL were tested in medium-term bioassays with nymphs of *Peucetia* sp. (Oxyopidae) from Madagascar. Alsystin 050 UL was also used in field trials in Mauritania, with *Thanatus* sp. (Philodromidae) as a monitor species. The end-points considered in the bioassays were mortality, predation rate and moulting frequency. In the field trials, relative and absolute abundance of *Thanatus* sp. were estimated. Technical-grade TFM had no toxic effect on *P. mirabilis,* nor did it affect predation or moulting. In the field, Alsystin 050 UL had no effect on *Thanatus* sp. at 25 g a.i./ha, but relative and absolute abundance, particularly of juveniles, were significantly reduced at 100 g a.i./ha. An initial toxicity was also observed in *Peucetia* sp. nymphs directly exposed to this formulation. It is suggested that this effect was solvent (methylpyrrolidone and methylnaphtalene) rather than TFM-induced. Alsystin 25 WP, which was administered indirectly via contaminated prey, did not harm *Peucetia* sp., providing further evidence that TFM is generally harmless to spiders.

Résumé. Des essais biologiques en laboratoire et des expérimentations à petite échelle sur le terrain ont été conduits pour étudier les effets du dérégulateur de croissance triflumuron (TFM) sur diverses espèces d'araignées d'Europe, de Mauritanie et de Madagascar. Les essais ont portés sur diverses formulations choisies en fonction du mode d'exposition. Du TFM au stade technique a été appliqué au cours d'essais à long terme au laboratoire sur des sous-adultes de *Pisaura mirabilis* (Clerck) [Pisauridae], une espèce européenne. L'Alsystin 50 WP et 050 UL a été testée au cours d'essais à moyen terme sur les nymphes de *Peucetia* sp. (Oxyopidae) de Madagascar. Des essais sur le terrain avec l'Alsystin 050 UL ont également été menés en Mauritanie sur *Thanatus* sp. (Philodromidae) en tant qu'espèce indicative. Les effets étudiés au cours de ces essais étaient la mortalité, le taux de prédation et l'incidence sur la mue. Les essais sur le terrain ont permis d'évaluer l'abondance relative et absolue de *Thanatus* sp. Le TFM au stade technique n'a pas été toxique pour *P. mirabilis* et n'a ni affecté son comportement prédateur ni son développement. Sur le terrain, l'Alsystin 050 UL n'a eu aucun effet sur *Thanatus* sp. à la dose de 25 g de m.a./ha, mais son abondance a été significativement réduite à la dose de 100 g de m.a./ha. Une toxicité initiale a également été observée sur les nymphes de *Peucetia* sp. exposées directement à cette formulation, mais elle devrait avoir été due aux solvants (méthylpyrrolidone et méthylnaphtalène) plutôt qu'au TFM. L'Alsystin 25 WP administrée indirectement au moyen de proie contaminée n'a pas été nocive sur *Peucetia* sp., ce qui apporte une preuve supplémentaire de la non-nocivité d'une manière générale du TFM sur les araignées.

Introduction

Recent research has confirmed the potential of insect growth regulators belonging to the chemical class of benzoyl-phenylureas (BPUs) as promising agents for barrier treatment to control hopper bands of migratory and desert locusts (Cooper et al. 1995; Scherer and Rakotonandrasana 1993; Wilps and Nasseh 1994). Since BPUs have been widely used as blanket sprays against forest pests in temperate zones, side-effects on non-target arthropods, especially insects and crustaceans, are relatively well known (Fischer and Lenwood 1992; Forster et al. 1993). However, when these agents entered the locust control scene in the 1990s, little knowledge existed about side-effects on non-targets in semi-arid and arid ecosystems. Moreover, as far as spiders are concerned, these are often neglected in environmental impact studies, despite their important role as polyphagous and ubiquitous predators in most terrestrial ecosystems (Wise 1993), and only a few guidelines for laboratory toxicity testing have been proposed so far (e.g. Hof et al. 1995).

BPUs interfere with chitin synthesis and thus mainly affect larval and immature life stages (Graf 1993; Reynolds 1987). Due to their long immature life stage and high frequency of moulting, spiders would appear to be a non-target likely to be susceptible to BPUs. Experimental evidence, however, is contradictory. Müller (1992) observed side-effects of triflumuron (TFM) on various Cape Verdean taxa. Tingle et al. (1996) found adverse effects of diflubenzuron (DFB) on araneids in a field trial in Madagascar. However, in a second trial one year later, results were not confirmed. Further evidence that spiders are not susceptible to BPUs has been provided by Everts and Jocqué (1990), KroKene (1993), Mansour and Nentwig (1988) and Peveling et al. (1994).

This paper summarises the results of bioassays and small-scale field trials conducted with spiders from three different biogeographic regions. The selected taxa represent characteristic and abundant species of the respective indigenous spider fauna. Depending on the desired mode of exposure, various formulations of TFM were laboratory-tested on sub-adult *Pisaura mirabilis* (Clerck) [Pisauridae] from Europe and nymphal *Peucetia* sp. (Oxyopidae) from Madagascar. In Mauritania, *Thanatus* sp. (Philodromidae) was used as an indicator species to monitor side-effects of high- and low-dose field applications of TFM (blanket spray). Tests on *Peucetia* sp. and *Thanatus* sp. were linked to seasonal (approx. three months) semi-field and field research activities on migratory and desert locusts (Scherer and Célestin 1996; Wilps and Diop 1996), while the bioassays with *P. mirabilis* were conducted in the scope of long-term (more than half a year) laboratory studies in Germany.

Material and methods

Bioassays with sub-adult Pisaura mirabilis

Age and origin of spiders
Sub-adult *P. mirabilis* of equal size were collected in the field near Saarbrücken, South-western Germany, in September 1993.

General outline of tests
Spiders (20 per treatment group) were maintained in individual plastic boxes (13 × 7 × 5 cm), the bottom covered with moistened sand, at 20–24 °C under a 12:12 h light:dark cycle. They were fed two 2nd to 3rd instar *Gryllus* sp. daily for 7 days and every 2nd day thereafter. Sixty days (topical application) or 67 days (ingestion) after test initiation, spiders were kept in a refrigerator at 1–5 °C in the dark for 62 days to simulate hibernation. Thereafter, they were maintained as before. Mortality and moulting frequency of survivors were monitored until 180 days post-treatment. As a sub-lethal end-point, the predation rate of survivors, i.e., the percentage of crickets killed and eaten (52 = 100%), was recorded for 46 days.

Test I. Topical application
Technical-grade TFM was dissolved in acetone at 0.625 µg, 0.125 g and 25g a.i./l. Two microlitres of these solutions was applied to the dorsal side of the cephalothorax with a Burkard microapplicator, corresponding to doses of 0.00125, 0.25 and 50 µg a.i./spider (field dose times 1/200, 1 and 200; estimate based on the approximate "ground area coverage", Jepson 1993). The unrealistically high dose was included against the background of no observed effects at doses between 0.00125 and 12.5 µg a.i./spider (spacing factor = 10) in a range-finding test (Köhne 1995, unpublished data). An untreated, an acetone-treated (vehicle) and a positive control (the same solutions/doses applied to the pronotum of ten 3rd instar *Gryllus* sp. per group) were included in this bioassay.

Test II. Exposure by ingestion
Third instar *Gryllus* sp. were treated as described above and subsequently fed to spiders on days 0, 5 and 10. Between feeding dates, spiders were starved to assure prey consumption. The assumption that TFM would be taken up *per os* was based on the fact that *P. mirabilis* thoroughly chews and kneads its prey prior to feeding.

Data analysis

Analysis of variance (ANOVA) and Kruskal-Wallis ANOVA were performed on moult and predation data. Since the design was not suitable for probit analysis, χ^2-analysis was performed to test differences in mortality (Zar 1974).

Bioassays with nymphs of Peucetia sp.

Age and origin of nymphs

Egg sacs were collected from *Opuntia* spp. near Betioky, South-western Madagascar, in May 1994. Tests started three days after the nymphs' emergence from the egg sac. All nymphs in each test series originated from the same egg sac to assure genetic homogeneity.

General outline of tests

Nymphs (20 per treatment group) were maintained together in test tubes ($\emptyset = 1.8$ mm; length = 180 mm), closed with cotton mesh, at ± 25 °C under natural (indoor) light:dark cycle. Starting 5 days after emergence, nymphs were fed termite larvae (10 per tube). Additional prey was provided whenever the number of live termites was < 3 per tube. Mortality was recorded daily for 12 days (test I) or 30 days (tests II and III). Each test was performed in triplicate, with new test solutions prepared in each series.

Test I: Contact + respiratory exposure (glass surface treatment)

Alsystin 050 UL was dissolved in acetone at concentrations of 20, 100 and 500 mg TFM/l. A volume of 0.5 ml was pipetted into tubes. These were evenly rotated by hand until the acetone had evaporated, yielding a final dose rate of 0.1, 0.5 and 2.5 µg a.i./cm^2 (field dose times 1/5, 1 and 5), and subsequently ventilated with an electric fan for 6 h prior to stocking. Control tubes were treated with acetone only.

Test II: Respiratory versus contact + respiratory exposure (paper surface treatment)

Alsystin 050 UL was dissolved in acetone at 500 mg TFM/l. A volume of 0.5 ml was pipetted on both sides of paper strips (45 × 175 mm), yielding a dose rate of 3.125 µg a.i./cm^2 on either side (sixfold field dose). Papers were air-dried at ± 25 °C for 12, 24 and 36 h. One half was coiled up longitudinally like a spiral, placed at the tube bottom and covered with cotton. The other half was rolled up transversely like a cylinder and slid into the tube, covering 80% of the interior glass surface and leaving a longitudinal window for observation. In the first situation, nymphs had no direct contact with papers but were exposed to solvent vapour (methylpyrrolidone and methylnaphtalene), whereas in the second, they were exposed to all solvent, vapour, and TFM.

Test III. Exposure through ingestion

In this test, a simple food chain (organic matter => detritivore => predator) was created to simulate pesticide uptake via prey. Termites were attracted to treated baits in the field. A bait consisted of eight carton discs (Ø = 106 mm) saturated with TFM (Alsystin 25 WP)-treated sugar solution (10%). Three concentrations were tested: 2, 20 and 200 µg a.i./g organic matter (dry weight), corresponding to 1, 10 and 100 times the maximum residual concentration to be expected in litter (Bayer, unpublished data). Control baits were only treated with sugar. Baits were put between two acrylic glass sheets (12 × 20 cm) and buried 10 cm deep in the soil. Once termite larvae had been attracted, the baits were dug out and stored in the laboratory, providing feed for several days. This process was repeated when more feed was needed. Dead termites found in 20 and 200 ppm baits indicated that TFM had actually been taken up. No dead termites were found in 2 ppm and control baits. However, termite mortality was not quantified.

Data analysis

A probit analysis was performed for mortality data from test I 24 and 48 h post-treatment, using an SPSS 5.0.1 statistical package. ANOVA was applied to arc-sine-transformed mortality data from tests II and III 30 days post-treatment. In most cases, conclusions could be drawn based on descriptive statistics.

Small-scale field trial

Site description

The trial was conducted near Akjoujt, western Mauritania, from December 1992 to January 1993. Four isolated patches (±0.25 ha) of dense (cover 50–70%) *Hyoscyamus muticus* (Solanaceae) vegetation were selected. The spider fauna mainly consisted of *Thanatus* sp. and *Peucetia viridis* (Blackwall).

Design, dose rate and application

The Before-After-Control-Impact- (BACI-) design was adapted in these trials, in which sampling dates are considered as pseudo-replicates in time (Stewart-Oaten et al. 1986). The sampling period was 42 days, 16 days pre-treatment (PRE) and 26 days post-treatment (POST). The latter was further divided into POST 1 (12 days) and POST 2 (14 days) to distinguish short- and medium-term effects. Two plots were sprayed with TFM (Alsystin 050 UL) at a dose rate of 25 g a.i./ha and 100 g a.i./ha, respectively, using hand-held Micro-Ulva spinning disk sprayers (orange nozzle, six batteries, flow rate: 40 ml/min). Each treated plot was paired with an untreated control plot.

Sampling methods and intervals

Relative abundance of *Thanatus* sp. was monitored using 16 pitfall-traps/plot ($\emptyset$ = 6.5 cm; preservation fluid: 0.5% formalin + detergent). Traps were grouped in four sets of four at an inter-trap distance of 10–15 m between and 1 m within sets. Absolute abundance was determined by counting spiders on four randomly selected individual *H. muticus* plants of equal size on each sampling date. To facilitate the search, plants were transferred to plastic bags, roots and subfoliar topsoil included, and stored in a deep-freeze to kill spiders prior to counting. Pitfall-traps were emptied and plant samples searched every second day.

Data analysis

Prior to statistical analysis, catch data for each sampling date were pooled, log (n + 1)-transformed, and the difference treatment minus control of transformed data calculated. Analysis of variance (ANOVA) followed by a Newman-Keuls (NK) multiple range test was performed to examine differences between phases PRE, POST 1 and POST 2.

Results

Bioassays with P. mirabilis

No dose-response-dependent effects of technical TFM on spiders were observed in tests I and II. The overall mortality was low ($\leq$30%) until the end of hibernation ($\approx$120 days), but relatively high ($\geq$40%) at the end of the bioassay (Tab. 1). However, differences between treatment groups were not significantly different at any time. Moulting also remained unaffected (Tab. 2). A slight decrease in predation activity was noted at a dose of 50 µg/spider (topical application). This difference was, however, not significant (p = 0.12). In contrast, 90–100% of all TFM-treated *Gryllus* sp. died nine days post-treatment (Tab. 1; degrees of freedom = 4, χ^2 = 18.2, p < 0.01). This result confirmed the principal effectiveness of TFM against a potential target insect.

Table 1. Bioassays with *P. mirabilis*. Percent cumulative mortality (M) at various points in time (1 at the beginning, 2 at the end of hibernation, 3 180 days post-treatment), all differences not significant at $p < 0.05$; mortality in positive control (*Gryllus* sp.) on day 9 post-treatment included, difference significant at $p < 0.01$

Test and mode of treatment		Treatment and dosage (µg a.i.)				
		No treatment	Vehicle-control	0.00125	0.25	50
I (topical)	M1	15	15	15	15	10
	M2	20	15	20	15	25
	M3	40	30	45	50	75
II (ingestion)	M1	10	0	30	10	10
	M2	15	5	30	20	10
	M3	45	60	45	65	45
Pos. control (top.)	M-*Gryllus*	40	50	90	100	100

Table 2. Bioassays with *P. mirabilis*. Mean number of moults (until 180 days post-treatment) and mean predation rate (until 46 days post-treatment) ±SD. All differences not significant at $p < 0.05$

Treatment and dosage (µg a.i.)	Number of moults	Predation rate (%)
	Test I – topical application	
No treatment	3.0 (0.6)	94.7 (2.3)
Vehicle-control	2.9 (0.5)	95.2 (2.2)
0.00125	2.8 (0.6)	95.0 (3.6)
0.25	3.3 (0.7)	96.1 (2.4)
50	3.4 (0.6)	91.6 (6.4)
	Test II – exposure via ingestion	
No treatment	4.4 (0.7)	95.5 (3.3)
Vehicle-control	4.1 (0.8)	95.5 (2.2)
0.00125	4.1 (0.8)	95.3 (4.4)
0.25	3.7 (0.5)	96.0 (2.4)
50	4.1 (0.5)	95.3 (3.0)

Bioassays with nymphs of Peucetia *sp.*

Test I

Alsystin 050 UL had a clear-cut initial toxic effect on *Peucetia* sp. The LD_{50} was 0.9 µg a.i./cm^2 (95%-confidence interval [CI]: 0.4–2.5) and 0.7 µg a.i./cm^2 (95%-CI: 0.3–4.4) after 24 and 48 h, respectively. Mortality remained nearly unchanged thereafter (Fig. 1), and no moult disruptures were observed. This indicates that the initial effect was not caused by TFM, in which case the response would have shown up with delay. After 6 h ventilation, solvents had not

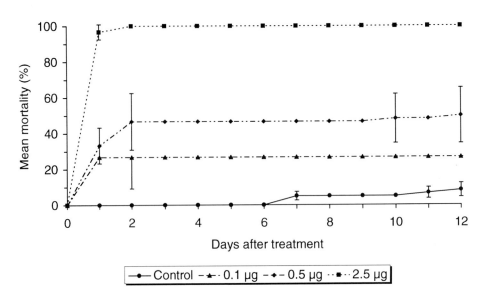

Figure 1. *Glass surface treatment.* Mean cumulative mortality in *Peucetia* sp. SD bars only shown once on each mortality level.

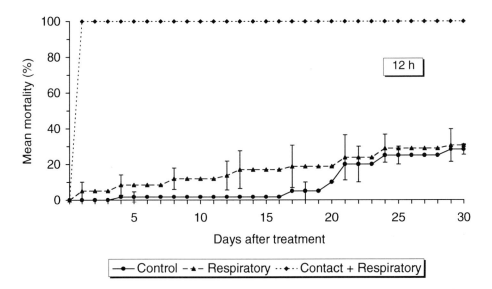

Figure 2. Paper surface treatment. Papers dried for 12 h. Mean cumulative mortality in *Peucetia* sp.; comment on SD bars, see Figure 1.

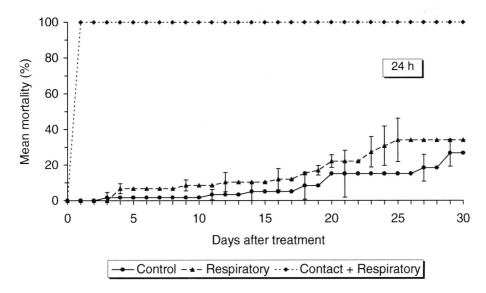

Figure 3. Paper surface treatment. Papers dried for 24 h. Mean cumulative mortality in *Peucetia* sp.; comment on SD bars, see Figure 1.

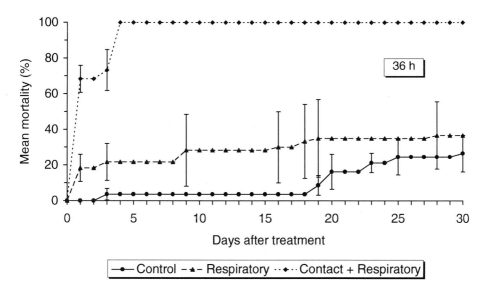

Figure 4. Paper surface treatment. Papers dried for 36 h. Mean cumulative mortality in *Peucetia* sp.; comment on SD bars, see Figure 1.

completely evaporated, and those nymphs dying within two days obviously had direct contact with these residues.

Test II

As in test I, Alsystin 050 UL was highly toxic to nymphs directly exposed to treated surfaces (Figs 2–4). Even when exposed to papers dried for 36 h, mortality increased to 100% within four days, indicating a strong residual activity of this formulation. In contrast, mortality in nymphs exposed to the solvent vapour only, though slightly elevated in all tests, did not differ significantly from controls.

Test III

Mortality in nymphs feeding on Alsystin 25 WP-baited termites did not differ significantly from controls ($p = 0.30$; Fig. 5).

Small-scale field trials

The majority of *Thanatus* sp. caught were in the juvenile stage. No adverse effects were detected at a dose rate of 25 g TFM/ha (Figs 6–7, Tab. 3). Both relative and absolute abundance in

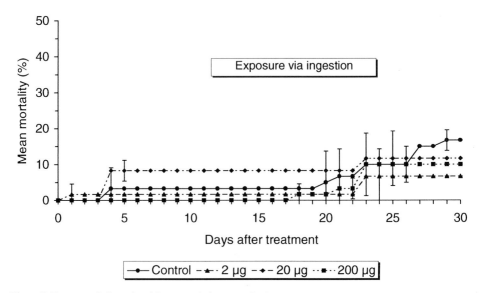

Figure 5. Exposure via ingestion. Mean cumulative mortality in *Peucetia* sp.; comment on SD bars, see Figure 1.

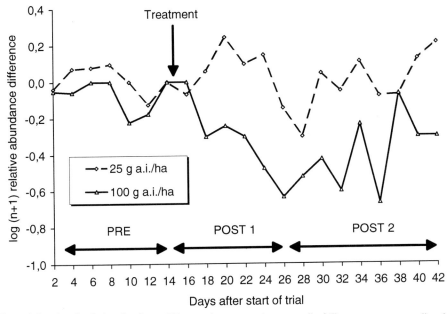

Figure 6. Log (n + 1) relative abundance difference (treatment minus control) of *Thanatus* sp. per sampling date.

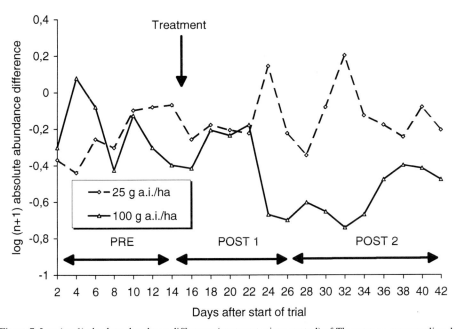

Figure 7. Log (n + 1) absolute abundance difference (treatment minus control) of *Thanatus* sp. per sampling date.

Table 3. Mean percent *Thanatus* sp. abundance in treated plots of paired untreated controls before (PRE) and after treatments (POST 1 and 2). Data detransformed from mean log (n + 1)-abundance differences

| | Mean percent abundance of paired untreated control (95% confidence interval) | | | |
| | Relative abundance | | Absolute abundance | |
Dose rate (a.i./ha)	25	100	25	100
PRE	101 (87 – 117)a	86 (73 – 102)a	59 (45 – 77)a	57 (40 – 81)a
POST 1	104 (64 – 169)a	39 (27 – 56)b	68 (45 – 101)a	37 (20 – 68)ab
POST 2	110 (86 – 140)a	43 (27 – 67)b	79 (58 – 109)a	28 (21 – 38)b

Data not sharing a letter are significantly different at $p < 0.05$

treated and control plots followed the same temporal course. In contrast, at 100 g a.i./ha, relative and absolute abundance were significantly lower (approx. one half of control) during the POST 2 phase than in the PRE phase (medium-term effect). Relative abundance was also significantly lower during POST 1 (short-term effect). However, these effects were mainly due to a post-treatment population increase in the control rather than a dramatic decline in the treated plot.

Discussion

Among the wide array of possible effects of BPUs on arthropods, moult disruptures and malformations of the cuticle are the most commonly reported (Retnakaran et al. 1985). In the present study, however, technical-grade TFM had no effect on *P. mirabilis*, irrespective of the dose and mode of exposure, and moulting frequency did not differ from controls even at a dose of 50 μg a.i. per individual. Similar bioassays with another European species, *Xysticus cristatus* (Clerck) [Thomisidae], confirmed the results reported here for *P. mirabilis* (Köhne 1995, unpublished data). Since the recommended field dose is only 50 g a.i./ha in locust control, and may reach a maximum rate of 300 g a.i./ha in army worm control (Bayer1993), the "initial environmental concentration" (Barret et al. 1994) is unlikely to reach critical values. Even in a worst-case scenario (e.g. direct exposure to spray at a dose rate of 1000 g a.i./ha), the quantity of TFM depositing onto an individual spider would not exceed 5 to 10 μg.

Contrary to technical-grade TFM, Alsystin 050 UL had an unexpected knock-down effect on *Peucetia* sp. nymphs which lasted for one to four days post-treatment (Figs 1–4). In test I, spiders either died shortly after the first contact with Alsystin 050 UL residues or survived until test termination. In test II, no spiders survived when directly exposed to papers treated 12, 24 or 36 h earlier. This effect was obviously not caused by TFM, in which case mortality would have increased more regularly over time. The results suggest that the toxicity was due to the solvents used in this formulation (methylpyrrolidone and methylnaphthalene), and that the low volatility of these combined carriers accounted for the residual effect. Unfortunately, no blanks of this formulation were available at the time of testing. Survival was shown not to be affected when spiders were exposed to the solvent vapour alone. This indicates that direct contact with treated surfaces was a prerequisite of Alsystin 050 UL toxicity. It also proves that the toxicity observed was not a laboratory artefact attributable, for example, to the impeded ventilation of test tubes.

With regard to the exposure of *Peucetia* sp. through ingestion, the real amount – if any – of TFM taken up via termites remains unknown. Since BPUs are generally not accumulated in insects, the net uptake by spiders would be a function of the elimination rate in their insect prey and the time elapsed until the prey is actually killed and fed upon. In this study, termites often survived up to two days before being attacked, and an effective metabolisation and excretion might already have taken place. In addition, chemical transformations caused by the digestion fluid as well as microfiltering (Foelix 1992) of TFM crystals may have hampered pesticide uptake. Despite these uncertainties, and based on the fact that this bioassay simulated a "real world" exposure regime, the results provided clear evidence that effects following consumption of contaminated prey can be precluded. This conforms well with previous results from bioassays in Mauritania, in which continuous feeding on houseflies which had been injected with up to 150 µg TFM (Alsystin 480 SC) did not affect survival and moulting of sub-adult *P. viridis* and *Thanatus* sp. (Peveling et al. 1994).

Thanatus sp. belongs to the group of "sit and wait" predators hiding in litter or vegetation in wait for prey. Thus direct collection of spray droplets as in web-building spiders is very unlikely. In the field trials in Mauritania, *Thanatus* sp. lived in close association with the densely foliated *H. muticus*. In this situation, *Thanatus* sp. was not affected by Alsystin 050 UL at 25 g a.i./ha, which is the lower limit of field doses recommended for locust control (Bayer 1993). However, an approximate 50% net decline relative to the control was observed at 100 g a.i./ha. Since the spray volume (2 l/ha) was four times higher in this application, spiders were more exposed to droplets and spray residues on the leaves, and it appears that – as in the bioassays – the effect was due to the acute toxicity and residual activity of the chemical carriers, which made up 95% of the total spray volume. Despite the effects observed, Alsystin 050 UL would only be classified as slightly harmful to spiders according to Hassan's hazard classification (1992). It is noteworthy that the manufacturer has meanwhile replaced the methylnaphthalene component in Alsystin 050 UL.

Chitin synthesis is considered a uniform process in all arthropods, and it is not understood why spiders, like most of the closely related mites (Graf 1993), are not susceptible to BPUs. Since the rate of metabolism and excretion is a key factor controlling the toxicity of BPUs to insects (Clarke and Jewess 1990), the hypothesis may be put forward that spiders eliminate BPUs more efficiently and are thus less susceptible than insects.

Acknowledgements
We are grateful to J. Everts and H. van der Valk, FAO-LOCUSTOX project, Senegal, for critical discussions. We are also grateful to Sow Demba Ousmane, Mauritania, and Dieudonné Andrianantenaina, Madagascar, who assisted in the field trials and bioassays, and R. Jocqué, Belgium, for the identification of Mauritanian spiders.

References

Barret KL, Grandy N, Harrison EG, Hassan S, Oomen P (eds) (1994) Guidance document on regulatory testing procedures for pesticides with non-target arthropods. Results from a joint BART, EPPO/CoE and IOBC worshop in conjunction with SETAC-Europe, held at IAC Wageningen, NL, 28–30 March 1994

Bayer (1993) Alsystin (BAY SIR 8514) – Technical information. Bayer AG, Leverkusen

Clarke BS, Jewess PJ (1990) The inhibition of chitin synthesis in *Spodoptora littoralis* larvae by fluflen-oxyron, teflubenzuron and diflubenzuron. Pesticide Science 28: 377–388

Cooper J, Dobson HM, Scherer R, Rakotonandrasana A (1995) Sprayed barriers of diflubenzuron (ULV) as a control technique against marching hopper bands of migratory locust *Locusta migratoria capito* (Sauss) (Orthoptera: Acrididae) in Southern Madagascar. Crop Protection 14: 137–143

Everts JW, Jocqué RC (1990) Ground-spiders. Pages 225–230 in Everts JW (ed) Environmental effects of chemical locust and grasshopper control – a pilot study. Rome: FAO

Fischer SA, Lenwood WH Jr (1992) Environmental concentrations and aquatic toxicity data on diflubenzuron (Dimilin). Critical Reviews in Toxicology 22 (1): 45–79

Foelix RF (1992) Biologie der Spinnen. Stuttgart: Thieme

Forster, R, Kampmann T, Kula C (1993) Gefährdungsabschätzung für eine Schwammspinnerbekämpfung mit chemischen und biologischen Pflanzenschutzmitteln in den Prüfbereichen Bodenfauna, Honigbiene und Nutzorganismen. Pages 203–217 in BBA (ed) Schwammspinner Kalamität im Forst – Konzepte zu einer integrierten Bekämpfung freifressender Schmetterlingsraupen. Mitteilungen aus der Biologischen Bundesanstalt für Land- und Forstwirtschaft 293. Berlin: Kommissionsverlag Paul Parey

Graf JF (1993) The role of insect growth regulators in arthropod control. Parasitology Today 9 (12): 471–474

Hassan SA (ed) (1992) Guidelines for testing the effects of pesticides on beneficial organisms: description of test methods. Bulletin IOBC/WPRS XV(3)

Hof A, Heimann, D, Römbke J (1995) Further development for testing the effects of pesticides on wolf spiders. Ecotoxicology and Environmental Safety 31: 264–270

Jepson PC (1993) Ecological insights into risk analysis: the side-effects of pesticides as a case study. Science of the Total Environment, Suppl 1993: 1547–1566

Köhne E (1995) Wirkungstests mit Triflumuron (Alsystin) an Araneae. Unpublished MSc thesis. Saarbrücken

KroKene P (1993) The effect of an insect growth regulator on grasshoppers (Acrididae) and non-target arthropods in Mali. Journal of Applied Entomology 116: 248–266

Mansour F, Nentwig W (1988) Effects of agrochemical residues on four spider taxa: laboratory methods for pesticide tests with web-building spiders. Phytoparasitica 16 (4): 317–326

Müller P (1992) Laborversuche und Testapplikationen mit Alsystin (480 SC und 250 OF) gegen *Oedaleus senegalensis* und andere Heuschrecken. Unpublished report to Bayer AG. Saarbrücken, Leverkusen

Peveling R, Weyrich J, Müller P (1994) Side-effects of botanicals, insect growth regulators and ento-mopathogenic fungi on epigeal non-target arthropods in locust control. Pages 147–176 in Krall S, Wilps H (eds) New trends in locust control. Schriftenreihe der GTZ 245. Rossdorf: TZ Verlagsgesellschaft

Retnakaran A, Granett J, Ennis T (1985) Insect growth regulators. Pages 530–601 in Kerkut GA, Gilbert LI (eds) Insect control. Comprehensive Insect Physiology, Biochemistry and Pharmacology 12. Oxford, New York: Pergamon Press

Reynolds SE (1987) The cuticle, growth and moulting in insects: the essential background to the action of acylurea insecticides. Pesticide Science 20: 131–146

Scherer R, Rakotonandrasana MA (1993) Barrier treatment with a benzoyl urea insect growth regulator against *Locusta migratoria capito* (Sauss.) hopper bands in Madagascar. Int J Pest Manag 39(4): 411–417

Scherer R, Célestin H (1996) Persistence of benzoylphenylureas in the control of the migratory locust *Locusta migratoria capito* (Sauss.) in Madagascar. This volume

Stewart-Oaten A, Murdoch WW, Parker KR (1986) Environmental impact assessment: 'pseudoreplication' in time? Ecology 67: 929–940

Tingle CCD, Raholijaona, Rollandson T, Gilbert Z, Romule R (1996) Diflubenzuron and locust control in SW Madagascar: relative abundance of non-target invertebrates following barrier treatment. This volume

Wilps H, Nasseh O (1994) Field tests with botanicals, mycocides and chitin synthesis inhibitors. Pages 51–79 in Krall S, Wilps H (eds) New trends in locust control. Schriftenreihe der GTZ 245. Rossdorf: TZ Verlagsgesellschaft

Wilps H, Diop B (1996) Field investigations on *Schistocerca gregaria* (Forskål) adults, hoppers and hopper bands

Wise DH (1993) Spiders in ecological food webs. Cambridge: University Press

Zar JH (1974) Biostatistical analysis. Englewood Cliffs: Prentice Hall

New Strategies in Locust Control
S. Krall, R. Peveling and D. Ba Diallo (eds)
© 1997 Birkhäuser Verlag Basel/Switzerland

Side-effects of insecticides on non-target arthropods in Burkina Faso

G. Balança and M.-N. de Visscher

CIRAD-GERDAT-PRIFAS, avenue du Val de Monferrand, B.P. 5035, F-34032 Montpellier Cedex 1, France

Summary. For two seasons the side-effects of three insecticides (lambda-cyhalothrin, malathion, pyridaphention) on non-target arthropods were studied in the course of various grasshopper control operations in northern Burkina Faso. This chapter sums up the results. It reveals the importance of certain factors which aggravate side-effects on the non-target fauna (type of insecticide, dosage, microhabitat). Ways of reducing the impacts of these factors are then proposed.

Résumé. Durant deux campagnes agricoles, les effets de trois insecticides (lambda-cyhalothrine, malathion, pyridaphention) sur les arthropodes non cibles ont été étudiés lors de diverses opérations de lutte contre les sauteriaux, au nord du Burkina Faso. Un résumé des résultats est présenté. L'importance de certains facteurs d'aggravation des effets sur la faune non cible est mise en évidence (nature de l'insecticide, dose utilisée, micro-habitat). Des propositions sont faites pour atténuer l'effet de ces facteurs d'aggravation.

Introduction

For several years chemical control of locusts and grasshoppers in the Sahel has been subjected to severe criticism because of major impacts on the environment and on non-target fauna. There-fore, efforts have been stepped up to evaluate adverse effects and to determine ways of limiting them. During the 1992 and 1993 seasons, side-effects of three insecticides on non-target arthro-pods (arachnids and 22 families or orders of insects) were studied in the course of various con-trol operations conducted by the Service de la Protection des Végétaux et du Conditionnement (DPVC) in the province of Yatenga, north-western Burkina Faso. Analysis of the results permitted us to test several hypotheses, and to gauge the importance of factors aggravating short- and medium-term ecotoxicological consequences of chemical control of grasshoppers. This chapter presents a condensed summary and a brief discussion of our field research. The methodology used and the complete results were the subject of another publication. (Balança and de Visscher 1995).

Materials and methods

In 1992 five grasshopper control operations were conducted. Two insecticides were used: lambda-cyhalothrin (two treatments in October) and malathion (three treatments in September and October). These applications were aimed principally at the Senegalese grasshopper (*Oedaleus senegalensis*, Krauss 1877) in millet fields and surrounding fallow land. In 1993 grasshopper density was low, and no ordinary control operations were organised. Therefore, applications were carried out on an experimental scale, the first in July using lambda-cyhalothrin, and the second and third in September and October, respectively, using pyridaphention. These experimental applications were performed in the same manner as ordinary control operations. Plot size varied from 15 to 300 ha. All insecticides were applied in the form of ULV (ultra low volume) formulations with battery-powered hand-held sprayers or motor-powered knapsack sprayers, either by DPVC staff or by trained farmers. Plots larger than 100 ha were treated with vehicle-mounted sprayers. In 1992 insecticide dose rates (see below) were those recommended for grasshopper control. However, in 1993, due to a handling error, one plot was overdosed by 100%.

Non-target arthropods were sampled by means of pitfall traps containing water, sweep-nets, and yellow dishes containing soap solution. Catches were sorted and classified according to family, genus and species. Relative abundance in treated plots of these taxa was calculated by dividing the number of individuals collected by the number obtained on the same day on the control plot. Variation with time of relative abundance is expressed as a percentage of the relative abundance measured just before the treatment. Raw data were log-transformed prior to statistical analysis to fit a normal distribution. All direct comparisons between treatments are based on the analysis of relative abundance of common taxa (joint occurrence) in treated and control plots of the respective year.

Results

Side-effects can be schematically divided into short-term (immediately visible) and medium-term. Medium-term effects are reflected by the degree of recolonisation visible three or four weeks post-treatment. Of those factors aggravating short-term effects, we focused on the type of insecticide, the dose rate and the microhabitat. Some of the results obtained are presented here.

Short-term effects

Side-effects on non-target arthropods of lambda-cyhalothrin applied at 20 g a.i./ha were compared to those of malathion at 480 g a.i./ha in 1992 and to those of pyridaphention at 250 g a.i./ha in 1993 (Tab. 1). In 1992 we discovered that malathion induced a significant reduction in a larger number of common taxa than did lambda-cyhalothrin (64% as compared with 36%). Crickets were the only insects significantly affected by malathion (67% reduction), while they seemed not to be sensitive to lambda-cyhalothrin. On the other hand, the mean reduction in relative abundance, irrespective of significance, was closely related for the two insecticides (maximum of 4% difference). In 1993 the proportion of common taxa significantly affected was the same for lambda-cyhalothrin and pyridaphention (86%), but the mean of all significant reductions in relative abundance was significantly different: 68% for lambda-cyhalothrin and 80% for pyridaphention. The immediate effects on grasshoppers varied little for the various products tested. They were slightly more pronounced than the observed side-effects on non-target arthropods.

In 1993 one plot was erroneously treated with pyridaphention at a dose rate double than recommended for grasshopper control (500 instead of 250 g a.i./ha). This error offered the opportunity to directly study the ecotoxicological implications of overdosing. With the exception of Tingidae (Heteroptera), Bruchidae (Coleoptera) and Hymenoptera, all of which

Table 1. *Summary* of immediate effects of malathion, lambda-cyhalothrin and pyridaphention in 1992 and 1993

Pesticide (dose rate)	1992		1993	
	Lambda-cyhalothrin (20 g a.i./ha)	Malathion (480 g a.i./ha)	Lambda-cyhalothrin (20 g a.i./ha)	Pyridaphention (250 g a.i./ha)
Percentage (%) of common non-target taxa significantly affected	36	64	86	86
(no. of common taxa affected/ no. of common taxa)	(4/11)	(7/11)	(6/7)	(6/7)
Mean reduction (%) in relative abundance of common non-target taxa (only taxa with significant reduction included)	91	89	68	80
Mean reduction (%) in relative abundance of common non-target taxa (all taxa)	56	60	56	67
Mean reduction (%) in relative abundance of grasshoppers	71	74	no grasshoppers	70

experienced a reduction of more than 96% even at a regular dose rate, arachnids and all other insect taxa studied in the course of the two experiments clearly showed a greater reduction at the double dose rate. The mean of significant reductions in relative abundance was 78% at 250 g a.i./ha and 93% at 500 g a.i./ha. This difference was significant at $p < 0.05$.

The importance of arthropod microhabitat occupation in relation to pesticide exposure and susceptibility can be evaluated by comparing pitfall-trap and sweep-net catches. The former are mainly composed of ground dwellers (e.g. tenebrionids, ants), while the latter are composed of herb dwellers (e.g. heteropterans, homopterans). During the two-year study, and based on all (pooled) samples, the overall percentage of taxa *significantly* reduced by various pesticides was lower in ground-dwelling (28%) than in herb-dwelling (63%) taxa. Likewise, mean reduction in relative abundance was significantly lower ($p < 0.01$) in pitfall-trap samples (57%) than in sweep net samples (75%). Separate analysis for arachnids and insects yields slightly different results: the difference is still significant for insects ($p < 0.01$), but not significant for arachnids.

Medium-term effects

These can be gauged by measuring the degree of recolonisation (recovery) of non-targets susceptible to pesticides following an initial population decline. Recovery of a population three or four weeks post-treatment can be expressed as a percentage of the relative abundance (definition see above) measured just before treatment. Recovery is not solely dependent on intrinsic species characteristics (susceptibility, fecundity, dispersal capacity), but also on external factors like the type of insecticide, the dose rate applied and the size of the plot treated. The time of treatment would equally interesting to consider. The later in the rainy season a treatment occurs, the more difficult recolonisation will be, because a number of species naturally reduce their activity in the dry season (diapause), which limits their capacity to recolonise a zone where the population has been reduced at the end of the rainy season. However, the insufficient number of similar treatments – with respect to insecticide, dose rate and plot size – at various points in time prevents us from testing this hypothesis.

In order to directly compare side-effects of two different insecticides in the medium term, recovery was estimated for two plots of approximately similar size (25 and 30 ha) treated with lambda-cyhalothrin and malathion, respectively, on October 21, 1992. Based on analysis of sweep-net samples, which comprised four insect families (Tettigoniidae, Alydidae, Bruchidae, Curculionidae) and arachnids, recolonisation in the lambda-cyhalothrin-treated plot (50%; 20 days post-treatment) was considerably lower than in the malathion sprayed plot (79%; 22 days post-treatment), but this difference was not statistically significant.

Table 2. Recolonisation (= percent post-treatment of pre-treatment relative abundance) of arachnids and insects 22 days (250 g a.i./ha) and 31 days (500 g a.i./ha) after treatment with pyridaphention

Insecticide		Pyridaphention	
Date of treatment		20.10.93	28.09.93
Dose rate (g a.i./ha)		250	500
	Arachnids	203	25
Pitfall-	Crickets	55	6
trap	Tenebrionidae	106	2
samples	Ants	31	104
	Diptera	19	114
Mean recolonisation (I)		*83*	*50*
	Arachnids	78	51
	Tettigoniidae	0	50
	Cicadellidae	45	125
Sweep-	Lygaeidae	82	60
net	Tingidae	175	6
samples	Bruchidae	96	28
	Chrysomelidae	565	46
	Curculionidae	310	0
	Wasps	47	48
	Diptera	78	86
Mean recolonisation (II)		*148*	*50*
Yellow	Arachnids	58	7
dish	Wasps	212	47
samples	Diptera	173	102
Mean recolonisation (III)		*148*	*52*
Mean recolonisation (I–III)		*130*	*50*
Recolonisation of grasshoppers		30	30

Comparison of recovery in the two plots treated with pyridaphention at single (250 g a.i./ha) and double (500 g a.i./ha) dose rates reveals great differences (Tab. 2). In 12 of 18 common taxa, recolonisation was substantially reduced in the overdosed plot. The mean 31 days post-treatment was only 50% as compared to 130% 22 days post-treatment in the plot sprayed at the recommended dose rate. Since the time gap between treatment and sampling was longer in the overdosed plot (31 versus 22 days), the difference might have been even greater on day 22 post-treatment. Differences in mean recolonisation are significant for sweep-net samples ($p < 0.05$) and for pooled pitfall-trap, sweep-net and yellow dish samples ($p < 0.01$). Grasshopper recolonisation was the same in both plots (30%).

The effect of plot size on arthropod recovery was analysed through comparison of sweep-net samples of two plots treated with malathion at equal dose rates (480 g a.i./ha),. but of quite different size (30 ha and 300 ha). For the six taxa included, mean recolonisation was significantly higher in the smaller plot (108%) as compared to the larger plot (14%) at $p < 0.05$, respectively 22 and 25 days after treatment.

Discussion

Differences in side-effects of lambda-cyhalothrin and organophosphates on non-target arthropods were generally minimal. The only significant difference concerned acute effects of lambda-cyhalothrin and pyridaphention. The effects of fenitrothion, an organphosphate reputed to be very toxic, were not examined in these studies. This insecticide is rarely used in Burkina Faso, particularly in cultivated areas and with hand-held sprayers.

The double dose rate of pyridaphention caused both a greater initial decline of non-target populations and a much reduced recovery one month post-treatment. Thus, overdosing seriously affected some populations to such an extent that recolonisation was hampered even in the longer term. The larger quantity will undoubtedly have taken longer time to drop below lethal environmental concentrations. Contrary to the recovery of non-targets, the reinvasion of grasshoppers was not affected by overdosing. It appears that overdosing can induce greater short-term and medium-term side-effects on non-target arthropods (or at least for a certain proportion) than on grasshoppers. Apart from economic reasons for respecting recommended dose rates, there are thus also sound ecological reasons for doing so. An attempt could even be made to vary dose rates in line with the sensitivity of target grasshoppers (and locusts) and their density. Since no treatments are undertaken until a certain threshold density is reached, which will depend on the grasshopper species and the state of the threatened crop, one option would be to adjust dose rates to the minimum required to efficiently reduce pest densities below damage thresholds.

Our results show that the ground vegetation cover constitutes a screen which protects ground-dwelling arthropods. The fauna inhabiting weeded fields is generally more exposed to chemicals and thus at a greater risk to be affected than that inhabiting fallow fields.

Some of ours results showed that a 10-fold increase in plot size resulted in a sevenfold reduction in non-target arthropod recolonisation within several weeks. Once again, with the goal of protecting beneficial arthropods, it is worthwhile to test the efficacy of a strategy of grasshopper control which spares plots of several hectares within treated zones as reservoirs for recolonisation.

Large-scale control operations often take place when *O. senegalensis* invades mature grain crops at the end of the rainy season. Since damage inflicted by this species to mature crops is relatively low, control does not always appear to be justified at this time of the season, even when aiming to reduce reproduction. Thus natural control of eggs by predators and parasitoids (Coleoptera, Diptera, Hymenoptera) could help reduce net reproduction, and chemical control would only be effected at the beginning of the following season, if hopper densities are high.

While still waiting for an ideal insecticide which is effective against locusts and grasshoppers, but safe to non-target arthropods, it is possible to take certain measures to limit adverse effects without hampering the protection of threatened crops. These elements could be incorporated into the principles of integrated locust and grasshopper control. Before this can be finalised, however, additional research is needed in collaboration with the plant protection services.

References

Balança G, de Visscher M-N 1995. Effets des traitements chimiques antiacridiens sur des coléoptères terrestres au Nord du Burkina Faso. Ecologie 26 (2): 115–126

Susceptibility of target acridoids and non-target organisms to *Metarhizium anisopliae* and *M. flavoviride*

C. Prior

The Royal Horticultural Society's Garden, Wisley, Waking, Surrey GU23 6GB, UK

Summary. *Metarhizium flavoviride* IMI 330189 is an insect pathogenic fungus from Niger with high virulence to acridoids (locusts and grasshoppers) and is under development by the LUBILOSA programme as a bioinsecticide. Strains with similar biochemical and molecular characteristics have been obtained from many countries in West and East Africa and also from Madagascar, Australia, Ecuador and Brazil. The strains are distinctive from the two previously described varieties and form a third subdivision of the species ("group 3"). IMI 330189 is virulent to a wide range of acridoid hosts under field conditions. Under laboratory conditions, the strain is infectious to honey-bees, although at the field doses used by LUBILOSA only 11% of test bees became infected. In tests carried out by FAO LOCUSTOX in Senegal, IMI 330189 was also infectious to *Bracon hebetor*, but control mortality was high, suggesting that the test protocol placed the insects under stress which may have rendered them more susceptible. IMI 330189 shows moderate virulence to termites and was not virulent to several species of beetle, weevil, coreid bugs, ants and cockroaches.

Résumé. Le programme LUBILOSA poursuit actuellement des travaux sur l'utilisation comme bio-insecticide de *Metarhizium flavoviride* IMI 330189, un champignon entomopathogène du Niger très virulent contre les acridiens (locustes et sauteriaux). Des souches présentant des caractéristiques bio-chimiques et moléculaires semblables ont été obtenues dans de nombreux pays d'Afrique de l'Ouest et de l'Est, ainsi qu'à Madagascar, en Australie, en Equateur et au Brésil. Ces souches différent des deux variétés décrites précédemment et constituent une troisième subdivision de l'espèce («groupe 3»). IMI 330189 est virulent pour un large groupe d'acridiens hôtes dans des conditions d'expérimentation sur le terrain. En laboratoire, la souche infecte les abeilles bien qu'aux doses employées sur le terrain par LUBILOSA seulement 11% des abeilles testées aient été infectées. Au cours d'essais menés par FAO LOCUSTOX au Sénégal, IMI 330189 a également infecté *Bracon hebetor*, mais la mortalité parmi les insectes témoins ayant également été élevée, on peut en déduire que le protocole des essais mettait les insectes dans une situation de stress et pouvait les avoir rendu plus sensibles. La virulence d'IMI 330189 sur les termites est modérée et elle est nulle sur différentes espèces de coléoptères, charançons, Coreidae, fourmis et cafards.

Introduction

Recent concerns over possible human health problems and environmental damage resulting from the large-scale application of chemical pesticides for locust and grasshopper control, as well as doubts about their efficacy (Anon. 1990), have led to proposals for alternative control strategies. However, most rely on the development of new technologies such as remote sensing and semiochemicals (van Huis 1992) which do not yet exist in implementable forms. It is likely, therefore, that control will continue to depend on pesticide spraying in the near future, and thus concerns about detrimental side-effects will be best addressed by improving the safety of the pesticides used.

Biological control based on pathogens formulated as biological pesticides is an alternative which offers more rapid prospects for implementation. Deuteromycete fungal pathogens are the most promising candidates for biopesticide development (Prior and Greathead 1989). As a result of the interest in these fungi as alternatives to chemical insecticides, the governments of Canada, the Netherlands, Switzerland, the United Kingdom and the USA have supported the research programme Lutte Biologique contre les Locustes et les Sauteriaux (LUBILOSA). This programme is executed by the International Institute of Biological Control (IIBC), the International Institute of Tropical Agriculture (IITA) and the Centre pour Agronomie, Hydrologie, Meteorologie (AGRHYMET), an institute of the Comité Inter-Etats pour la Lutte contre la Sécheresse dans le Sahel (CILSS); (LUBILOSA formerly cooperated with the Département de Formation en Protection des Végétaux (DFPV), now a part of AGRHYMET-CILSS) (Prior et al. 1992). The LUBILOSA programme concentrates primarily on the genus *Metarhizium*.

The genus *Metarhizium*: current taxonomic status

The genus *Metarhizium* is placed in the Deuteromycotina: Moniliales and contains two species virulent to acridoids, *M. anisopliae* var. *anisopliae* and *M. flavoviride*. The genus has been regarded by some workers as a single species, *M. anisopliae*, containing numerous varieties (var. *album*, var. *flavoviride* etc.) including some as yet uncharacterised (Milner et al. 1994): however, this revision has not yet been formally proposed.

Isolates of *M. flavoviride* that have been studied in detail fall into three morphological groups:

Group 1 isolates with pale green conidia from North European Coleoptera and soil, including the type of *M. f.* var. *flavoviride* Gams and Rozsypal;

Group 2 isolates with smaller, pale green conidia from Homoptera in South-East Asia, including the type of *M. f.* var. *minus* Rombach, Humber and Roberts;

Group 3 isolates with dark green conidia from acridoids in West Africa, Tanzania, Madagascar, Australia, Brazil and the Galapagos Islands studied by the LUBILOSA programme.

St. Leger et al. (1992) noted that *M. flavoviride* isolates from Europe, the Philippines and the Galapagos Islands (corresponding to groups 1, 2 and 3 above) were genetically distinct, and additional biochemical and molecular taxonomic studies indicate that group 3 isolates form a distinctive taxon (Bridge et al. 1993; Bidochka et al. 1994). Recent studies using PCR-RAPD (P. Bridge, personal communication) and rDNA sequencing (F. Driver, R.J. Milner, J.W.O. Ballard and J. Curran, personal communication) have further determined that this taxon may be sufficiently distinct from groups 1 and 2 to merit a new varietal name "var. *acridum*" (Milner et al. 1994), but no attempt has been made yet to validate this name as a formal taxon.

Virulence of *Metarhizium* genotypes to acridoids

The LUBILOSA programme has accumulated many *Metarhizium* isolates from both acridoid and non-acridoid hosts. Acridoids have yielded predominantly *M. flavoviride* group 3, but also some *M. anisopliae*; none have been *M. flavoviride* group 1 or 2. More than 160 isolates have been screened for virulence to *S. gregaria* by topical application of a measured dose of conidia (Bateman et al. 1992) since the programme began in 1989. Experience with the application of this screening method to both *S. gregaria* and other acridoid species in Benin and Niger has shown that *S. gregaria* is relatively susceptible to infection by some isolates of *Metarhizium anisopliae* and all isolates of *M. flavoviride* group 3, but not to *M. a.* var. *majus* or *M. f.* var. *flavoviride* or var. *minus* (groups 1 and 2).

The dose used for screening by the LUBILOSA programme is higher than would be applied during field treatment (75,000 conidia per adult insect, equivalent to approx. 37,000 conidia per gram of body weight). At this dose, virulent isolates kill 50% of the test insects in 4–5 days. The screening programme has revealed a continuous gradation of virulence from isolates where all insects are dead within 4 days to isolates where no mycosis is evident after >10 days. The isolate first selected for investigation, IMI 330189 (Prior et al. 1992), has been included in many of the screens as a standard for comparison. The mean average survival time (AST) for 26 tests on this isolate is 4.4 days (SD 0.45) (R.P. Bateman, M. Carey and D. Moore, unpublished results). More than 20 isolates of *Metarhizium* spp. are as virulent as this standard, and the majority of these are *M. flavoviride* group 3, collected exclusively from acridoid hosts.

All *M. f.* group 3 isolates are highly virulent to *S. gregaria*, but *M. anisopliae* has unpredictable virulence. Isolates obtained from acridids in Oman and Pakistan, gryllids in Australia and a tettigonid in Brazil all had low or no virulence to *S. gregaria*, whereas isolates from acridids in Ethiopia and Australia had high virulence. However, isolates from coleopterans in the USA, Côte d'Ivoire, India and Taiwan, a hemipteran in Trinidad and soil in Benin and Cameroon also had high virulence. Many of the screens using these non-acridoid isolates showed high levels of non-mycosis mortality, with little or no sporulation on the cadavers. By contrast, virulent acridoid isolates of *M. anisopliae* and most *M. flavoviride* group 3 usually sporulated on the cadavers.

M. f. group 3 isolates show moderate to high virulence to the pyrgomorphid *Zonocerus variegatus* in West Africa. There is some evidence from screens and field tests that isolates from acridids are less virulent to this pyrgomorphid pest than pyrgomorphid isolates, though the reverse does not seem to be the case (I. Godonou and C.J. Lomer, personal communication).

Virulence of IMI 330189 to non-target arthropods

IMI 330189 is the *M. flavoviride* group 3 strain chosen by LUBILOSA for field testing under the registered tradename Green Muscle. The available data on host range for this strain are tabulated here (Tab. 1). Experiments were carried out by: IITA, Benin; LOCUSTOX, Senegal; IIBC, UK; Rothamsted Experimental Station, UK; CSIRO, Australia; CATIE, Costa Rica. With the exception of field observations on myrmeleonid spp. and an unidentified tettigonid sp., all data were obtained under laboratory conditions. Except in the experiments on *Phyllophaga* sp. and termites, acridids were used as positive controls in all experiments, and the doses used caused high mortality.

IMI 330189 appears to be highly virulent to many acridoids, including most of the important pest species, but shows low virulence to other families in the Orthoptera or in most other orders. The infections in hymenopterans require comment. Data presented by LOCUSTOX for six experiments on *Bracon hebetor* showed that control mortality (blank oil treatment) was 52–80% compared with 84–100% for the *Metarhizium*-treated insects. Sporulation (the check for infectivity) ranged from 32–100% in the treated insects. The results indicate that IMI 330189 is infectious to *B. hebetor* under these experimental conditions, although the high control mortality suggests that the treated insects may have been under stress, which would increase their susceptibility. In tests on *Apis mellifera*, a realistic field dose killed 11% of the test bees and all the test locusts, compared with a control consisting of a fenitrothion-pyrethroid insecticide mixture which killed all test bees at a dose slightly under the realistic field dose (the dose was sub-lethal to locusts). Doses of *M. flavoviride* equivalent to twice the expected field dose resulted in 30% mortality of bees and a 20-fold higher dose killed 87%. Infections were confirmed at all doses from both oil and water formulations (Ball et al. 1994). Laboratory experimental systems place stress on social insects such as bees, and further tests are planned to see if infection occurs under field conditions.

Table 1. Arthropod host range data for IMI 330189

Host	Susceptibility
Orthoptera: Acrididae	
Schistocerca gregaria	High
Locusta migratoria	High
Locustana pardalina	High
Chortoicetes terminifera	High
Oedaleus senegalensis and *O. nigeriensis*	High
Kraussaria angulifera	High
Diabolocatantops axillaris	High
Acorypha glaucopsis	High
Aiolopus simulatrix and *A. thalassinus*	High
Phaulacridium bivittatum	High
Hieroglyphus daganensis	Moderate
Cataloipus cymbiferus and *C. fuscocoerulipes*	Moderate
Homoxyrrhepes punctipennis	Moderate
Orthoptera: Pyrgomorphidae	
Zonocerus variegatus	Moderate
Pyrgomorpha cognata	Moderate
Orthoptera: Gryllidae	
Teleogryllus commodus	Very low
Orthoptera: Tettigonidae	
Unid. sp.	None
Coleoptera: Curculionidae	
Neochetina eichhorniae	None
Coleoptera: Tenebrionidae	
Pimelia sinensis	None
Trachyderma hispida	None
Tenebrio molitor	Low
Coleoptera: Coccinellidae	
Hyperaspis notata	None
Coleoptera: Scarabaeidae	
Phyllophaga spp.	Low
Heteroptera: Coreidae	
Clavigrella shabadi and *C. tomentosicollis*	None
Hymenoptera: Formicidae	
Tapinoma sp.	None
Hymenoptera: Encyrtidae	
Epidinocarsis lopezi	None
Hymenoptera: Braconidae	
Bracon hebetor	Moderate (see comments in text)
Hymenoptera: Apiidae	
Apis mellifera	Low (see comments in text)
Isoptera: Termitidae	
Coptotermes and *Nasutitermes* spp.	Moderate
Dictyoptera: Blattidae	
Blatta sp.	None
Neuroptera: Myrmeleonidae	
Unidentified spp.	Low

Conclusions

Metarhizium flavoviride IMI 330189 appears to be a member of a highly distinctive, well-characterised genotype known only from acridoids and with low virulence to other arthropods in laboratory tests. In host range tests by LUBILOSA and collaborators, high virulence seems confined to the Acridoidea, although other families in the Orthoptera have not yet been tested. Outside the order Orthoptera, IMI 330189 has shown only low or moderate infectivity to some species in the Isoptera, Coleoptera and some Hymenoptera. Hemiptera, Dictyoptera and other Coleoptera and Hymenoptera were not infected. The infections in Hymenoptera were unexpected and may be at least partly an artefact of laboratory experiments. These insects are difficult to maintain in laboratory conditions. In *A. mellifera*, infectivity was low at field doses, but was dose related. In *B. hebetor*, infectivity was high, but control mortality was also very high. Thus, although there is no doubt that IMI 330189 can infect these species, at least some of the susceptibility may be due to stress imposed by laboratory conditions. Goettel and Johnson (1992) noted a similar situation in studies on the infection of leafcutter bees by *Beauveria bassiana* in Canada.

To elucidate host range fully, arthropods should be subjected to a centrifugal testing programme similar to that used in weed biocontrol to test phytophagous insects and plant pathogens. Centrifugal testing of microbial pest control agents is recommended by Agriculture and Agri-Food Canada (Anon. 1993). Before this can be done, an arthropod taxonomy must be agreed as a basis for test organism selection. We are not aware of any cases where centrifugal testing has been tried in a rigorous way with arthropods and pathogens such as *Metarhizium*. At present, it can only be stated that for IMI 330189 and probably for other group 3 isolates, high virulence appears limited to the Acridoidea.

Acknowledgements
Projet LUBILOSA is an international collaborative research programme. Project staff who have contributed to the data and ideas presented here include Y. Abraham, R. Bateman, D. Batt, M. Carey, D. Moore, P. Shah (IIBC); P. Byrne, O.K. Douro-Kpindou, I. Godonou, J. Langewald, C. Lomer, A. Paraïso, J. Sagbohan (IITA); C. Kooyman and Z. Ouambama (AGRHYMET-CILSS). We also acknowledge the contributions of J. Waage (IIBC), D. Greathead and M. Thomas (Imperial College, London University, UK) P. Bridge and R. Paterson (International Mycological Institute, UK); R. Milner, J. Staples and F. Driver (CSIRO, Australia); H. van der Valk and cooperators (LOCUSTOX, Senegal); B. Ball, B. Pye and N. Carreck (Rothamsted Experimental Station, UK); M. Goettel, J. Irvin and D. Johnson (Agriculture and Agri-Food Canada); M. Bidochka and R. St. Leger (Boyce Thompson Institute, USA); S. Smith and P. Shannon, CATIE, Costa Rica.

References

Anon. (1990) A plague of locusts. Office of Technology Assessment, Special Report OTA-F-450. Washington, DC, US Government Printing Office, p 129

Anon. (1993) Regulatory Proposal: Registration Guidelines for Microbial Pest Control Agents. Pro93-04, Plant Industry Directorate, Agriculture and Agrifood Canada, p 55

Ball BV, Pye BJ, Carreck NL, Moore D, Bateman RP (1994) Laboratory testing of a mycopesticide on non-target organisms: the effects of an oil formulation of *Metarhizium flavoviride* applied to *Apis mellifera*. Biocontr Sci Technol 4: 289–296

Bateman RP, Carey M, Moore D, Prior C (1992) The enhanced infectivity of *Metarhizium flavoviride* in oil formulations to desert locusts at low humidities. Ann Appl Biol 122: 145–152

Bidochka MJ, McDonald MA, St. Leger RJ, Roberts DW (1994) Differentiation of species and strains of entomopathogenic fungi by random amplification of polymorphic DNA. Curr Genet 25: 107–113

Bridge PD, Williams MAJ, Prior C, Paterson RRM (1993) Morphological, biochemical and molecular characteristics of *Metarhizium anisopliae* and *M. flavoviride*. J Gen Microbiol 139: 1163–1169

Goettel MS, Johnson DL (1992) Environmental impact and safety of fungal biocontrol agents. Pages 356–361 in Lomer CJ and Prior C (eds) Biological control of locusts and grasshoppers. CAB International, UK

Milner RJ, Driver F, Curran J, Glare TR, Prior C, Bridge PD, Zimmermann G (1994) Recent problems with the taxonomy within the genus *Metarhizium*, and a possible solution. Pages 109–110 in Proceedings of the VIth International Colloquium on Invertebrate Pathology and Microbial Control, Montpellier, Society of Invertebrate Pathology

Prior C (1989) Biological control of locusts: the potential for the exploitation of pathogens. FAO Plant Prot Bull 37: 37–48

Prior C, Lomer CJ, Herren H, Paraïso A, Kooyman C, Smit JJ (1992) The IIBC/IITA/DFPV collaborative research programme on the biological control of locusts and grasshoppers. Pages 8–20 in Lomer CJ and Prior C (eds) Biological control of locusts and grasshoppers. CAB International, UK

St. Leger RJ, May B, Allee LL, Frank DC, Staples RC, Roberts DW (1992) Genetic differences in allozymes and in formation of infection structures among isolates of the entomopathogenic fungus *Metarhizium anisopliae*. J Invertebr Pathol 60: 89–101

van Huis A (1992) New developments in desert locust management and control. Proc Exper Appl Entomol, NEV Amsterdam 3: 2–18

New Strategies in Locust Control
S. Krall, R. Peveling and D. Ba Diallo (eds)
© 1997 Birkhäuser Verlag Basel/Switzerland

Effects of anti-locust insecticides in surface waters in the Sahel: a summary of five years of research

J. Lahr[1] and A.O. Diallo[2]

[1]FAO, Projet GCP/SEN/041/NET (LOCUSTOX), B.P. 3300, Dakar, Senegal
[2]Ministère de l'Agriculture, Direction de la Protection des Végétaux, Projet GCP/SEN/041/NET (LOCUSTOX), B.P. 20054, Thiaroye, Senegal

Summary. Water is scarce in the Sahel, and its quality is therefore vital to the economy, human populations and wildlife. Aquatic invertebrates and fish play an important role in different types of aquatic ecosystems in the region. Results of field experiments carried out over the past few years indicate that several insecticides used in locust control have considerable adverse effects on non-target aquatic animals in these waters at recommended application rates. The seriousness of the impact varies between different products and between permanent and temporary waters. Following these observations a start was made to develop laboratory-based toxicity tests with aquatic species typical for waters in the Sahel. Some initial results obtained with invertebrates captured in temporary ponds suggest that the acute effects observed in the laboratory can be extrapolated to the field. The text discusses how these results may be applied.

Résumé. L'eau est peu abondante dans le Sahel et pour cette raison sa qualité est un facteur clé pour l'économie, les populations et la vie sauvage. Les invertébrés aquatiques et les poissons jouent un rôle important dans les différents écosystèmes aquatiques dans la région. Les résultats d'expériences de terrain, exécutées pendant les dernières années, ont indiqué que plusieurs insecticides utilisés dans la lutte antiacridienne ont des effets néfastes considérables sur la faune aquatique non-cible dans ces eaux quand ils sont appliqués à la dose recommandée. L'ampleur de l'impact varie selon les différents pesticides et selon les types d'eau: permanents ou temporaires. Suivant ces observations le développement des tests de toxicité au laboratoire avec des espèces typiques des eaux de Sahel a été commencée. Quelques premiers résultats, obtenus avec les animaux capturés dans les mares temporaires semblent indiquer que les effets aiguës observés au laboratoire peuvent être extrapolés au terrain. La façon dont ces données peuvent être utilisées est discutée dans le texte.

Introduction

The aquatic environment and locust control

Water is of primal importance in arid areas like the Sahel region, where bodies of water of different types are used for transport, fishing, irrigation and as a source of drinking water for the human populations and their livestock. The aquatic habitats also attract a good number of wild animals, and their abundance is a key factor for animal survival in the dry season. Several wet zones of the region are considered to be of regional or even global importance, especially for water birds. A large number of nature preserves in the Sahel consist of swamps or estuaries, or contain ponds and other types of aquatic environments.

Surface waters are not intentionally targeted during control operations against desert locusts and grasshoppers. Nevertheless, when insecticides are applied in the vicinity of water bodies, contamination can occur in several ways. The largest bodies of water such as lakes, rivers, flood plains and estuaries may be exposed to pesticide drift carried by the wind, while in abundant small bodies of water, such as swamps, irrigation systems and small ponds, contamination can be direct. Especially when aerial treatments are conducted, it is extremely difficult to locate small bodies of surface water in advance or to interrupt the treatment when a pond is detected just ahead in the area to be treated.

Aquatic organisms in general, and invertebrates in particular, are very sensitive to insecticides. Even though water bodies make up a small proportion of the overall surface of the Sahel region relative to land, effects of contamination can be devastating in this environment. In view of the importance of waters and their great vulnerability, the LOCUSTOX project has given very special attention to the potential effects on bodies of freshwater of the insecticides currently employed in locust and grasshopper control. These aquatic studies are the first to be conducted within the framework of locust control. This article is a summary of a series of publications, to be published at a later date.

The research strategy

Although during its pilot phase in 1989 a study of fish was made as a part of the programme, it was decided to focus aquatic research within the LOCUSTOX project on aquatic invertebrates first. This group of organisms is particularly sensitive to insecticides and also has the advantage that it is easy to study. Among these invertebrates one finds macrocrustaceans (decapods and large branchiopods), microcrustaceans or zooplankton (cladocerans, copepods and ostracods), and aquatic and semi-aquatic insects (notably hemipterans, coleopterans, ephemeropterans, dipterans, dragonflies and damselflies). The selection of invertebrates as a target group is also due to the fact that they constitute a source of food for (semi-)aquatic vertebrates such as birds and fish and that certain species contribute to regulating algal populations. Fish will again become the object of research in the near future because of their economic importance.

The strategy of experimental research adopted, as summarised by Lahr and Diémé (1992), starts with field trials. The application of insecticides on aquatic sites permits the study of effects in a worst-case scenario: a direct and complete contamination at operational dose rates recommended for locust control (FAO 1992, 1995, recommends methods and dose rates of insecticides for the control of desert locusts). These studies were performed to identify indicator species revealing effects under the natural conditions of the ecosystems concerned, and to show the development and dynamics over time of different populations following the insecticide applications.

After the field trials, preliminary laboratory tests were carried out with the most promising indicator species in order to gauge their potential for the development of acute toxicity tests. We are currently performing laboratory tests with two species characteristic of temporary ponds. Currently, these animals are captured in the field, but in the future rearing methods will be developed for several suitable species.

During the pilot phase of the project the type of water studied was permanent water. In view of the risk of direct contamination by aerial treatments and their importance in the rainy season in arid zones, temporary ponds were investigated during the second phase of the project (1991–1994). Their ecology and the biology of the species living there are poorly known.

Location of sites and experiments conducted

Four large irrigation basins (15–30 ha) situated in sugar cane plantations around Richard-Toll in northern Senegal were treated in a large-scale field trial in 1989. We determined that these basins contained fauna resembling that of the Senegal River and its tributaries, most notably with respect to fish and crustaceans. Individual basins were treated with chlorpyrifos, fenitrothion and diflubenzuron.

An appropriate site for the study of temporary ponds has been found at Nioro du Rip, in central Senegal. These ponds are fed by rainfall and are abundant during and shortly after the rainy season, from July to November. They do not exceed 1.5 ha in size and are fairly shallow. Experimental treatments were carried out with fenitrothion, diflubenzuron, deltamethrin and bendiocarb.

Two species from temporary ponds were selected for the laboratory tests: *Streptocephalus sudanicus* (Branchiopoda, Anostraca, Streptocephalidae) and *Anisops sardeus* (Hemiptera, Notonectidae). These fairy shrimps and backswimmers constitute the majority of the macroinvertebrates captured in these ponds.

Results and discussion

At operational dose rates used in locust control two organophosphates, chlorpyrifos and fenitrothion, provoked considerable noxious effects in the irrigation basins. Both caused acute mortality in different macroinvertebrates and reductions of certain populations, which sometimes lasted for several weeks (Lahr 1990). The detrimental long-term effect on the numerous and important freshwater shrimps was significant. The insect growth regulator (IGR) diflubenzuron had less effect on the macroinvertebrates, but it was possibly more noxious for the zooplankton than were the organophosphates. Chlorpyrifos elicited mortality in small fish (Banister 1990), and *Porogobius schlegelii* (Gobiidae) has been shown to disappear completely from treated irrigation basins.

In temporary ponds, particularly diflubenzuron and deltamethrin caused long-term effects (Lahr and Diallo 1993, unpublished data). In *Streptocephalus* spp. (Anostraca, Streptocephalidae) the effects lasted until the ponds dried up some time after the end of the rainy season. Deltamethrin also caused reductions in the populations of different species of backswimmers (Hemiptera, genus *Anisops*) and in one cladoceran (*Ceriodaphnia* sp., Daphniidae). In the cladocerans the effects lasted several weeks, but the adult populations of the backswimmers recovered in the course of a week. Fenitrothion also had effect on *Anisops*, but it was less noxious for anostracans and the zooplankton. The only important effects of bendiocarb in the temporary ponds was the suppression of the populations of cladocerans for some weeks. The few significant reductions occasionally observed in backswimmers after application of this compound were, however, of short duration and may have occurred by chance.

The fauna of temporary ponds is characterised by populations specifically adapted to survival during the dry period. The dormant eggs of *Streptocephalus*, for example, require a period of desiccation before they can hatch. This phenomenon explains why eradicated populations cannot recover during the same rainy season. In contrast, *Diaphanosoma* sp. (Cladocera, Sididae), another producer of dormant eggs, recovered during the same rainy season after treatments with fenitrothion and bendiocarb. This species thus seems to be capable of both continuous and discontinuous reproduction. The prolonged effect of diflubenzuron on this species (until the end of the rainy season) may be attributable to the persistence of this product.

An augmentation of populations of *Paradiaptomus rex* (Copepoda, Diaptomidae) after the applications of fenitrothion and diflubenzuron was probably related to the disappearance of *Streptocephalus* spp. or *Diaphanosoma* sp., which may well be competitors for the same food sources (algae, microbes or yeasts).

The difference in the period required for recovery between adult and larval populations of *Anisops* confirms that the rapid recolonisation by adults is due to their capability to fly and thus to immigrate from untreated areas. The nymphs, which recover less rapidly, are wingless.

In conclusion, it has been shown in field experiments that of the four insecticides tested at dose rates recommended for locust control, all elicited adverse effects on certain populations of aquatic organisms. The application of insecticides in the vicinity of wet zones should be done with the greatest possible care in order to avoid contaminating surface waters. A choice of the product to be applied on the basis of an understanding of the potential risk posed to aquatic ecosystems would reduce the possibility of noxious effects on non-target fauna in these areas.

The effects of the insecticides tested varied, depending on the different products and the types of ecosystems. Some of the most suitable indicator species in the aquatic environment in the Sahel include (small) fish and freshwater shrimp for permanent waters, and fairy shrimp and backswimmers for temporary ponds.

The field trials have provided much information which could not have been obtained solely with research in the laboratory or from a literature survey. Nevertheless, the first series of laboratory tests with *Streptocephalus sudanicus* and *Anisops sardeus* gave results which correspond well with the effects observed in the field. The LOCUSTOX project will continue the development of rearing and test methods with these two species. The possibilities of tests with small fish (juveniles of *Oreochromis niloticus*) and freshwater shrimp (*Palaemonetes africanus* or *Caridina africana*), two other groups of indigenous organisms, will also be studied.

Organisms to be used in the toxicity tests being developed are representative of arid ecosystems. The results can be used in three ways. First of all, they permit us to predict the possible impact on populations in the field. Second, the rapid and easy execution of the tests will allow us to compare the relative toxicity of a much larger range of products than would be possible using field tests. These data can be included in risk analysis of products for registration purposes. Finally, in combination with models for the deposition and drift of spray droplets during ultra low volume (ULV) spraying, test data could be used to define buffer zones.

Acknowledgements
The LOCUSTOX project is a programme of the Food and Agriculture Organisation of the United Nations (FAO) and the Direction de la Protection des Végétaux (DPV) of Senegal. The studies mentioned here have been financed by the governments of the Netherlands, Senegal and the United Kingdom.

References

Banister K (1990) Chapter V. Fish. Pages 99–118 in Everts JW (ed) Environmental effects of chemical locust and grasshopper control. A pilot study, report of Project ECLO/SEN/003/NET LOCUSTOX, FAO, Dakar, Senegal
FAO (1992) The desert locust guidelines IV. Control. FAO, Rome, Italy
FAO (1995) Evaluation of field trial data on the effectiveness of insecticides against locusts and grasshoppers. Report to FAO by the Pesticide Referee Group, 19–21 September 1994, Rome, Italy

Lahr J (1990) Chapter IV: Aquatic invertebrates. Pages 67–98 in Everts JW (ed) Environmental effects of chemical locust and grasshopper control. A pilot study, report of project ECLO/SEN/003/NET LOCUSTOX, FAO, Dakar, Senegal

Lahr J, Diémé E (1992) Le projet Locustox, un programme de recherche écotoxicologique sur l'impact de la lutte antiacridienne en Afrique sur l'environnement. Pages 77–87 in Balança G, de Visscher MN (eds) Méthodes de recherche en écologie des traitements antiacridiens en Afrique. CIRAD-GERDAT-PRIFAS, Montpellier, France

Lahr J, Diallo AO (1993) Effects of experimental locust control with fenitrothion and diflubenzuron on the aquatic invertebrate fauna of temporary ponds in central Senegal. Report no 93/3, Project ECLO/SEN/003/NET LOCUSTOX, FAO, Dakar, Senegal

Environmental impact

Poster contributions

New Strategies in Locust Control
S. Krall, R. Peveling and D. Ba Diallo (eds)
© 1997 Birkhäuser Verlag Basel/Switzerland

Diflubenzuron and locust control in south-western Madagascar: relative abundance of non-target invertebrates following barrier treatment

C.C.D. Tingle[1], Raholijaona[2], T. Rollandson[3], Z. Gilberte[3] and R. Romule[3]

[1]*Environmental Sciences Department, Natural Resources Institute, Central Avenue, Chatham Maritime, Kent ME4 4TB, UK*
[2]*Research Unit, Anti-locust Centre, B.P. 3, Betioky-Sud, Toliara, Madagascar*
[3]*University of Toliara, Toliara 601, Madagascar*

Results are presented of environmental monitoring associated with large-scale trials to test the efficacy of the insect growth regulator (IGR) Dimilin (diflubenzuron) used in barrier treatments for control of the migratory locust (*Locusta migratoria capito* (Sauss.)) in Madagascar (Cooper et al. 1995). The aim of the study was to assess the impact of diflubenzuron barriers on the relative abundance of non-target invertebrates and the duration of any effects detected, in order to determine the environmental acceptability of this form of locust control at the operational level. Identical sampling techniques were used in two different areas (20 km^2 and 5 km^2, respectively), separated by about 300 km, during two consecutive years, with treatments applied at different times of year. Sweep netting was used to gain a preliminary characterisation of the vegetation-inhabiting invertebrate faunal composition, and to sample those invertebrates most directly at risk from spraying. Results show that faunal composition is similar at the order and family level for the two areas, but quite different at the species level. Short-term monitoring shows that the majority of invertebrates sampled either occurred in numbers too small to evaluate statistically or showed no evidence of effects during the months immediately following treatment, even within spray barriers. However, data for 1993 show marked changes in relative abundance of non-target grasshoppers (Acrididae) with evidence of possible effects on spiders and heteropteran bugs within spray barriers (Tab. 1). Data for 1994 show a severe negative impact on lepidopteran larvae within barriers, lasting for over three months, but show no evidence of changes in relative abundance within the inter-barrier spaces. No effects were detected on non-target grasshoppers (probably because most were already adult by the time of treatment). Possible impacts on spiders and Heteroptera require further investigation, but analysis at family level suggests that any effects are minor and short-lived (Tab. 1).

In the short term, it appears that diflubenzuron barriers can be regarded as a relatively environmentally friendly method of locust control (Keith 1992; van der Valk and Kamara 1993; Balança and de Visscher 1994; Ostermann 1996), but a risk to both Lepidoptera and grasshop-

Table 1. Statistical significance of analysis of variance (ANOVA) on relative abundance of non-target fauna in different treatment areas for the Bemalo (unsprayed; within spray barriers) and Antanimieva (unsprayed; within spray barriers; between spray barriers) study sites: (i) two-way ANOVA for post-treatment period; (ii) ANOVA for individual sample dates both pre- and post-treatment with duration of differences at each level of significance, between treatments. Post-treatment sampling spanned two months in 1993 and three months in 1994

Bemalo 1993

Taxon	Two-way ANOVA Interaction time vs treatment	Pre-treatment (duration in weeks) <1	2	3+	Post-treatment (duration in weeks) <1	2	3+
Araneae	*	*			*	n.s.	n.s.
Araneidae							
Oxyopidae			NO DATA				
Salticidae							
Gryllidae	n.s.	n.s.			n.s.	n.s.	n.s.
Non-target Acrididae	**	n.s.			***	**	*
Psocoptera	n.s.	n.s.			n.s.	n.s.	n.s.
Cicadellidae	n.s.	n.s.			n.s.	n.s.	n.s.
Heteroptera	**	n.s.			*	n.s.	n.s.
Lygaeidae							
Miridae			NO DATA				
Pentatomoidea							
Lepidoptera (larvae)	n.s.	n.s.			n.s.	n.s.	n.s.
Braconidae	n.s.	n.s.			n.s.	n.s.	n.s.

Antanimieva 1994

Taxon	Two-way ANOVA Interaction time vs treatment	Pre-treatment (duration in weeks) <1	2	3+	Post-treatment (duration in weeks) <1	2	3+
Araneae	n.s.	*	n.s.	n.s.	n.s.	n.s.	n.s.
Araneidae	n.s.	n.s.	n.s.	n.s.	*	n.s.	n.s.
Oxyopidae	n.s.	***	n.s.	n.s.	n.s.	n.s.	n.s.
Salticidae	*	**	n.s.	n.s.	***	n.s.	n.s.
Gryllidae	n.s.	n.s.	n.s.	n.s.	n.s.	n.s.	n.s.
Non-target Acrididae	n.s.	n.s.	n.s.	n.s.	n.s.	n.s.	n.s.
Psocoptera	n.s.	n.s.	n.s.	n.s.	*	n.s.	n.s.
Cicadellidae	*	n.s.	n.s.	n.s.	**	n.s.	n.s.
Heteroptera	n.s.	n.s.	n.s.	n.s.	n.s.	n.s.	n.s.
Lygaeidae	n.s.	*	n.s.	n.s.	n.s.	n.s.	n.s.
Miridae	n.s.	**	n.s.	n.s.	*	n.s.	n.s.
Pentatomoidea	n.s.	n.s.	n.s.	n.s.	**	n.s.	n.s.
Lepidoptera (larvae)	**	*	n.s.	n.s.	*	**	***
Braconidae	n.s.	n.s.	n.s.	n.s.	n.s.	n.s.	n.s.

n.s. = not significant; * $P<0.05$; ** $P<0.01$; *** $P<0.001$.

pers has been identified, dependent on timing of treatment. Further analysis is under way to assess the magnitude and ecological implications of this risk. Assessment of the environmental acceptability of diflubenzuron barrier treatments must await results of longer-term monitoring, which suggests that effects may still be found a year after treatment.

References

Balança G, de Visscher M-N (1994) Les effets sur les araignées et les insectes non-cibles des traitements chimiques contre les criquets ravageurs. Rapport annuel sur la deuxième campagne de relevés (Burkina Faso, juillet à novembre 1993) D.494, CIRAD-GERDAT-PRIFAS, Montpellier, France. X+61 pp

Cooper JF, Coppen GDA, Dobson HM, Rakotonandrasana A, Scherer R (1995) Sprayed barriers of diflubenzuron (ULV) as a control technique against marching hopper bands of migratory locust *Locusta migratoria capito* (Sauss.) (Orthoptera: Acrididae) in southern Madagascar. Crop Protection 14(2): 137–143

Keith JO (ed) (1992) Effects of experimental applications of malathion and dichlorvos on populations of birds, mammals and insects in southern Morocco. Morocco Locust Project Research Report. Denver Wildlife Research Centre, USA 83 pp

Ostermann H (1996) Aspects écotoxicologiques des IGRs: comparison des effets d'un insecticide organophosphoré et d'un insecticide dérégulateur de croissance utilisés dans la lutte anti-acridienne sur les arthropodes non-cibles dans le sud-ouest de Madagascar. In Scherer R. (ed) La lutte antiacridienne à Madagascar. Antananarivo, Madagascar: GTZ (in press)

van der Valk HCHG, Kamara O (1993) The effect of fenitrothion and diflubenzuron on natural enemies of millet pests in Senegal (the 1991 study). LOCUSTOX Project Progress Report ECLO/SEN/003/NET. Dakar, Senegal. 37+VIII pp

New Strategies in Locust Control
S. Krall, R. Peveling and D. Ba Diallo (eds)
© 1997 Birkhäuser Verlag Basel/Switzerland

Impact of deltamethrin on the parasitic locust fly, *Wohlfahrtia pachytyli*

N. Saffer[1], S.A. Hanrahan[1] and H.D. Brown[2]

[1]*University of the Witwatersrand, Zoology Department, P.O. Wits 2050, Johannesburg, South Africa*
[2]*Plant Protection Research Institute, Pretoria, South Africa*

The locust fleshfly, *Wohlfahrtia pachytyli*, is a common facultative parasite of newly moulted or damaged brown locusts (van Schalkwijk 1939; Greathead 1963). Casual field observations have shown that *W. pachytyli* larviposits regularly on brown locust hoppers treated with a pyrethroid, deltamethrin, and completes its development. Laboratory studies confirm these observations. *W. pachytyli* shows no significant difference in breeding cycle patterns when bred on sprayed or unsprayed locusts. Lethal dose (LD) values were established for *W. pachytyli* adults, the brown locust, *Locusta pardalina*, and another Sarcophagid, *Sarcophaga inequalis*. The results (in μg a.i./g body weight) are shown in the table below:

	LD_{50}	LD_{90}
W. pachytyli	0.4709	1.3600
L. pardalina	0.0688	0.2555
S. inequalis	0.0175	0.0325

W. pachytyli showed a highly significant increased tolerance to deltamethrin when compared with both *L. pardalina* and *S. inequalis*.

Conclusion

These results show a highly anomalous response by *W. pachytyli* to deltamethrin, which appears to be a tolerance rather than a resistance to this toxin. This knowledge could be creatively exploited to provide a more effective control strategy against the brown locust.

References

Greathead DJ (1963) A review of the insect enemies of Acridoidea (Orthoptera). Trans Roy Entomol
    Soc 114: 437–517
van Schalkwijk HAD (1939) The status of *Wohlfahrtia euvittata* Vill. (Diptera, Sarcophagidae) as a para-
    site of the brown locust. J Entomol Soc S Afr 2: 18–35

New Strategies in Locust Control
S. Krall, R. Peveling and D. Ba Diallo (eds)
© 1997 Birkhäuser Verlag Basel/Switzerland

The dissipation of certain insecticides in the environment of the Sahel

B. Gadji

Locustox Project/FAO, B.P. 3300, Dakar, Senegal

The persistence of several insecticides recommended by the Food and Agriculture Organisation of the United Nations FAO) for locust control was tested in Senegal. The insecticides tested were fenitrothion and diflubenzuron (trials in 1991 and 1992), bendiocarb (1992–1993) and deltamethrin and chlorpyrifos (1993). The trial plots were fields of millet and temporary ponds in the region of Nioro du Rip (in southern Senegal), as well as pastures in the vicinity of Richard Toll (in northern Senegal). These two sites were chosen for their contrasting climatic conditions. At Nioro du Rip, rain falls from July to September, with relatively low temperatures of 25 to 35 °C and a continuous alternation between sun and clouds. Richard Toll, in contrast, has only sparse rainfall and nearly continuous sunshine, with temperatures of at least 40 °C.

Ultra low volume (ULV) formulations were used and the treatments were made with a micro-ULVA sprayer at the following, generally recommended, dose rates:

Chemical	Commercial name	Rate
Fenitrothion	Sumithion 500	450 g/ha
Diflubenzuron	Dimilin 450	60 g/ha
Bendiocarb	Ficam 40	100 g/ha
Chlorpyrifos	Dursban 240	240 g/ha
Deltamethrin	Decis 10	15 g/ha

After treatment, samples of leaves and heads of millet, of soil, of *Boscia senegalensis* (a shrub), *Tribulus terrestris* (a herb) and of water were taken on site over a two-week period, to monitor the dissipation of the insecticide with time. Various meteorological factors were also monitored in parallel.

Analyses using gas chromatography for most of the insecticides and HPLC (high-performance liquid chromatography) for diflubenzuron made it possible to detect the residue one hour after treatment and to calculate the half-life for each chemical. Comparison of the results with

FAO/WHO standards made it possible to establish the period of delay related to the use of each chemical tested.

Many results were obtained. The most notable concerned fenitrothion (an organophosphate). With this chemical, the initial residue, as observed one hour after treatment, was of the order of 50 mg a.i./kg fresh vegetation. The breakdown of this chemical in the dry environment of the Sahel appears to depend very much on climatic conditions. At Richard Toll, in a more arid environment and in the absence of rain, the half-life varied between 25 and 40 h. At Nioro du Rip, in the first year, when the total rainfall until the last samples were taken did not exceed 20 mm, the half-life was 18 h. It was no more than 6 h in the second year, with a cumulative rainfall of 190 to 254 mm. The amount of rainfall therefore seems to have a major impact on the persistence of fenitrothion in the environment of the Sahel. In temporary ponds, fenitrothion had a breakdown curve strongly resembling that observed on vegetation, with an initial average deposit of ca. 80 µg a.i./l and a half-life of up to 60 h.

Diflubenzuron, from the benzoylurea family, was deposited at the rate of 40 to 50 mg a.i./kg of fresh vegetation. Its persistence was greater than that of fenitrothion. The half-life varied between 100 and 150 h in a humid zone and 50 h in a dry zone. In the temporary ponds, the initial deposit, one hour after treatment, was, on average, 20 µg a.i./l of water. Samples taken 24 h after treatment gave no results on analysis.

Bendiocarb was tested in a trial at Richard Toll. In a plot where the vegetation was almost entirely based on *T. terrestris*, the half-life of the chemical was between 11 and 23 h. A trial in the ponds showed that the chemical was split between the water and solid particles in suspension (particles with a concentration of 0.3 to 0.5 g/l of water). One hour after treatment, there was, on average, 15 µg a.i./l in the water and 24 µg a.i./g in the solid particles in suspension.

Chlorpyrifos ethyl was tested in plots of millet. The initial deposit found was 32 mg a.i./kg of fresh leaves. The half-life appeared to be relatively independent of rainfall and ranged from 28 to 45 h.

Deltamethrin was tested during the winter (wet) season. Four treatments were carried out in plots of millet in the region of Nioro du Rip and five treatments in temporary ponds. The average half-life in the millet plots was 98 h, with the initial deposit varying between 1.2 and 2.2 mg a.i./kg of vegetation. In the pond waters, the chemical was not detected, even only 1 h after the treatment. In contrast, it was found on the solid particles in suspension at an average of 0.3 mg a.i./kg of particles.

Studies carried out in parallel in the soils gave lower deposits, of the order of 1 mg a.i./kg of soil. However, the half-lives found were often very much higher than those found in the vegetation.

Environmental impact

Working group

Results and recommendations of the working group *Environmental impact*

H. van der Valk (Chairman) and R. Peveling (Secretary)

The working group acknowledged that the harmful effects of control must be limited as much as possible without compromising the battle against acridoid pests. Two tools which can be used to achieve this objective are ecotoxicological research and environmental monitoring. If the advantages and drawbacks of a control method or strategy are to be assessed, acceptability criteria for its adverse effects on the environment are essential. It is clear that at present no such criteria exist. One of the aims of research must be to quantify adverse effects and to make the data available to decision-makers. Although these criteria are not constant and may change, it is important that they be defined as soon as possible. Information, training and legislation are the essential intermediate elements in ensuring that the results of research and monitoring are effectively applied. Figure 1 shows the various links between research and monitoring.

Current knowledge in African locust areas			
Aquatic ecosystems	Fish		+
	Invertebrates		++
	Algae		0
Terrestrial ecosystems	Mammals		0
	Birds		+
	Reptiles		0
	Invertebrates	Pollinators	·0
		Predators & Parasitoids	++
		Detritivores	+
	Soil microflora		+

0 = negligible; + = moderate; ++ = more or less detailed

Research

The knowledge acquired through research over recent years (see table above) was discussed briefly in order to identify gaps and priority areas. The following criteria were applied to define priorities for research: ecological function, lack of ecotoxicological information, sensitivity to insecticides, economic significance. In addition, it was noted that knowledge of the arid and semi-arid ecosystems affected by anti-locust treatments is extremely limited in terms of taxonomy, biology and ecology. The research topics which deserve more detailed attention are:

Terrestrial ecosystems

Beneficial arthropods:

⇒ pollinators

⇒ natural enemies of acridoid pests

⇒ soil microfauna

Vertebrates:

⇒ reptiles

⇒ birds

Aquatic ecosystems

⇒ fish

Studies should be directed towards the ecological roles of these organisms rather than confined to species abundance. The variability over time of the effects of insecticides on the environment must be studied in greater detail. Isolated ecosystems in the desert environment (oases, wadis) deserve particular attention on account of the poor prospects they have of being recolonised. Research results should lead to practical recommendations for choosing insecticides, application methods and control strategies. These recommendations should be tested under operational conditions before being made generally available.

Monitoring

The working group identified three types of monitoring or environmental follow-up for anti-locust treatments:

⇒ technical follow-up of spraying, relating to applied dosage, spraying quality and adherence to safety instructions

⇒ ecological follow-up:

first level: operators' health, field evidence of acute effects on non-target fauna (search for animal carcasses), residue sampling, effectiveness of treatment

second level: large-scale testing of research recommendations and potential long-term effects

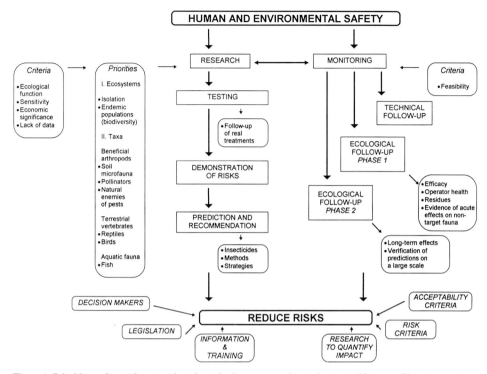

Figure 1. Priorities and steps in research and monitoring to assess the environmental impact of locust control.

Technical and first-level ecological follow-up can already commence using simple methods which have already been tried and tested. The working group considered that this follow-up should be an integral part of locust control operations. A small team with two vehicles, a health officer, a spraying technician and a biologist could carry out this type of follow-up at very reasonable cost. On the other hand, the ecological follow-up methods of the second level have yet to be developed. The ecological follow-up methods used in experimental research cannot all be applied to the monitoring of real-life anti-locust treatments on account of a variety of constraints (too short a time between the decision to treat and the possibility of studying it). Moreover, as yet there are either no bioindicators (organisms or ecological functions) or biomarkers (biochemical parameters) available, or else they do not suit the ecosystems affected by anti-locust treatments.

Economics of locust control and crop loss assessment

Economics of desert locust control

S. Krall[1] and C. Herok[2]

[1]*Deutsche Gesellschaft für Technische Zusammenarbeit (GTZ) GmbH, P.O. Box 5180, 65726 Eschborn, Germany*
[2]*Humboldt-Universiät zu Berlin, Luisenstraße 56, 10099 Berlin, Germany*

Summary. The desert locust, *Schistocerca gregaria* (Forskål), is an extremely mobile pest. It is not uncommon for swarms to travel hundreds of kilometres. Damage caused by desert locusts can be devastating, although – owing to the insect's mobility – it is never uniformly distributed. This makes it extremely difficult to precisely ascertain crop losses. Attempts to study the economic impact of desert locusts also run up against certain limits. Microeconomic calculations cannot be performed, and even macroeconomic studies conducted at the level of the national economy do not permit many conclusions to be drawn. Truly useful results are only yielded by regional studies that take account of the locusts' movements across national borders. This paper highlights the current situation, in which the lack of reliable figures makes cost-benefit calculations a difficult task. In this paper, an attempt is made to take available figures on swarms and hopper bands, the costs of control measures and potential damage as the basis for a novel approach to gauging economic aspects of desert locust control. Possible backup measures for collecting data are also sketched.

Résumé. Le criquet pèlerin, *Schistocerca gregaria* (Forskål) constitue un fléau extrêmement mobile. Il n'est pas inhabituel pour des essaims de parcourir des centaines de kilomètres. Les dommages causés par le criquet pèlerin peuvent être dévastateurs, mais ne sont jamais uniformément répartis – en raison justement de l'extrême mobilité des acridiens. Il est donc quasiment impossible d'évaluer avec précision les dommages causés aux cultures et l'étude de l'impact du fléau en termes économiques se heurte à certaines limites. Des calculs au niveau microéconomique ne sont guère réalisables et même des études menées sur le plan national au niveau macroéconomique ne permettent pas d'en tirer des conclusions intéressantes. Seules des études régionales tenant compte du fait que les acridiens franchissent les frontières politiques peuvent amener des résultats véritablement utiles. Cet article montre combien il est malaisé d'établir des analyses coûts-avantages en raison du manque de données chiffrées fiables. Il essaie également de montrer comment les chiffres disponibles sur les essaims et les bandes larvaires, ainsi que les données sur les coûts des mesures de lutte antiacridienne et les dommages potentiels peuvent servir à évaluer par une nouvelle approche les aspects économiques de la lutte contre le criquet pèlerin. L'article présente également quelques méthodes pour améliorer la fiabilité des données collectées.

Introduction

The desert locust, *Schistocerca gregaria* (Forskål), poses an ever-present threat to African agriculture (Steedman 1990). Desert locusts are difficult to manage and control because of the unpredictability of outbreaks and upsurges and because the insects are extremely mobile. Add to this the fact that locusts make the transition from the solitarious phase, in which they live as separate individuals, to the gregarious swarming phase in semi-desert areas. In such areas, monitoring the insects necessitates an enormous and therefore also costly logistical effort. The difficulties are often compounded by the remoteness and ruggedness of the terrain and by violent conflicts (Krall 1995; van Huis 1994).

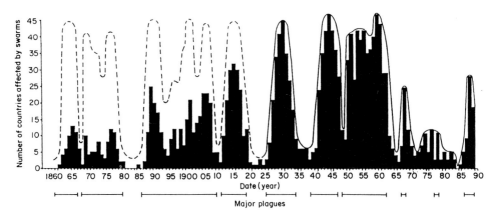

Figure 1. Numbers of countries reporting either bands or swarms during a year. Broken lines denote estimated values (according to Symmons 1992)

As a result, outbreaks and early upsurges are often not noticed until it is too late and therefore rarely suppressed. For this and other reasons, it is still virtually impossible even today to prevent desert locust plagues. Yet the last 35 years have not seen any extremely destructive, long-lasting plagues of the kind that occurred with frequency in earlier decades (Fig. 1), a number of which were thoroughly documented. The reasons for this are not yet known. It may be due to successful control measures of the kind that became feasible in the 1960s, involving application of dieldrin, a highly effective, persistent insecticide. But climatic, geographical, anthropogenic and/ or natural causes may also play a role, like those held responsible for the disappearance of the problems previously caused in the Sahel by the African migratory locust (*Locusta migratoria migratorioides*, Reiche and Fairmaire).

Due to the behavior of the desert locust, which differs completely from that of nearly all other pests, it has not been possible to apply the classical methods of cost-benefit analysis to control measures. No attempts have been made to systematically ascertain crop losses caused by desert locust attacks. For the most part, the same decades-old figures have been cited over and over again. Only a few surveys have been carried out during the last 10 years, and these have not come up with enough data for reliable calculations (Launois 1994). Surprisingly, while everyone is currently trying to cut down on pesticide use in integrated pest management programmes, the chemical control of the desert locust has not even been subjected to a cost-benefit analysis. Studies of this kind did not begin until very recently (Herok and Krall 1995).

The difficulties involved in addressing economic issues

The classical methods used to study economic aspects of crop protection activities take either a microeconomic or a macroeconomic approach. A given measure can be considered at the farm level, and its cost and benefits can be calculated. This is useful when the aim is to persuade farmers of the economic feasibility of individual crop protection measures. Economists, however, are more interested in the macroeconomic situation; as a rule, this involves studies at the level of the national economy.

When dealing with the desert locust, however, both approaches are problematic. Microeconomic studies are not very useful, since desert locust plagues occur so irregularly and in such widely differing forms from region to region that virtually nothing of relevance can be concluded for any given farm. A survey conducted in Niger in 1991 (Krall 1994) provided some indication of the significance of desert locusts at the individual farm level. Farmers were asked which was the principal pest afflicting their pearl millet. If this question was formulated very generally, then 57% of those questioned named the desert locust. If the same question focussed on growing seasons, however, then the majority cited other pests. This demonstrates that although farmers consider the desert locust to be a spectacular and dangerous pest, they actually experienced it once or only a few times during their lifetime.

It follows logically from this that combating plagues is not the job of individual farmers. Instead, national crop protection services take care of this in cooperation with regional organisations like the Desert Locust Control Organisation for Eastern Africa (DLCO-EA), an association of seven East African countries. This is a good example of how the desert locust eludes the classical macroeconomic approach, which is typically restricted to a single country.

Take, for instance, the case of Mauritania. Agriculture does not play a major role in the economy of this West African country, in contrast to other countries of the Sahel zone. Two-thirds of its land area is desert, and agriculture is intensively practiced only along the Senegal River in the south of the country. When desert locust plagues occur, large numbers of swarms regularly occur in Mauritania. They usually enter from the east, and reproduce within the country. During the 1993 upsurge alone, over 100 small, medium-sized and large swarms were sighted in Mauritania (Wilps, personal communication). These swarms typically did not inflict any major damage, however, as many of them flew off towards the north to Morocco and Algeria, westward to the Atlantic Ocean, or – less frequently – towards the south, to Senegal (van Huis 1994). This has to do with the prevailing wind directions, among other things. Only 9 out of every 10 swarms pose a serious threat to the country's own agricultural sector, according to information provided by the Mauritanian crop protection service (Galledou, personal communication). They do, however, pose a major threat to the northern Maghreb, where a number of high-value agricultural crops are grown.

Taking a macroeconomic approach to this problem (i.e., considering this country in isolation), one would have to conclude that controlling desert locusts is not economically worthwhile for Mauritania. But if the scope of the study is enlarged to include Algeria and Morocco, completely different results will be obtained. This example shows that there is little point in performing the analyses at the level of the national economy. Macroeconomic approaches only make sense for an entire region, which in this case embraces at least the entire Sahel and the Maghreb. The difficulties involved are obvious – after all, we are talking here about a dozen or so independent states and a land area three times the size of Western Europe.

Yet these difficulties, as daunting as they are, are compounded further by the fact that the available figures, in other words the basis for performing calculations of all kinds, are extremely inadequate (Herok and Krall 1995). If we wish to consider environmental impacts as well (at the meta level), then we are quickly forced to enter the realm of pure speculation.

Bases for economic calculations

Three main groups are affected by problems related to desert locusts, on either the cost or the benefit side:
- farmers
- afflicted countries
- donor countries

In 1986–89 alone, the donor countries contributed about US$275 million, thus meeting a substantial share of the costs for monitoring and controlling desert locusts (OTA 1990).

A wide variety of factors play a role. On the cost side, for example, expenditures are incurred for equipment, consumables and materials for monitoring and control measures, acquiring information, medical care, functioning of international organisations and environmental damage. On the benefit side, we have, among other things, reduction of crop and quality losses, reduction of foreign exchange expenditures on food imports, training effects and strengthening of crop protection services.

It is difficult to validate these factors, however; environmental impacts are a case in point. Time preferences can also be validated in different ways. On the one hand, benefits ought to be forthcoming more or less in the same year in which most of the costs are incurred: control measures prevent losses. On the other hand, there can also be long-term positive effects attributable to effective control or equipment that is originally brought in to combat locusts but is subsequently used for other purposes. Account must also be taken of the fact that certain expenditures continue between the occurrence of plagues, such as the fees and contributions that must be paid in foreign exchange to regional or supraregional international organisations. Because of this, it would appear to be appropriate to apply the capital value method, or alternatively to determine the internal rate of return. All of these calculations, however, rely upon the availability of substantiated data.

Data for economic calculations

After the relevant factors have been identified, figures need to be assigned to them. A thorough review of the available data reveals that there is a particularly acute lack of figures on potential and actual benefits. The information on damage is, when available at all, too outdated (Tab. 1) or too imprecise to be used for cost-benefit analyses (Tab. 2).

Table 3 attempts to provide a brief overview of the costs and benefits for the years 1986 to 1993. A desert locust plague occurred during this time period (in 1987–88).

Table 1. Crop losses caused by locusts. (based on Steedman 1990)

Year	Country	Amount of crop eaten by the desert locust
1944	Libya	7,000,000 grapevines; 19% of total vine cultivation
1954	Sudan	55,000 tonnes of grain
1957	Senegal	16,000 tonnes of millet, 2000 tonnes of other crops
1957	Guinea	6000 tonnes of oranges
1958	Ethiopia	167,000 tonnes of grain, which is enough to feed 1,000,000 people for a year
1962	India	4000 hectares of cotton (value £300,000)

Table 2. Estimated yield losses between 1986 and 1993

Country	Loss as percentage of total production	Regional maximum
Chad	No value	80%
The Gambia	No value	70%
Mauritania	No value	60%
Senegal	3%	-
Sudan	cereals <5%, total <1%	76%

Table 3. Available data on costs and benefits of desert locust and grasshopper control (US$) (1986–1993)

Costs		Benefits	
		Farmers	
Pesticides and equipment	0	Gained yields	?
Working time	0	Improved quality	?
Health hazards	?	Inputs	?
Subtotal	**?**	**Subtotal**	**?**
		Affected countries	
		Crop protection service	
Pesticides	?	Foreign exchange	?
Equipment	?	Support for crop protection services	?
Transport	?	Balance-of-payments effect	?
Operating costs	?	Educational effect	?
Personnel	?	Image	?
Subtotal	44,322,254	Taxes	?
		Military	
Equipment and personnel	?		
		Government	
Loans	?		
Contributions to internat. aid	2,187,000		
Contributions to internat. institutions	644,300		
Environmental effects	?		
Subtotal	**2,831,300**	**Subtotal**	**?**
		Donors	
Pesticides	69,000,000		
Equipment and training	?		
Transport and operating costs	?		
Personnel	?		
Subtotal	**295,247,000**	**Subtotal**	**?**
Total costs	**342,400,554**	**Total Benefits**	**?**

Possibilities for economic assessment of costs and benefits

The example given above makes it plain that no useful results can be achieved today using macroeconomic study methods, since for the most part there is a lack of concrete figures. There are, however, possibilities for getting a grip on the problems despite these gaps in the data. The

Table 4. Crop equivalents of control costs (in tonnes/ha of sorghum)

Year	Control costs	Sorghum equivalent (in t)		Sorghum equivalent in ha Yield = 500 kg/ha	
		World market	Local market		
	(in mill. US$)	110 US$/t	300 US$/t	110 US$/t	300 US$/t
1986	50.2	456,363	167,333	912,726	334,666
1987	35.8	325,454	199,333	650,908	398,666
1988	102.8	934,545	342,667	1,869,090	685,334
1989	98.7	897,273	329,000	1,794,546	658,000
1990	16.9	153,636	56,333	307,272	112,666
1991	8.4	76,364	28,000	152,727	56,000
1992	6.7	60,909	22,333	121,818	44,667
1993	22.9	208,181	76,333	416,364	152,667
Total	342.4	3,112,725	1,221,332	6,225,451	2,442,666

simplest way is to compare the known costs against the equivalent food losses which would have had to be prevented to yield a kind of break-even point. This can be done on the basis of either world-market prices or local prices. An argument in favor of applying world-market prices is that most of the expenditures required for desert locust control call for foreign exchange to be spent (e.g. to buy pesticides, sprayers, vehicles etc.).

Table 4 lists these values for the years 1986–93. The equivalent amounts of sorghum are given both in tonnes and in terms of land area in hectares, which would have had to be destroyed merely to offset the costs.

It is of course no easy matter to interpret such figures. Hopefully, however, they will motivate agricultural statisticians to compare them with the actual situation. The question arises, for example, whether it is realistic to suppose that between 24,000 and 62,000 km^2 of millet or sorghum fields could have been totally destroyed during the mentioned years. The answer can be yes or no, but either way it might encourage better collection of data on crop losses caused by desert locusts.

Another possibility is more complex, and involves the use of model calculations to approximate potentially prevented losses. Bullen (1969) devoted an enormous effort in the 1960s to working out a crop vulnerability index (CVI). This was based on data on all major field and tree crops grown throughout the entire region, rounded out by data on swarms and hopper bands provided by the Anti-Locust Centre in London and the Food and Agriculture Organisation of the United Nations (FAO), and defined crops potentially subject to attack from desert locusts. This yielded relative CVI figures that provided an indication of where to expect the greatest damage and crop losses. Bullen concluded that 50% of the anticipated losses would occur in the Indo-Pakistan region, 23% in north-western Africa, 13% in the Middle East, 11% in East Africa and 2% in West Africa.

In the following, another possible approach, developed by Herok and Krall (1995) and similar to Bullen's model, will be considered. It is based on the same type of data on locust swarm and hopper band frequency used by Bullen for the calculation of CVIs, as well as agricultural production data for the potentially affected African countries. The chief differences are that (1) more recent data were included and (2) Herok and Krall pooled the values of each country's agricultural production. This yielded figures expressing potential crop losses as absolute monetary values instead of relative values as in Bullen's model. Based on an assessment of swarm size, the extent of damage and the efficacy of control, the potentially preventable damage was evaluated, expressed as absolute monetary values, while distinguishing among different cases (Fig. 2).

These values were compared to control costs, which could be assessed relatively precisely for the last few years, and calculated net positive or negative benefits. The costs for the years 1986 to 1993 are listed in column 2 of Table 4. In a number of cases, it proved impossible to make a clear distinction between costs for grasshopper and desert locust control, since many of the campaigns conducted during these years were directed against both groups. Because of this difficulty, only the total control costs are listed here.

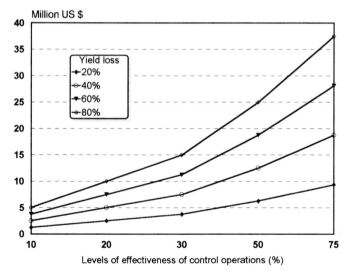

Figure 2. Potentially preventable annual yield losses with desert locust control in Africa (in mill. US $) (according to Herok and Krall 1995)

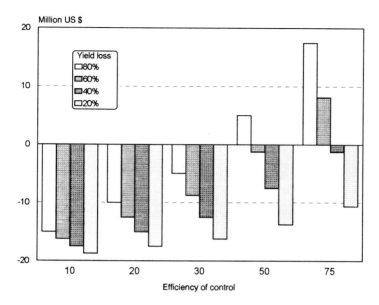

Figure 3. Net benefit of desert locust control in Africa (cost/year = US$20 million)(according Herok and Krall 1995)

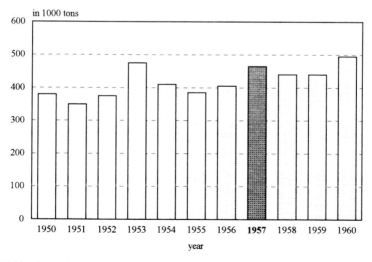

Figure 4. Yields of cereals in Senegal between 1950 and 1960 (desert locusts caused considerable damage in 1957)

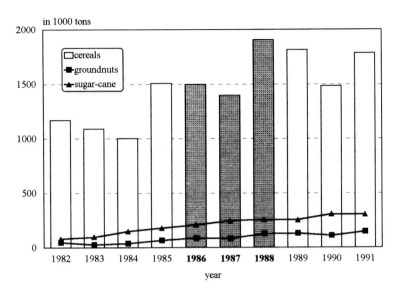

Figure 5. Yields of cereals in Mali between 1982 and 1991 (desert locust plague 1986–88)

The average value for each of the eight years studied is US$42.8 million. Even deducting 50% for grasshopper control, some US$20 million remains. Based on this assumption, Figure 3 shows the net benefits for different damage levels and efficiency factors of control measures. A positive net benefit only results if one assumes extensive damage and highly effective control, with an efficiency factor of at least 50%.

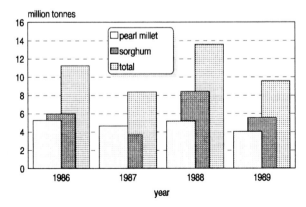

Figure 6. Yields of cereals in the Sahel between 1986 and 1989 (major desert locust plague year in 1988)

Do locusts cause famines?

In lectures and the media, references abound to famines caused by desert locusts. Some speak of thousands of deaths. Needless to say, these reports are unfounded. Nevertheless, we considered it important to find out whether the available figures on agricultural production in recent decades actually provide any indication of emergency situations of this kind. We therefore investigated a number of different cases to establish whether the statistics provide evidence of food shortages (Figs 4–6).

In all three cases it can be seen that there have not been any significant yield losses in years with locust plagues. In 1988 there were even above-average harvests both in Mali and throughout the Sahel zone. We were unable to analyze the years prior to 1950, as insufficient data were available for them.

One frequently cited argument is that desert locusts have a deleterious impact on rangelands. No reliable data whatsoever exist to back up this claim in the case of the Sahel, however. Studies in Paraguay (Wilhelmi 1995) showed that, in the case of the field locust *Staurorhectus longicornis* (Giglio-Tos), a decline in meat and milk production is improbable unless severe damage is inflicted over a lengthy period of time.

On the other hand, livestock-keeping nomads living in the Sahel frequently complain that they are affected by the adverse effects of locust control campaigns. A number of times, apparently, cattle have been killed by insecticides sprayed to combat locusts. In some cases this was the result of unintentional direct spraying of animals by aircraft, and in other cases was caused by ingestion of contaminated forage from treated areas (Anonym 1987).

Discussion

Owing to the extremely unsatisfactory data situation, it is impossible to perform cost-benefit analyses using real data. In order to remedy this problem as quickly as possible, national crop protection services should regularly survey the effectiveness of control measures and inflicted damage. In the case of control measures, this is definitely feasible; methods exist for measuring their efficacy. The task is more difficult where damage is concerned. Quantitative measurement methods are only available for certain cases (Pantenius and Krall 1993). Such methods still need to be developed for most crops. For the time being, there is no way to avoid getting subjective assessments. But information of this kind is still better than none at all.

As we have seen, all of the calculation models available today have shortcomings. Either they are extremely time-consuming to use, like the method proposed by Bullen (1969), or – like that of Herok and Krall (1995) – rely upon a number of assumptions. Nevertheless, the latter method is the only available approach capable of dealing with the sheer size of the region under study and the special nature of the complex problems associated with the desert locust.

Although Bullen did not arrive at a very precise comparison of costs and benefits, he does deserve credit for having identified which regions are most at risk. His writings reveal that two-thirds of the expected damage in Africa is concentrated in the Maghreb, and within that region primarily in Morocco and Algeria. In other words, in monetary terms it is not primarily smallholders who profit from the control campaigns conducted in the Sahel as a whole – it is the growers of high-value crops in the Maghreb who benefit. To date there has been no real evidence of damage to rangeland having any seriously adverse effects on livestock farming. Yet livestock animals have been killed a number of times as a result of insecticides used to control locusts. It may thus be concluded that locust control does not have any positive effects on livestock raising. In 1970 Bullen compared locusts and grasshoppers with other agricultural pests, concluding: "Thus locusts and grasshoppers, even at their worst, constitute only a very small proportion of the overall crop protection problem." He continued: "It is therefore important that the status of locusts and grasshoppers as crop pests should be defined in relation to crop losses caused by other insects. Has man been emotionally blinded by the spectacle of locust invasions and deluded into believing that they are pests of major importance?"

Particularly in view of the substantial expenditure involved and the need for equipment and so forth, it is increasingly questionable whether and to what extent, controlling desert locusts is worthwhile. This conclusion was drawn 25 years ago, but had few consequences, since for quite a while thereafter no additional plagues occurred. Bullen's work was therefore forgotten, and failed to exert any influence on the large-scale control campaigns conducted in the late 1980s and early 1990s.

It was not until these campaigns were well under way that the issue whether cost-intensive control measures make economic sense was again addressed. The model developed by Herok and Krall (1995) attempts, for the first time, to compare the potentially preventable damage with the actual cost of control measures. Their study concludes that the strategy being pursued today does not make economic sense in terms of costs and benefits. Although this model only constitutes an initial approximation and involves a number of estimates, it nevertheless ought to prompt a reconsideration of the currently applied locust control strategy. Relatively uncoordinated combating of swarms and hopper bands like those typical today should be abandoned. A strategically concerted effort is essential. Within this context, the focus should be on protecting crops. Control measures in the most remote areas should be thoroughly reconsidered in the light of the population dynamics of the desert locust, which is characterized by the natural collapse of plagues. Nor is it realistic to expect that outbreaks and even upsurges can be suppressed during their early stages, considering the rugged terrain and the security situation in many countries.

Initial studies have shown that no famines have been caused by locust plagues during the last five decades. It may very well be possible for regionally limited shortages to occur, but these can be offset by appropriate distribution policies at the national level. Growers of high-value crops may suffer serious economic losses, but even if these cannot be prevented by control measures, they can at least be compensated by a suitable insurance system.

We do not wish to create the impression that the desert locust problem should be addressed from a purely economic standpoint, expressing everything in monetary terms. Major human and social components also deserve attention.

Besides political considerations, one of the most important of these is maintaining a reliable supply of locally produced food at the village level; this cannot simply be replaced by food aid, a point that future studies need to take into account. Conversely, neither should attention center on social aspects to the complete exclusion of economic issues. They must nevertheless be taken into consideration when interpreting data of all kinds. Most important, however, the database must be improved. This is the only way to obtain useful results that can be used to persuade those in charge of locust control to modify their strategies.

References

Anonym (1987) Campagne de lutte antiacridienne 1986/87, Bilan et perspectives. Ministère de l'Agriculture et de l'Elevage, Ouagadougou, Burkina Faso

Bullen FT (1969) The distribution of the damage potential of the desert locust (*Schistocerca gregaria* Forsk.). Anti-Locust Memoir 10, Anti-Locust Research Centre, London

Bullen FT (1970) A review of the assessment of crop losses caused by locusts and grasshoppers. Proc Int Study Conf Current and Future Problems of Acridology, London, 163–169

Herok C, Krall S (1995) Economics of desert locust control. Roßdorf: TZ-Verl-Ges, 70 pp

Krall S (1994) Importance of locusts and grasshoppers for African agriculture and methods for determining crop losses. In Krall S, Wilps H (eds) New trends in locust control. Roßdorf: TZ-Verl-Ges

Krall S (1995) Desert locust in Africa – a disaster? Disasters, The Journal for Disaster Studies and Management 19(1): 1–7

Launois M (1994) Les dégâts des criquets pèlerins en Mauritanie et au Sénégal. Sahel PV Info no 64: 6–17

Office of Technology Assessment (OTA) (1990) A Plague of locusts. Special Report, US Congress, Washington

Pantenius U, Krall S (1993) A new method for determining yield losses caused by damage to the heads of pearl millet (*Pennisetum glaucum* (L.) R. Br.) due to diseases and pests. J Plant Diseases and Protection 100 (5): 522–529

Steedman A (ed) (1990) Locust handbook. Chatham: Natural Resources Institute

Symmons P (1992) Strategies to combat the desert locust. Crop Protection 11: 206–212

Van Huis A (1994) Can we combat the desert locust successfully? Proc Seminar Wageningen, Netherlands, 6–11 Dec 1993, 11–17

Wilhelmi F (1995) *Staurorhectus longicornis* (Giglio-Tos), an acridid grasshopper pest species on pasture land in the Central Chaco, Paraguay. Eschborn: GTZ, pp 55

New Strategies in Locust Control
S. Krall, R. Peveling and D. Ba Diallo (eds)
© 1997 Birkhäuser Verlag Basel/Switzerland

Yield losses on pearl millet panicles due to grasshoppers: a new assessment method

S.A. Kogo[1] and S. Krall[2]

[1]*Direction de la Protection des Végétaux, P.O. Box 323, Niamey, Niger*
[2]*Deutsche Gesellschaft für Technische Zusammenarbeit (GTZ) GmbH, P.O. Box 5180, 65726 Eschborn, Germany*

Summary. In cooperation with the crop protection directorate of the Niger, experts working within the framework of a technical cooperation programme assisted by the Deutsche Gesellschaft für Technische Zusammenarbeit (GTZ) have developed a method of estimating yield losses in pearl millet, *Pennisetum glaucum* (L.) R. Br. The method had to be as simple as possible so that rural extension workers could use it without external supervision, the role of the national crop protection directorate being restricted to carrying out the subsequent data analysis. Using this method, losses caused by a range of crop pests (diseases, birds, insects) can be estimated. In the case of grasshoppers, the data collected showed that, at the regional level, average losses occurring between 1992 and 1994 did not exceed 9% and were, in most cases, well below 2%.

Résumé. En coopération avec la Direction de la Protection des Végétaux du Niger, des experts de la Deutsche Gesellschaft für Technische Zusammenarbeit (GTZ) ont mis au point une méthode pour évaluer les dégâts occasionnés sur le mil à chandelle, *Pennisetum glaucum* (L.) R. Br. La méthode devait être aussi simple que possible afin que les vulgarisateurs agricoles puissent l'utiliser sans supervision externe, le rôle de la Direction Nationale de la Protection des Végétaux se limitant à réaliser l'analyse de données subséquente. Cette méthode permet d'estimer les dégâts causés par différents ennemis des cultures (maladies, oiseaux, insectes). En ce qui concerne les acridiens, les données recueillies ont montré qu'au niveau régional les pertes subies en moyenne entre 1992 et 1994 n'excédaient pas 9% et étaient dans la plupart des cas nettement inférieures à 2%.

Introduction

Methods used to measure yield losses due to pests or diseases are usually very expensive and can only be carried out with the use of a great deal of extra equipment, manpower and time. For this reason, these methods are usually restricted to one pest and one region. It is therefore not really possible to use this sort of study to collect countrywide data on yield losses. Nevertheless, it is vital to assess yield losses over a large area in order to be able to quantify the potential damage that pests can cause in crops.

Within the framework of cooperation between the Niger and Germany, the Deutsche Gesellschaft für Technische Zusammenarbeit (GTZ) worked together with the Plant Protection Directorate of the Niger to set up and develop a methodology to assess the damage caused by different pests on panicles of pearl millet (*Pennisetum glaucum* (L.) R. Br.) (Pantenius and Krall 1993).

The objective of applying this method was to carry out studies over the whole of the Niger to evaluate and quantify the impact of pests and diseases on panicles of pearl millet. Particular attention was given to grasshoppers, as they are seen as major pests by the crop protection services of all the countries in the Sahel.

Methods

General points

Estimates of crop losses at harvest were based on a large number of observations of millet panicles made in farmers' fields. The study looked at pests and diseases, particularly grasshoppers, that affected, directly or indirectly, the panicles of millet. The present study deals only with the effect of acridians. Results concerning other pests and diseases are published elsewhere (Krall et al. 1995).

Data collection

The studies were carried out in 20 to 25 *arrondissements* of 6 *départements* (Tillaberi, Dosso, Tahoua, Maradi, Zinder and Diffa). Only in one *département* (Agadez) was no data collected, because the area is mainly desert. In each *arrondissement* data from at least three villages and three fields per village with a total of 195 to 287 fields per year were assessed.

Each field selected measured at least 60 × 60 m and was about to be harvested. A plot of 30 × 30 m 15 steps from the border was marked out in each field for the collection of general data, especially plant stand and the level of damage (Fig. 1).

In order to assess the level of damage, 30 panicles of millet per field were chosen at random. These 30 panicles had to be a representative sample of the field that was being assessed and to be chosen from all over the field. For this reason, one panicle per planting hill was assessed. It was therefore necessary to have 30 planting hills containing panicles with yield potential (panicles at the milky, pasty or ripe stages).

The selection of the planting hills as well as of the panicles had to be completely random. The method chosen to achieve this was as follows (Fig. 2). It begins at point A in the plot with the choice of a planting hill in the first row by taking four steps. The next planting hill is chosen from the next row by taking four steps and looking for a planting hill containing panicles within reach and with yield potential. The term *yield potential* means that the panicles will later be

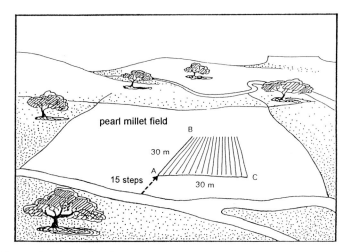

Figure 1. Marking out the observation plot.

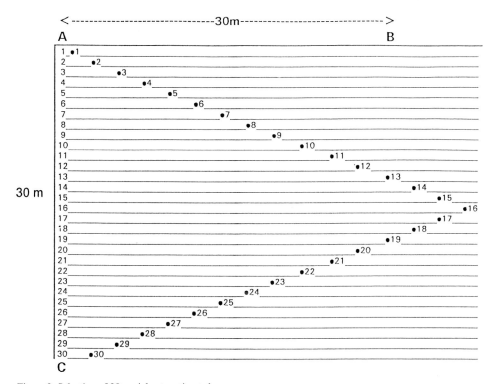

Figure 2. Selection of 30 panicles to estimate losses.

harvested by the farmer, whereas panicles in flower or not yet in flower will not reach maturity and are not considered as having yield potential.

Moving on to the next row, again four steps are taken. The selection can continue outside the plot boundaries, provided the field is big enough, until half the number of panicles have been selected or until a minimum distance has been reached with respect to the edge of the field. The selection continues then in the opposite direction until 30 panicles have been examined. In order to ensure that the panicles are really chosen at random, the person making the selection keeps their head down while taking the four steps along the row, so that the panicles are not within the field of vision.

At the site of the planting hill, a stalk with panicle is grasped without looking, i.e., with the person's head lowered or turned away. A panicle with yield potential having been selected, it is then examined to see if it is damaged. A single panicle can show several types of damage or symptoms, caused either by a single pest at different growth stages of the panicle or attributable to different pests. The person carrying out the study should be familiar with the symptoms of the different types of damage and be able to identify the cause of the damage. However, in a number of cases it is not possible to decide on the exact cause of the damage. For this reason it is necessary to make a catalogue of the types of damage that can be found and then divide these into different categories of damage. The 'grasshopper' category is subdivided into two groups:

- Grasshoppers – early damage: this group comprises all types of damage to the panicle between heading and the milky stage. At the time of carrying out the study, this damage is manifested by the complete destruction of the spikelets and milky grains and therefore by patches without grains.
- Grasshoppers – late damage: this second group comprises all types of damage occurring after grain development at the pasty or full maturity stages. In this situation the grains are usually only partially damaged, revealing their white interior.

To identify the different types of damage and divide them into the various categories, the reader is referred to a reference booklet that has been prepared for this purpose (Krall and Dorow 1993).

Establishing the size of the area damaged and its location

In order to assess the damage caused to panicles of millet by pests, and grasshoppers in particular, both sides of the panicle need to be examined. The type of damage on each side must be identified.

It is the responsibility of the person carrying out the study to decide what percentage of each side of the panicle has the same symptoms or has been damaged by the same pests. If the whole side of a panicle has been attacked, it is enough to record this as 100%. If, on the other hand, only part of the panicle has been damaged and this in an irregular pattern, it is much more difficult to estimate the area involved. In this situation it is necessary to begin by comparing the damaged area with the undamaged area to decide on the percentage attacked.

To make the task easier for the person carrying out the work, four assessment keys have been prepared of the different general types of damage not related to one specific species, to be used as a reference in estimating the size of the damaged area on the panicle (Fig. 3).

In cases where there are several damaged areas, care must be taken that the total of the percentages noted does not exceed 100% and the remainder is in fact equal to the area of undamaged panicle. It should be noted that although an area of a panicle may be damaged, it does not necessarily follow that there will a total loss of grains. For example, grasshopper attacks on ripe millet panicles will result in losses of 50% because the grains are only partially damaged and the remaining grains might still be used for human or animal consumption. On the other hand, attacks at the flowering or milky stages will result in total destruction by inhibiting the formation of the grains. The areas damaged will show, at the time of harvest/assessment, a loss of 100%.

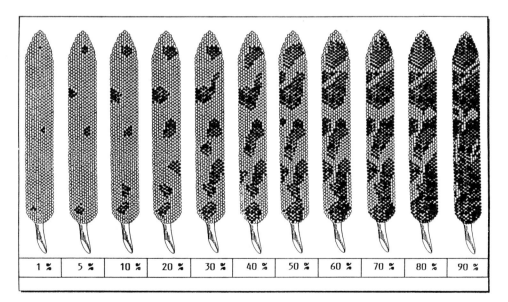

| 1 % | 5 % | 10 % | 20 % | 30 % | 40 % | 50 % | 60 % | 70 % | 80 % | 90 % |

Figure 3. Key for assessing damage on millet panicles (part of a series of four keys showing different types of damage).

Results

From 1992 to 1994, regular assessments of yield losses were carried out at the national level. All relevant factors were taken into account, including diseases and pests. Figure 4 shows the damage caused by grasshoppers to pearl millet heads for each *département*.

The average national damage level for the years 1992 to 1994 was 1.4%. It can be seen that only the *département* of Diffa had relatively high average losses (8.9%) in 1993. In all the other *départements*, for the three years under consideration, the level was less than 3% on average and, for most of them, was well below this – the lowest figure was 0.03% for Diffa in 1994. In 1994, harvest losses due to acridians were close to zero.

If individual field data are pooled in classes from zero to >20% yield loss, more than 70% of the fields are without any loss or less than 1% (Fig. 5). On the other hand, yield losses of about 20% and even higher occur in a number of fields.

Losses are not equally distributed, and the national average or even the average per *département* does not necessarily show considerable local damage. A breakdown of the data into *arrondissements* (Fig. 6) demonstrates that yield losses were nearly 10% in the *arrondissement*

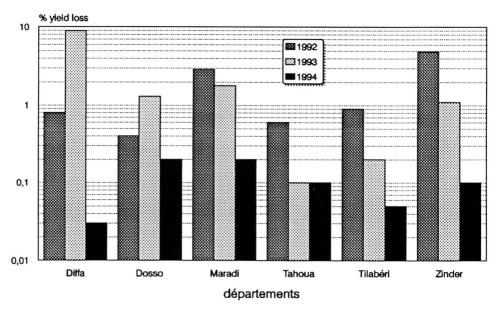

Figure 4. Yield loss on pearl millet due to grasshoppers (the Niger, 1992 = 281 fields, 1993 = 287 fields and 1994 = 195 fields).

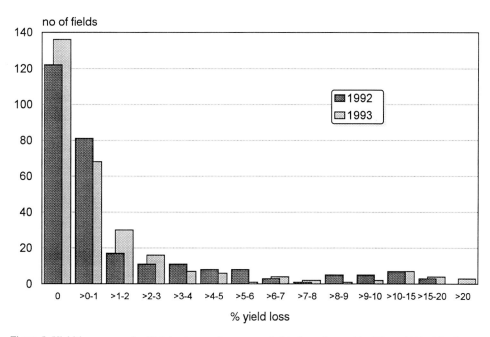

Figure 5. Yield loss on pearl millet due to grasshoppers pooled in loss classes (the Niger, 1992=281 fields, 1993=287 fields).

Tanout, whereas the average in this *département* (Zinder) was only 5% and on the national level only 1.7%.

Discussion

The method described uses comparatively simple means to assess losses on pearl millet over a large area. Damage and losses due to digging up seeds after sowing and defoliation have not been included, as the assessments were only made on pearl millet panicles at harvest time. Total losses due to acridians during the whole growing season may then in reality be higher than the results shown in the diagram in Figure 4. On the other hand, damage at harvest time is more serious for the farmer than is damage to young plants.

The data presented give useful reference points about the damage that these pests can cause. As local damage can be hidden behind national averages we advice that data be analysed on an

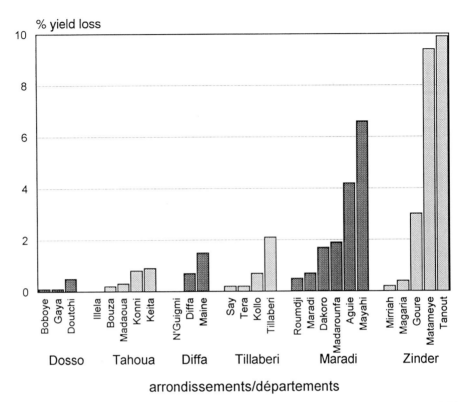

Figure 6. Yield loss due to grasshoppers in the Niger, 1992, broken down into arrondissements (n = 287 fields).

arrondissement basis. Also, the method can be used to target specific grasshopper attacks in a given zone with a high number of fields evaluated.

To reduce the incidence of mistakes or inaccuracies in the assessments, it is essential to have a large amount of data available and ensure that staff collecting data receive training, because simple evaluation involves detailed analysis providing exact figures.

High yield loss due to grasshoppers often seems to be limited to a few outbreak areas. The national average shows for the three years that it was not an important pest. Control operations should be envisaged only when heavy outbreaks occur and insecticides and sprayers are immediately available to the farmer.

References

Krall S, Dorow E (1993) Brochure de référence sur les dégâts causés aux épis de mil. Third ed. Eschborn: GTZ, 35 pp

Krall S, Youm O, Kogo SA (1995) Panicle insect pest damage and yield loss in pearl millet. Pages 135–145 in Nwanze KF, Youm O (eds) Panicle insect pests of sorghum and pearl millet: proceedings of an international consultative workshop, 4–7 October 1993, ICRISAT Sahelian Center, Niamey, The Niger

Pantenius U, Krall S (1993) A new method for determining yield losses caused by damage to the heads of pearl millet (*Pennisetum glaucum* (L.) R. Br.) due to diseases and pests. J Plant Diseases and Protection 100 (5): 522–529

New Strategies in Locust Control
S. Krall, R. Peveling and D. Ba Diallo (eds)
© 1997 Birkhäuser Verlag Basel/Switzerland

Comparison of the costs of barrier and blanket treatments using insect growth regulators in Madagascar

W. Zehrer

Deutsche Gesellschaft für Technische Zusammenarbeit (GTZ), Projet Protection des Végétaux, Bureau GTZ, B.P. 869, Antananarivo, Madagascar

Summary. Insecticides represent the greatest cost factor in the control of locusts and grasshoppers in Madagascar. By using insect growth regulators in barrier treatment, control costs can be reduced by half. For example US$2.30/ha could be saved if 4000 ha were treated by this method (at the 1992 exchange rate). It has been demonstrated that one person can cover 500 ha per day with one Micro-ULVA sprayer. In Madagascar ground treatment is especially interesting, as it can be executed quickly and is cheaper and simple to organise. Thus it should take preference over aerial treatments in most situations.

Résumé. Parmi l'ensemble des coûts de la lutte antiacridienne, les acridicides représentent la partie la plus impor-tante, suivis par les frais d'application. En utilisant les dérégulateurs de croissance, pour des traitements en barri-ère, les coûts pourraient être réduits de moitié. Pour le cas d'un traitement de 4.000 ha, on pourrait économiser 2,30 US$/ha (cours de change de 1992, 1 US$ = 1,864 FMG). En ca qui concerne Madagascar, cette méthode est surtout intéressante pour les traitements terrestres qui sont effectués beaucoup plus rapidement. Il a démontré qu'un agent peut protéger 500 ha par jour avec un appareil Micro-Ulva. Ainsi, une grande partie des traitement aériens pourraient être remplacée par des traitement terrestres.

Introduction

On average 60,000 ha are treated for migratory locusts (*Locusta migratoria capito* Saussure 1884) and red locusts (*Nomadacris septemfasciata* Serville 1838) in Madagascar every year. The cost of this control, of which insecticides represent the greatest proportion followed by contingent expenses, is an extremely heavy burden for the country.

Until 1989 dieldrin was used as an insecticide in Madagascar. During the campaign of 1981/82, hopper bands of *L. migratoria* were treated with dieldrin over more than 600,000 ha on the Horombe plateau. In this instance the Service de la Lutte Antiacridienne benefited by the rapid deployment of resources made possible through the technique of barrier treatment. Aerial treatment with barrier spray width of 100 m (every 1000 m) almost certainly prevented an inva-sion as the first generation was eliminated.

After 1989 dieldrin was banned in Madagascar, and no other insecticides with such long persistence were available. The destruction of the remaining 45,000 l of dieldrin in England was financed by Germany. Only insect growth regulators (IGR) with a completely different mode of action were known for their long persistence. However, during this period no experiments were carried out with this group of insecticides.

This chapter describes the results of five years of experience with three IGRs. Costs derived from blanket treatment were extrapolated to barrier treatment and compared. In addition costs of ground and aerial operations were compared.

Difficulties encountered in the economic evaluation of locust and grasshopper control

Locust control activities are rarely analysed in terms of costs, an exceptional situation in the area of plant protection and perhaps explained by the following points.

- Costing of crop losses to migratory locusts is extremely difficult, since it is not possible to anticipate the dynamics and movement of the populations. For example, if locusts (*L. migratoria capito*) are not controlled in their breeding areas in the south-west of Madagascar, an area of more than 1000 km to the north may be invaded. However it is impossible to relate the losses of the rice crop in the north-west and centre of the island during the following years to this invasion.
- A major portion of the pesticides is financed and provided by donors. Consequently the true value of this aid is not always appreciated by the responsible administrators or by the field officers performing the control operations in the recipient countries.

The red locust (*N. septemfasciata*), like the migratory locust, belongs to the category of "national disasters" in Madagascar. Except in years of rapid reproduction, the red locust, with one generation per year, is just one pest among many others and causes localised damage to maize and rice crops only. On the other hand, migratory locusts become very mobile as soon as they enter the gregarious phase, threatening the whole country except for the humid east coast. Thus, efforts by technicians to strike the red locust off the list of national disasters have failed, and farmers continue to demand that the locust control centre control the red locusts in their scattered maize fields, at enormous cost to the service. These treatments continue for political rather than economic reasons.

Recently it has become more difficult for countries at risk to obtain foreign aid for locust control. Scarce funds are earmarked for regions outside Africa. To obtain funds in this situation donors need reassurance regarding

- the economic viability of locust control measures,
- the safety and safe handling of products by training technicians applying the products,
- low environmental hazards.

The last point is becoming more important. For example, in case of an emergency, USAID is prepared to finance only IGRs for Madagascar.

Costs of treatment

According to a study carried out by Bauer and Walter (1992), the annual cost of the Plant Protection Service in Madagascar has increased to FMG 1,157 million (at the 1992 exchange rate) on average. This sum includes operating costs and salaries, and 960 million solely for insecticides. This trend is supported by looking at the actual costs of a treatment (Tab. 1).

Table 1. The example of Tanandava treating 700 ha

Item	Costs in FMG
Insecticides	60,900,000
Aircraft hire	24,520,000
Personnel – allowances	270,000
Salaries (six days)	180,000
Vehicles – fuel	190,000
Depreciation	1,450,000

Regarding Table 1 the following should be pointed out:
• The costs of insecticides represent two-thirds of the total.
• Aircraft rental is the second most important expenditure.
• All the other costs are negligible, including allowances for field officers.
• Travel expenses (0.3% of total costs) are always a critical point, since they are not covered by donors.

In general, salaries and depreciation of equipment (vehicles, spraying equipment) are not included, because salaries of officials are paid directly by the government and the equipment is provided by donors. For the vehicles, the only cost estimated is that of fuel. This is why these figures do not appear again in Tables 2 to 5.

Possible ways of cutting costs

Costs of insecticides

- Persistent insecticides suitable for barrier treatment should be used. This avoids repeated treatments. In Madagascar, considerable experience has been gained with two IGRs, Alsystin (triflumuron) and Dimilin (diflubenzuron), for which the price and the efficacy at different dosages are known. In barrier treatment, they are less expensive than traditional insecticides. In most cases a dose of 5 g a.i./ha has been used, but proved not to be sufficiently effective under all circumstances, therefore a dose of 10 g a.i./ha is recommended. With the persistence of these products, a second treatment against the newly hatched hoppers is not required for up to three weeks. In 1992 in Madagascar this procedure would have saved a considerable percentage of total costs.
- As far as possible, pesticide concentrates should be purchased. They can be diluted with locally available materials, and the reduced packaging will save transport costs. In the case of propoxur, one tonne of 80% a.i. can be diluted into 16 tonnes of 5% for application. Powders can be used by field officers with little experience. Similarly, liquid products can be mixed with diesel oil purchased locally for aerial ultra low volume (ULV) application at half a litre per hectare or, following the recommendations of the FAO (Food and Agriculture Organization of the United Nations), at one litre per hectare.

Table 2. Operation at Bekily: 9000 ha treated (barriers of 100 m spaced at 1000 m)

Item	Barrier treatment (extrapolation)	Blanket treatment (actual treatment)
Duration of treatment	1 day	3 days
Products used	900 l Alsystin 050	4500 l Diazinon 90%
Flying hours		
Spray aircraft	1 h 42 min	13 h 24 min
Guidance aircraft	1 h 53 min	14 h 00 min
	Costs in FMG	
Aircraft hire	2,459,976	17,219,832
Allowances	39,000	135,000
Insecticide	34,560,000	78,300,000
Fuel	115,200	194,400
Total costs	37,174,176	95,849,232
Costs per hectare	4130	10,649

Costs of aircraft

- Avoid the use of guidance aircraft. In Madagascar there is only one company renting spraying aircraft. Because of this monopoly, the plant protection directorate incurs relatively high costs when aerial treatment is required during major invasions. This company still uses guidance aircraft, which could be avoided if the spraying aircrafts were equipped with GPS (global positioning system). Costs could be reduced by 30–40% (Tabs 2 and 3).

Costs of treatment

- By practising barrier treatment costs can be cut by 80%, though this calls for the use of more persistent products. The treated barriers cover only one-fifth or one-tenth of the area to be protected (Tab. 5).

Comparison of total costs of aerial barrier and blanket treatments

The costs of the two types of treatment in 1992 are presented in Table 2.

The blanket treatment was carried out on 7 March and again on 30 March 1992, because new hoppers hatched in the meantime. If persistent products like IGRs had been used, the second

Table 3. Operation at Tanandava: 7000 ha treated (barriers of 100 m spaced at 1000 m)

Item	Barrier treatment (extrapolation)	Blanket treatment (actual treatment)
Duration of treatment	1 day	6 days
Products used	700 l Alsystin 050	3500 l Diazinon 90% and Sumithion 100
Flying hours		
Spray aircraft	2 h 14 min	
Guidance aircraft	9 h 23 min	13 h 33 min
		20 h 49 min
Costs in FMG		
Aircraft hire	7,379,928	21,524,790
Allowances	39,000	270,000
Insecticide	26,880,000	60,900,000
Fuel	180,000	324,000
Total costs	34,478,928	83,018,790
Costs per hectare	4,925	11,859

treatment would not have been necessary, because when hoppers appeared the product from the first treatment would still have persisted on the vegetation.

The figures are not consistent between the tables because of variable conditions: contract with aerial spraying company, stand-by periods for the aircraft, size of areas and the distances to air strips. However it is obvious from Tables 2 and 3 that the cost of barrier treatment with IGRs at 5 g a.i./ha is less than half that of blanket treatment, mainly by reducing expenditure on insecticides and aircraft rental.

The most economic aerial treatment

The costs can be reduced further if lower but realistic prices are used for insecticides. A theoretical recalculation of the 7000 ha treatment at Tanandava is presented in Table 4.

Costs in Table 5 are based on the price of diesel in Madagascar and of Dimilin 450 in February 1995 and the following conditions:
- A guidance aircraft is not required.
- Within-barrier treatment is at a rate of 0.5 l/ha.
- Ratio of the barrier to the entire unsprayed area is 1:10.
- Dimilin 450 mixed with diesel oil is used.
- Flight time between treatment area and air strip is 15 min.

Comparison between ground blanket and barrier treatment

As barrier treatment is more rapid than blanket treatment, ground teams can treat larger areas. This reduces the need for aerial treatment and thereby costs, which is of particular interest to Madagascar.

In this example (Tab. 5) the IGR Alsystin 050 UL was applied in barrier treatment at 7 g a.i./ha (overall dose rate). The table compares the costs between ULV spinning disk sprayers and a spraying unit with ULV equipment for blanket treatments and barrier and blanket treatments using spinning disk ULV sprayers.

Table 4. Extrapolated costs of barrier treatment with Dimilin 450 at a dosage of 5 g active ingredient per hectare at Tanandava

Items	Costs in FMG	Remarks
Aircraft hire	2,000,000	
Allowances	39,000	Insecticide must be mixed with diesel oil
Insecticide	16,200,000	
Fuel	390,000	
Total costs	18,629,000	
Costs per hectare	2,662	(US$1.50)

Table 5. Costs of actual operation at Soamanga: 460 ha

Item	Barrier treatment	Blanket treatment	
	Micro-ULVA	Micro-ULVA	Solo Port 423 Apparatus
Treatment duration	1 day	8 days	5 days
		Costs in FMG	
Insecticide	2,515,000	4,002,000	4,002,000
Vehicle fuel	14,000	14,000	14,000
Apparatus costs:			
Batteries	80,000	240,000	-
Fuel	-	-	150,000
Allowances	28,000	224,000	160,000
Total costs	2,637,000	4,512,000	4,326,000
Costs per hectare	5,734	9,809	9,406

Conclusion

Our experience in Madagascar and the findings of Dobson et al. (1996) clearly show that the costs of controlling locusts and grasshoppers by barrier treatment on the ground is always less than by aerial treatments. The situation is different if a large area has to be treated, if the region is inaccessible or when very limited time is available. Furthermore, the costs of barrier treatments are always substantially lower than blanket treatments even at 10 g a.i./ha of Alsystin 050 UL, irrespective of whether treatments are via the ground or the air. Further advantages of barrier treatments are the speed of operation, their simple organisation, a more efficient use of materials and, last but not least, a reduced impact on the environment (Tingle et al. 1996). Preference thus should be given to ground over aerial treatment and to barrier treatment in all situations.

References

Bauer and Walter (1992) Developpement et introduction d'un système de suivi et evaluation et économie de la lutte antiacridienne. Rapport de consultation à demande du "Projet Protection Intégrée des Cultures et des Denrées Stockées à Madagascar" de la Deutsche Gesellschaft für Technische Zusammenarbeit GmbH (GTZ) "Protection des végétaux", PARTICIP GmbH, Consultants für Entwicklung und Umwelt, Wehingen, RFA, 30 pp

H Dobson, J Cooper, A Rakotonandrasana and R Scherer (1997) Economics and practicalities of migratory locust hopper band control using barriers of insect growth regulator. This volume

CCD Tingle, Raholijaona, T Rollandson, Z Gilberte and R Romule (1997) Diflubenzuron and locust control in south-western Madagascar: relative abundance of non-target invertebrates following barrier treatment. This volume

New Strategies in Locust Control
S. Krall, R. Peveling and D. Ba Diallo (eds)
© 1997 Birkhäuser Verlag Basel/Switzerland

Economics and practicalities of migratory locust hopper band control using barriers of insect growth regulator

H. Dobson[1], J. Cooper[1], A. Rakotonandrasana[2] and R. Scherer[3]

[1] *Natural Resources Institute, Central Avenue, Chatham Maritime, Kent ME4 4TB, England*
[2] *Cellule de Recherche, Centre Antiacridien, Betioky-Sud, Madagascar*
[3] *Projet Protection des Végétaux GTZ, Bureau GTZ, B.P. 869, Antananarivo, Madagascar*

Summary. Migratory locusts are a serious pest in Madagascar, and chemical control is carried out with varying degrees of success by finding, and spraying, hopper bands and swarms with conventional insecticides. An alternative strategy is barrier spraying, i.e., applying persistent insecticides onto widely spaced strips of vegetation, but use of the product with which this technique was developed, dieldrin, has been discontinued due to environmental and human health hazards. Insect growth regulators (IGRs) such as diflubenzuron are persistent, yet have a relatively low non-target environmental impact, and are safe to humans due to their mode of action (disrupting chitin synthesis). The application method used in a successful large-scale IGR barrier trial in Madagascar is described briefly, and the logistical and economic merits of this and other techniques are compared using a spreadsheet model. When hand-held spinning disk sprayers are used for IGR barrier spraying at a spacing of 600 m, a team with four sprayer operators can achieve a work rate of almost 900 ha/day at a cost of around US$1.7/ha. The case is made that this manual application is preferable to aircraft barrier spraying for infested areas of less than 10,000 ha, since it costs less, produces a more uniform deposit and allows farmer participation in strategic locust control.

Résumé. Le criquet migrateur constitue un fléau grave à Madagascar. La lutte chimique consistant à localiser les bandes larvaires et les essaims puis à les traiter en épandant des insecticides conventionnels ne remporte que des succès relatifs. Le traitement en barrière consistant en des applications d'insecticides rémanents sur des bandes de végétation largement espacées les unes des autres est une méthode alternative à envisager, sans toutefois utiliser la dieldrine, substance avec laquelle cette technique a justement été mise au point, en raison de ses effets nocifs sur l'environnement et sur la santé humaine. Les dérégulateurs de croissance (DC) tels que le diflubenzuron sont certes persistants, mais n'ont qu'une incidence relativement faible sur le milieu non-cible et n'affectent pas la santé humaine en raison de leur mode d'action (perturbation de la synthèse de la chitine). L'article décrit brièvement la méthode d'application utilisée dans un essai d'épandage de DC en barrière à Madagascar et compare au moyen d'un modèle de tableur les avantages logistiques et économiques de cette technique par rapport à d'autres méthodes. A l'aide de pulvérisateurs manuels centrifuges, une équipe de quatre opérateurs appliquant des DC en barrière avec des espacements de 600 mètres peuvent traiter près de 900 hectares par jour à un coût d'environ 1,7 $ US par hectare. Il apparaît que l'application manuelle est supérieure aux épandages aériens en barrière pour les surfaces contaminées inférieures à 10 000 hectares en raison de son moindre coût, du fait que le produit se dépose de manière plus uniforme et que les agriculteurs participent ainsi eux-mêmes à la lutte antiacridienne.

Introduction

The migratory locust, *Locusta migratoria capito* (Saussure, 1884), is a major constraint to agricultural production in the south-west of Madagascar (Farrow 1974). Populations can multiply rapidly and become gregarious in favourable conditions due to the potential development of three generations during the rainy season between October and April. During outbreaks, hopper bands cause damage to rice and maize crops in the south-west and, if not controlled, can lead to devastating swarms of adults that may migrate northwards to the large rice-growing areas in the middle-west and the highlands. Since swarms may originate in one area and migrate to another, the migratory locust is treated as a national problem where strategic control, i.e. area-wide population reduction, is preferable to crop protection.

Control is carried out each season: farmers employ traditional mechanical methods such as beating or burning the hoppers or digging trenches in their path, but this can only ever be a crop protection measure and is not likely to have a significant impact on the total population in the region nor prevent swarms escaping to other areas. Control is also carried out by staff of the Direction Protection des Végétaux (DPV) who spray and dust hopper bands with ground-based equipment and, if the scale of the problem escalates, spray bands and swarms from aircraft using conventional contact insecticides. Successful large-scale hopper band control can reduce the frequency and scale of aerial operations against hopper bands and swarms and reduce the level of crop damage in the treated area and elsewhere. However, as with the desert locust, the greatest constraint to successful control of migratory locust hopper bands is one of logistics due to the extent and nature of the target distribution (Symmons 1992); finding and spraying all of the bands in a large but patchy infestation, especially those in areas far from agricultural land or settlements, is so time-consuming as to be impossible. The lack of sufficient manpower, vehicles or systematic search strategy means that most bands are probably not even detected. In heavy infestations the only practical option has been to mark out large blocks thought to contain many hopper bands and to blanket-spray the blocks from aircraft with conventional insecticides.

Insect growth regulator barriers applied by hand: a new approach to control

In 1994, a large-scale trial was carried out to test the efficacy and practicability of a technique with potential practical, logistical, environmental and economic advantages. The technique called barrier spraying involves applying a persistent stomach poison to widely spaced strips of vegetation so that marching hopper bands encounter them, feed on them and are killed before they fledge. Up until the mid-1980s, dieldrin was the insecticide of choice for use in barrier spraying because of its long-term efficacy – several weeks under tropical conditions – and it gave good results when sprayed in Madagascar as a barrier in 1981 (Skaf, personal communication). However, the use of dieldrin has now been discontinued in most countries because it accumulates in biological systems (WHO 1989) and is a hazard to operators (WHO hazard class 1b).

If barrier spraying is to be acceptable from environmental and human health standpoints, a new type of product is required.

The product used in this trial is a benzoylurea insect growth regulator (IGR) called Dimilin (diflubenzuron). This class of compound interferes with chitin synthesis and thus kills at the next moult, since the new exuviae cannot be formed. Dimilin is relatively persistent on vegetation with a half-life in Sahelian conditions of around 15 days (Sissoko 1991; Gadji 1993), although it is quickly broken down by micro-organisms on contact with the soil (Nimmo et al. 1984) and is relatively insoluble in water. It has a relatively low toxicity to mammals (including humans), fish and birds. The nature of the distribution of IGRs in barrier spraying (widely spaced strips), their principle route of entry (ingestion) and the mode of action (disrupting moulting) make them somewhat selective against highly mobile, phytophagous, chitinous organisms such as locusts. Initial results of ecotoxicological assessments in Senegal indicate that non-target effects are likely to be less when barrier spraying with IGRs than when using conventional pesticides. In Madagascar, only a few invertebrate groups showed adverse impacts of diflubenzuron barrier spraying for locust control, even within the treated barriers (Tingle et al. 1996).

Summary of trial method

The trial was carried out as part of a collaboration between the DPV, the Deutsche Gesellschaft für Technische Zusammenarbeit (GTZ) and the Natural Resources Institute (NRI) of the Overseas Development Administration (ODA), and is reported in detail in Cooper et al. (1995). Building on the experience of previous laboratory trials (Coppen 1994), field persistence trials (Sissoko 1991; Gadji 1993), small-scale blanket spray trials (Rhind 1991) and barrier trials (Scherer and Rakotonandrasana 1993), the application parameters were set nominally at 50-m-wide barriers, 600-m barrier spacing and a dosage within the barrier of 90 g a.i./ha using a volume application rate (VAR) of 0.83 l/ha. This equates to an overall dosage over the 2000-ha block of 7.2 g a.i./ha.

Applications were made by a team of seven people: a navigator/supervisor to plot the course of the spray team, four sprayer operators (sufficient to treat the barrier in one pass without having to revisit it) and two porters to carry additional spray product and equipment. The porters each carried around 15 l of Dimilin – sufficient for the team to apply two whole barriers (each 4 km long) so that the supply vehicle could remain at one edge of the plot. This vehicle, with driver, was used to carry the team to and from the spray site and to act as a supply vehicle to replenish the porters' stocks of IGR at the edge of the block. Operators wore protective clothing and used hand-held ultra low volume (ULV) spinning disc sprayers (Micron Micro-Ulva). Porters carried one spare sprayer and field equipment including measuring cylinder, stop watch, funnels, portable insecticide containers, prismatic compass, anemometer, vibrating needle tachometer, note pad, flags to mark the barrier ends, tools, spare batteries, protective clothing and soap and water for washing. Subsequent field trials have shown that a hand-held global positioning systems (GPS) provides an even easier and more accurate means of navigating the barriers and avoids the need to mark the barrier ends with flags before application.

Sprayer operators walked at a comfortable speed of around 1.25 m/s using a 12-m track spacing and an emission height between 0.5 and 1.5 m depending on the strength of the wind – the sprayer was held higher in lighter winds to ensure that the drops were carried over a sufficient downwind swathe. The sprayer operators moved in a line one downwind of another, but in staggered formation to avoid exposure to the spray emitted upwind (Fig.1). As soon as one sprayer ran out of spray liquid, everyone stopped while the porters refilled the reservoir bottles.

A significant practical advantage of using hand-held sprayers compared with vehicle-mounted sprayers quickly became apparent in their ability to cover areas with obstacles such as rocky outcrops, streams or rice paddies. Also, since ULV spraying normally depends on overlapping the swathes from several successive passes, the cumulative deposit from four portable sprayers

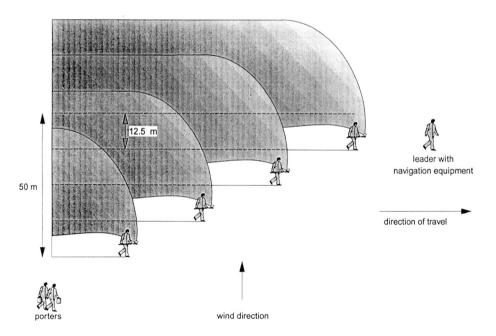

Figure 1. Configuration of spray team to avoid operator exposure to insecticide.

is more uniformly distributed over the barrier than the single swath produced by an aircraft pass.

Effects of diflubenzuron were observed three days after treatment. Bands showed reduced displacement, and good control of both bands and scattered hoppers was achieved from exposure to one barrier treated with 93.7 g a.i./ha.

Modelling the logistics of barrier and blanket spraying

In order to make comparisons between this and other application methods, a spreadsheet was produced to model theoretical costs and work rates of barrier and blanket spraying with different types of equipment. Sprayers considered were: hand duster, motorised knapsack duster, lever-operated knapsack sprayer (LOK), ULV hand-held spinning disk sprayer, motorised ULV knapsack airblast sprayer, ULV vehicle-mounted drift sprayer, ULV vehicle-mounted airblast sprayer and ULV aerial sprayer.

Tables 1 and 2 list the basic rates, costs, assumptions, symbols and formulae used in the calculations, and Tables 3 and 4 show calculated work rates and costs for the different methods of treating a 10 km × 10 km plot. The input values, including block size, can be changed to investigate their effect on the performance of different application methods. Other data assumptions for individual sprayer types such as track spacing and refill times are given in the Microsoft Excel spreadsheet, which is available from the authors.

Results of the model

Tables 3 and 4 show that a hand-held ULV sprayer is capable of a work rate over seven times that of low-volume knapsack sprayers, while a vehicle-mounted airblast sprayer can work up to six times faster than a hand-held ULV sprayer and an aircraft almost 100 times faster. If four hand-held ULV sprayers are used together as a team, the work rate advantages of vehicles and aircraft are reduced to factors of 1.5 and 25 respectively. In addition, the constraints of access to difficult terrain for vehicle sprayers and the logistical demands of aerial spraying mean that delay and extra expense have to be offset against these advantages (see conclusions).

For barrier spraying, total costs per hectare of the different options are similar because the product is the largest cost component. However, when this is excluded and operational costs are compared, low-volume knapsack sprayer application costs five times as much, vehicle spraying

Table 1. Data and assumptions used in the calculations

The block is square. Length/width of block (km)	10
Barrier spacing (km)	0.6
Barrier width (km)	0.05
Area barrier treated (km^2)	100
Actual area of barriers (km^2)	8.83
Number of barriers	18
Cost of vehicle hire/day (incl fuel) US$	50
Cost of spray aircraft hire/hour (incl fuel) ($)	500
Cost of formulated IGR/litre ($)	22
Cost of petrol/diesel per litre ($)	0.5
Cost of set of sprayer batteries ($)	2
Life of set of sprayer batteries (h)	10
Spray vehicle fuel used/hour (l/h)	5
Knapsack mistblower consumption/hour (l/h)	0.9
Vehicle-mounted sprayer fuel used/hour (l/h)	1.8
Cost of ULV insecticide/litre ($/l)	10
Cost of dust formulation/kg ($/kg)	3
Farmers/labourers daily rate (US$/day)	2
DPV staff salary + field allowance (US$/day)	4.25
Number of hours of spraying carried out during a working day	5
Fuel (petrol and diesel fuel oil) cost (US$/litre)	0.5
Knapsack sprayer fuel consumption (l/h)	0.8
Vehicle sprayer fuel consumption (for motorised airblast machines) (l/h)	5
Time added for each aircraft turn to reach the start of next pass/barrier (s)	40

For blanket spraying, start one track spacing upwind of downwind edge.

For barriers start at downwind edge and put last barrier at upwind edge.

Turn time for ground sprayers is the time taken to travel the inter-pass distance at spraying speed.

Barriers are sprayed by teams with a sufficient number of sprayers to complete them in one combined pass without the need to revisit the barrier.

The same number of operators as that used for the barrier spraying is used for the blanket spraying.

Ferry time is the time for the one-way journey from spray site to refill site.

Sprayers in a team can ferry and fill simultaneously.

Vehicle hire costs covers non-spraying fuel costs (transport, ferrying of materials etc.).

Aircraft applied barrier is 50 m wide – in fact the IGR is likely to be spread over a wider swathe with a lower dosage.

Low-volume application (50 l/ha) is a water-based emulsifiable concentrate formulation, with the concentrate costing the same as the formulated ULV IGR ($22/l). This is an assumed figure and costs can vary with amount purchased and where it is retailed.

Filling time for aircraft includes taxiing after landing and before take-off.

Time and costs for demarcation of the target area are not included.

costs over 30% more and aerial spraying costs 50% more per hectare than a team with four hand-held ULV sprayers.

Table 2. Formulae used in the calculations

Calculation	Symbol	Blanket	Barrier spraying
Number of barriers	N_b		$\dfrac{b+1}{t}$
Number of passes	N_p	$\dfrac{b \times 1000}{t}$	$\dfrac{N_b \times w}{t}$
Total distance	d	$N_p \times b + b - t$	$N_p \times b + b$
Total spray time	T_s	$\dfrac{d}{u}$	$\dfrac{d}{u}$
Additional time for turning (aircraft)	T_t	$\dfrac{(N_p - 1) \times k}{3600}$	$\dfrac{(N_b - 1) \times k}{3600}$
Total refill/taxi time	T_r	$\dfrac{f \times V \times a \times 100}{e \times 60}$	$\dfrac{f \times V \times y \times 100}{e \times 60}$
Total ferry time	T_f	$\dfrac{2 \times z \times V \times a \times 100}{e \times 60}$	$\dfrac{2 \times z \times V \times y \times 100}{e \times 60}$
Work rate for individual sprayer	R_i	$\dfrac{a \times 100}{(T_s+T_t+T_r+T_f)}$	$\dfrac{a \times 100}{(T_s+T_t+T_r+T_f)}$
Work rate for team	R_t	$R_i \times g$	$R_i \times g$

Symbols: a = area treated (km^2); b = length of side of square spray block (km); N_p = no. of spray passes; N_b = no. of barriers; y = surface area of barriers within block (km^2); t = track spacing (km); d = distance travelled (including spraying and walking between spray passes) (km); u = speed (km/h); s = barrier spacing (km); w = barrier width (km); T_s = total spray time (h); T_t = total turning time (h); T_r = total refill/taxi time (h); T_f = total ferry time (h); R_i = work rate of individual sprayer (ha/h); R_t = work rate of spray team; V = volume application rate (l/ha); e = tank capacity; f = time for single refill and taxi; z = time for one ferry to and from site; g = number of sprayers operating simultaneously; k = additional time at turns (for aircraft only)

Table 3. Blanket spraying with conventional insecticides. Work rates and costs for each sprayer type

Parameters (Costs in US$)	Symbol	Hand duster	Knap motor duster	LV knap LOK	ULV hand drift	ULV knap drift	ULV vehic. drift	ULV vehic. blast	ULV aerial drift
Work rate for one sprayer (ha/h)	RI	2.10	4.20	0.50	3.90	9.70	15.30	27.30	379.60
Team work rate (ha/h)	R_t	10.58	8.36	8.23	15.70	19.42	30.67	27.29	379.61
Team work rate ratio to spinning disk		0.67	0.53	0.52	1.00	1.24	1.95	1.74	24.18
Team operational costs/h		25.00	24.05	40.00	13.70	14.05	40.10	28.50	25.10
Team operational costs/ha		2.36	2.88	4.86	0.87	0.72	1.31	1.04	0.07
Insecticide costs per sprayed ha		15.00	15.00	8.33	8.33	8.33	8.33	8.33	8.33
Total treatment costs/ha		17.36	17.88	13.20	9.20	9.05	9.64	9.37	8.40

Table 4. Barrier spraying with IGRs. Work rates and costs for each sprayer type

Parameter(Costs in US $)	Symbol	LV knap LOK	ULV hand drift	ULV knap blast	ULV vehic. drift	ULV vehic. blast	ULV aerial drift
Work rate for one sprayer (ha/h)	RI	5.90	44.70	105.8	167.00	292.80	4169.50
Team work rate (ha/h)	R_t	94.10	178.90	211.70	334.10	292.80	4169.50
Team work rate ratio to spinning disk		0.53	1.00	1.18	1.87	1.64	23.30
Team operational costs/h		40.00	14.30	15.40	40.10	29.40	525.10
Team operational costs/ha		0.43	0.08	0.07	0.12	0.10	0.13
Insecticide costs per sprayed ha		1.62	1.62	1.62	1.62	1.62	1.62
Total treatment costs/ha		2.04	1.70	1.69	1.74	1.72	1.74

Table 5 compares cost and work rate of blanket spraying and barrier spraying using hand-held ULV sprayers at various different barrier spacings. The comparison is valid, since blanket spraying is often carried out on large blocks of hopper band-infested habitat due to the difficulty of finding and treating the individual bands. The data show that with a barrier spacing of 600 m, the work rate for barrier spraying with hand-held ULV sprayers will be around 11 times that for blanket spraying with the same equipment. Cost per barrier-treated hectare is also less than 20% of the cost for full-coverage spraying with conventional insecticide. It also shows that with wider barrier spacing (a real possibility requiring further testing), the work rate and cost advantages of barrier spraying are even greater.

Table 5. Comparison of barrier and blanket spraying at different spacings using hand-held spinning disk sprayers (*)

Type of treatment	Barrier spacing (m)	Barrier width (m)	% of area sprayed	Team work rate	Team time to spray 100 km^2 (h)	team cost/treated ha ($/ha)
blanket	n/a	n/a	100	15.7	637	9.2
barrier	600	50	8.3	179	56	1.7
barrier	1000	50	5	290	35	1.06
barrier	2000	50	2.5	524	19	0.58
barrier	5000	50	1	1018	9.8	0.29

(*) Area = 100 km^2; track spacing = 12 m; speed = 4.5 km/h; number of sprayers = 4; full coverage product = fenitrothion; barrier product = diflubenzuron

Conclusions

IGR barrier spraying is an effective and economic technique for large-scale hopper band control and is relatively safe to operators and the environment. IGRs cannot completely replace conventional insecticides, which must be available to deal with adults which have escaped control as hoppers and, due to the slow action of IGRs, to kill locust hopper bands posing an immediate threat to crops. Since IGRs do not accumulate in the insect in the same way as dieldrin did, the parameters of barrier width, barrier spacing, dose and application accuracy may be critical factors.

Hand-held ULV sprayers are an efficient and practical method of applying IGR barriers. Capital outlay is small, the technology is simple and self-contained, and farmers can be trained as operators in a day to a level where they can spray safely under the supervision of a more highly trained team leader. This provides employment for rural labour and allows beneficiaries to participate in the strategic control process. A team with four operators using hand-held ULV sprayers can barrier spray an area of over 900 ha in a day (assuming a 5-h spraying day) and will produce a more uniform deposit over the barrier than vehicles or aircraft. This is the most economic and practical choice for IGR barrier applications in Madagascar on medium infestations up to 10,000 ha (11 days' work for one team). Although ULV vehicle sprayers may in theory be able to work much faster than portable sprayers, this advantage may be outweighed by the problems of access and mobility over difficult terrain – in these conditions the vehicle work rate would be very low when all the delays are taken into account. Aircraft do not suffer these access problems and have a work rate around 20 times that of a team with four hand-held ULV sprayers. However, they have operational costs around 50% more per hectare (excluding cost of product), they do not produce as uniform a deposit, they require considerable logistical support such as landing strips and ground marker parties, and there may be delays while the aircraft is contracted and brought to the infested area. Aircraft may be a more appropriate choice for larger infested blocks (>10,000 ha), especially where infestations are in remote and inaccessible areas or where rapid treatment of fledging hoppers is required.

IGR barrier spraying with hand-held ULV sprayers may be suitable for control of other locust species, including the desert locust, but the practicalities would need to be assessed in large-scale trials. The open terrain more typical of desert locust habitats would make navigation easier, but the typically hotter conditions and remote locations might shorten the ground team's effective spray window to the extent that the faster work rates of vehicles or aircraft are required.

The spreadsheet model provides a simple means of exploring the theoretical costs and work rates of the various locust application and control options – different values for basic spray parameters, input costs and assumptions can be entered to model different locust control scenarios. However, the data must be assessed along with the constraints of real control operations, which may have a large influence on actual cost, work rate and practicability.

References

Cooper JF, Coppen GDA, Dobson HM, Rakotonandrasana R, Scherer R (1995) Sprayed barriers of diflubenzuron (ULV) as a control technique against marching hopper bands of migratory locust *Locusta migratoria capito* (Saussure.) (Orthoptera: Acrididae) in Southern Madagascar. Crop Protection 14 (2): 137–143
Coppen GDA (1994) The use of benzoylphenyl ureas as novel insecticides for the control of locusts and grasshoppers. PhD thesis: University of Southampton
Farrow RA (1974) Comparative plague dynamics of tropical *Locusta* (Orthoptera: Acrididae). Bull Ent Res 64: 401–411
Gadji B (1993) Déposition et dégradation du fénitrothion et du diflubenzuron sur végétation et dans les mares temporaires. Rapport du project FAO-Locustox (Sénégal) ECLO/SEN/003/NET
Nimmo WB et a1. (1984) The degradation of diflubenzuron and its chief metabolites in soils - part 1: hydrolytic cleavage of diflubenzuron. Pestic Sci 15: 574–585
Rhind D (1991) MSc thesis on the control of grasshoppers with dimilin in Sahelian grassland
Saussure H(1884) Prodromus Oedipodiorum insectorum ex ordine Orthopterorum. Mem Soc Phys Hist nat Geneve 28 (9): 1–20
Scherer R, Rakotonandrasana A (1993) Barrier treatment with a benzoyl urea insect growth regulator against *Locust migratoria capito* (Sauss) hopper bands in Madagascar. International Journal of Pest Management 39(4): 411–417
Sissoko M (1991) M Phil thesis on persistence of dimilin in Sahelian grassland
Symmons PM (1992) Strategies to combat the desert locust. Crop Protection 11: 206–212
Tingle CD, Raholijaona, Rollandson T, Gilberte Z, Romule R (1996) Diflubenzuron and locust control in SW Madagascar: relative abundance of non-target invertebrates following barrier treatment. This publication
WHO (1989) Aldrin and dieldrin. Environmental Health Criteria 91. WHO, Geneva, Switzerland, 355pp

Management strategies

New Strategies in Locust Control
S. Krall, R. Peveling and D. Ba Diallo (eds)
© 1997 Birkhäuser Verlag Basel/Switzerland

Desert locust control strategies

P. Symmons

Brooklands, Bishops Frome, Worcestershire WR65BT, UK

Summary. The problems of combating desert locust upsurges change as an upsurge develops. The initial outbreak occurs with little warning and so must be fought by attacking nymphal infestations with the resources on hand. The ultra low volume nymphal target blocks are difficult to define at all stages of an upsurge. Theoretical analysis suggests that the resources that might be expected to be available are unlikely to be sufficient to destroy more than a small part of the nymphal populations. Swarm control, which is possible against the later stages of an upsurge, should be more efficient and more effective. There are no estimates of the effectiveness of campaigns at any stage based on sampling. There is an urgent need for field research to test the theoretical analyses. The assessment of the practical value of recent research must take account of the problems currently faced in combating upsurges with chemical pesticides.

Résumé. Les problèmes de la lutte contre les infestations de Criquet pèlerin changent au fur et à mesure que s'amplifient ces infestations. Les premières pullulations surviennent souvent inopinément et devraient être combattues en attaquant les infestations de larves avec les moyens dont on dispose. Or, il est difficile quelle que soit la situation acridienne de déterminer les blocs qui feront l'objet d'un traitement en ULV des larves. Une analyse théorique peut amener à penser que les moyens dont on peut espérer pouvoir disposer soient insuffisans pour détruire plus qu'une petite partie des populations de larves. Le contrôle des essaims qui est possible à des phases plus avancées de l'invasion devrait être plus efficace et efficient. Il n'existe pas d'estimations basées sur des échantillonnages qui permettent de mesurer l'efficacité des campagnes de lutte aux différentes phases. La recherche sur le terrain devrait de toute urgence tester les analyses théoriques. L'évaluation de la valeur pratique des recherches récentes devra tenir compte des problèmes actuels de la lutte chimique contre les invasions acridiennes.

Introduction

When considering strategies to combat the desert locust it is essential to remember that a plague arises from an upsurge, which is a sequence of successful breedings over a number of generations. The first breeding giving rise to clear gregarious behaviour is usually referred to as an outbreak. It is also necessary to bear in mind the characteristics and requirements of ultra low volume (ULV) application, and especially the need to treat relatively large blocks when attacking nymphs.

Intervention stage

We might in theory choose to attack an upsurge at one of three stages:
- at the initial outbreak stage;

- during the middle stage of upsurge development;
- at the late upsurge/early plague stage.

I will consider mainly the first and last of these.

The current official strategy is plague prevention. This is normally taken to mean attacking the outbreak, or the early upsurge, effectively enough to prevent the upsurge developing. If that fails, as has been the case of late, campaigns are mounted against the developing upsurge. If those campaigns fail to halt the upsurge, action must be taken to combat the late stages of the upsurge or the early stages of the plague. In recent years campaigns have been prosecuted at all three stages. But against which stage are campaigns likely to be most successful?

The argument that the lack of a major plague during the last 30 years shows prevention to have been successful is to confuse correlation with cause. A valid case would need evidence of successful campaigns based on field sampling. But no such evidence exists. Until such evidence becomes available, we must rely on calculations using plausible inputs.

It is of the greatest importance to decide at what stage of an upsurge control is likely to have the greatest impact. If we rely on outbreak control to prevent plagues, we shall be ill-prepared to combat upsurges and plagues if our reliance proves to be ill-founded. It is oversimple to assume that the fewer locusts early in an upsurge, the easier the control. It is also essential to decide the likely impact of control against the different stages of locust development, which means essentially comparing adult with hopper control.

Adult control versus ULV hopper control

Adult control is limited to swarms; swarm control is difficult unless the swarms are cohesive and persistent. So swarm control is largely restricted to the later stages of an upsurge.

Although ULV hopper control can be practised at all upsurge stages, it suffers from two drawbacks, either one of which is probably crippling. These are the difficulty of detecting and marking a treatment block, and the large area that would need to be sprayed, even if good targets could be defined.

ULV hopper target block detection and demarcation

Gregarious hopper infestations, either the patches of an outbreak or the later-stage bands, are sought on the ground, usually by vehicle. The patches can only be seen if within a few tens of metres of the vehicle, and the bands from perhaps 100 m or so. The first problem is to define a block, by remembering where infestations were seen in a limited and probably irregular traverse (Fig. 1). Even if that is accomplished, there remains the difficulty of deciding whether the outlined block is densely infested enough to make it worth spraying.

These problems have worried me for more than 20 years, but I have no ready solution. I am told "local knowledge" and "experience" provide the answer. That is difficult to accept without sampling support. A theoretical solution would be to divide the country into standard-sized control blocks and sample each under a sequential scheme to reach a decision either to treat or to leave. That is now technically possible with global positioning devices, but the process would be extremely tedious. Moreover, there might well be a good target straddling the boundary between two blocks, even though neither block reaches the control infestation threshold.

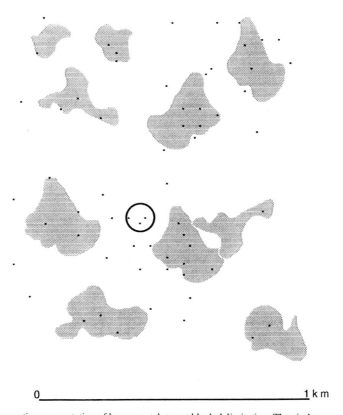

0_____1 k m

Figure 1. Diagrammatic representation of hopper patch target block delimitation. The circle represents the detection radius. Moving the circle would simulate search. The patches (represented by the dots) within the circle at any given time would be the only ones visible. The task is to outline a block containing many "patches" on the basis of a limited amount of "search". The shaded areas represent green vegetation but have no other significance.

Area needing treatment by ULV treatment

The second drawback to ULV hopper control is the area that needs to be treated.There are no direct estimates, so the problem must be approached theoretically. That is best done by considering the likely adult progeny without control and working back to the hoppers. There are a number of estimates of densities of swarms; a commonly accepted mean figure is $50/m^2$ (Pedgley 1981). There are also some density estimates for mid-instar bands (Ashall and Ellis 1962); densities varied, but most were below $100/m^2$. This suggests it would take at least $0.5 km^2$ of band to make $1 km^2$ of swarm. There are no published estimates of the percentage of infestation in band block targets. However, the late Rafik Skaf estimated the infestation in a good target as 5% (R. Skaf, personal communication). If we accept that figure as an average, swarm spraying would be some 10 times more efficient than band block treatment. In fact, the advantage of swarm spraying might well be much greater. Joyce (1971) claims it would need $2.5 km^2$ of band to make $1 km^2$ of swarm, which would make swarm spraying 25 times more effective than ULV band spraying. Moreover, there would be some late instar and fledgling mortality. Furthermore, band target blocks are unlikely to average as much as 5% infestation, and mid-instar bands are likely to average less than 100 insects/m^2. On the other hand, swarms in flight are thought to occupy a larger plan area than when settled, but even that may well be more than offset by the efficiency with which flying insects collect small drops of pesticide.

However, it is not merely a matter of efficiency but of scale. An early plague infestation might comprise $1000 km^2$ of swarm requiring for treatment at the most 50,000 l of a pesticide effective against bands at 0.5 l/ha. To treat the blocks containing the bands giving rise to that area of swarm, assuming those blocks could be found and marked, would probably require between 0.5 and 1.25 million l of similar pesticide. That would be too much to fund, too much to apply and pose too great an environmental risk to be acceptable.

The control requirements should be less with an outbreak, but the deployment difficulties would be greater. An outbreak is likely to take place within an area covering many tens of thousands of square kilometres. Outbreaks require heavy and widespread rain. Outbreaks cannot be forecast ahead of the rain, so they must be fought with the resources on hand. That, in general, means treating hoppers with vehicle-mounted sprayers.

Outbreak hopper populations comprise both "patches" and scattered hoppers. A patch might on average cover about $10 m^2$ and contain, say, 2000 mid-instar hoppers. To produce enough adults to form $10 km^2$ of swarm with a mean density half that of plague swarms would require roughly 300 million mid-instar hoppers. That would suggest some 75,000 patches, if half the hoppers were scattered. There are no estimates of the number of patches in blocks deemed to be worth controlling, and it is not easy to guess what a plausible figure might be. I suggest tentatively 200 patches per square kilometre as an average. That would mean treating nearly 400 km^2 to account for all the patches. The pesticide needed would be relatively modest, but the vehicle requirements would be substantial. A track spacing of 35 m, a sprayer speed of 10 km/h (FAO 1994) with a 4-ha block and 1 min turn at the end of each track, gives a treatment rate of approximately 20 ha/h. Assuming that rate is halved to allow for redeployment between treatment blocks and there is 4 h of spraying per day gives a work rate of 40 ha per operating day. If the sprayer operates on 20 days within a campaign, one sprayer could in theory treat about 8 km^2. That would suggest that at least 50 vehicle sprayers would be needed for the campaign. To that number must be added support vehicles and almost certainly extra vehicles for survey and search. Would such a force be available at such short notice? Even with such a force, some of the patches would be untreated because they would lie outside the best laid out blocks, and most of the scattered hoppers would escape.

Treating individual hopper aggregations

Treating individual bands and patches requires little pesticide but is time-consuming. A team might treat at most 50 patches or 4 ha of band in a day. That would indicate a need for, at the least, some 75 teams to deal with an outbreak consisting of 75,000 patches, assuming 20 operating days for a team in the campaign, and even more to combat a late upsurge or early plague infestation. Treating individual bands and patches is efficient but is not likely to be very effective.

Treating all of a suspect breeding area

During the late 1950s large areas were treated with widely spaced tracks of dieldrin to control hoppers, on the basis of the distribution of laying swarms. The technique is usually called barrier spraying, although in fact the pesticide was spread patchily over much of the area. Insect growth regulators (IGRs) are like dieldrin in being persistent but are not cumulative in their effect, as dieldrin is. To be most effective one would suppose an insect would need to ingest a lethal dose of an IGR before detoxification starts. Uptake would be affected by feeding behaviour, by the width of the barrier, by the speed of band movement, by the vegetation density, by the deposit and the deposit profile across the barrier. A precise control of barrier width and deposition, and of barrier spacing, would be needed. Moreover, a treatment that might work in one situation might well fail in another. However, recent laboratory studies suggest that IGRs may act in a partially cumulative manner, with the greatest effect resulting from uptake spread over some days. That might remove some of the doubts about IGRs as a dieldrin replacement for band treatment.

To treat the whole area made green by the outbreak rain might mean treating many thousands of square kilometre; that is not feasible with a contact pesticide. But barriers would be difficult to use against outbreak hopper populations because of the lack of information about the distribution of laying and the short time available between the rain which creates the conditions for laying and the hoppers that are to be controlled. There is also the possible risk to the environment of treatment over very large areas, even with an IGR.

Mid-upsurge campaigns

I have tried to examine the difficulties of campaigns against the desert locust by considering outbreak and late upsurge/early plague campaigns. An upsurge is a continuum. The intermediate situations are difficult to categorise. There may still be many patches, but there will also be bands.There will be a smaller percentage of scattered hoppers and scattered adults than with the outbreak. Swarms will be larger and more cohesive and so present better targets. But there will be a mixture of types of infestation: patches, small bands, medium-sized bands, adult groups, small low-density swarms and medium-sized higher-density swarms.

A strategy?

I do not believe we are in a position to decide on a strategy, although I think there is a basis for questioning the current claimed strategy on both practical grounds – Does it work? – and on theoretical grounds – Can it work? There is an urgent need for research to put the analyses I have outlined in this note on a sound basis. The studies would be neither difficult nor expensive; I have submitted on outline proposal to various potentially interested parties.

Currently donors are asked for large inputs to create large organisations that, it is claimed, will prevent plagues, plagues that would otherwise cause great crop loss and great hardship. Is the case an honest one? Is it sensible? Is it reasonable?

I believe the truth is more likely to be something like this. The funds to create large organisations will not be provided. The large organisations, even if formed, would not be maintained.

Even if the organisations were maintained, they would be ineffective when needed through long periods of underemployment. But most critically, even if none of this were so, there is every reason to suppose plagues would still occur.

I would, in any case, approach matters from the other end. What activities could we reasonably expect to support both organisationally and financially and, very important, where? We then should be realistic about the likely outcome of what could reasonably be supported. Essentially, I believe small locust units in key recession countries is all we can hope to maintain. These should be able to detect outbreaks and upsurge breedings, and perhaps retard an upsurge. But plagues would occur from time to time. I believe organisations capable of terminating a plague at its start can be created quickly and at relatively small cost if there is proper contingency planning and if the recession activity is maintained.

Relevance to the conference

Any new finding, if it is to be practically useful, must take account of the realities of desert locust behaviour, on the one hand, and the realities of organisation, security, logistics and funding, on the other.

Can the new approach be operated by the small units, which is the most that might reasonably be expected to be maintained? Will the innovation lead either directly or indirectly to us being able to find the populations that should be attacked more quickly? Is there a new method to help us find and delimit the ULV hopper targets? Or will a new method of suppression avoid the hopper target search problems associated with ULV pesticide application? Will a new method of control be logistically, organisationally and technically easier than ULV spraying? Will it be cheaper and safer?

For example: A biopesticide may be safer than a chemical spray, but it is just as difficult to apply. Again, will some new agent spread through a population when the population does not mix much? Could a pheromone trap for mature adults work when very large suspect areas must be seeded with traps cheaply, within a few days and usually with very little warning?

I doubt if there are any new strategies for desert locust control. But one would hope research might help us to do effectively what we now largely fail to do, and to do that cheaply and safely.

References

Ashall C, Ellis PE (1962) Studies on numbers and mortality in field populations of the desert locust
  (*Schistocerca gregaria* Forskal). Anti-Locust Bull no 38, Anti-Locust Research Centre, London
FAO (1994) The desert locust guidelines. IV. Control. Rome
Joyce RJV. In Gunn DL, Rainey RC (1971) Strategy and tactics of control of migrant pests. Phil Trans
  R Soc Lond B 287:
Pedgley D (ed) (1981) Desert locust forecasting manual,Vol 1, Centre for Overseas Pest Research
  London

New Strategies in Locust Control
S. Krall, R. Peveling and D. Ba Diallo (eds)
© 1997 Birkhäuser Verlag Basel/Switzerland

Can we prevent desert locust plagues?

A. van Huis

Department of Entomology, Wageningen Agricultural University, P.O. Box 8031, Wageningen, Netherlands

Summary. For centuries people in Africa have been catching locusts not only to protect their crops but also to eat. In the beginning of this century locusts were controlled by mechanical means. When persistent insecticides and advanced application methods became available, emphasis shifted towards obtaining overall population reduction. The three strategies reflect the time of intervention during the development of a plague: upsurge prevention, upsurge elimination and plague elimination. The technical means available determine the strategies to be followed. Dieldrin was crucial in the upsurge prevention strategy. Ultra low volume (ULV) applications seem more effective for the upsurge elimination strategy, as spraying in demarcated blocks is more effective when more of the population occurs in gregarious units. During plague elimination swarms and hoppers are controlled wherever and whenever possible. Theoretical calculations on the impact of chemical control during outbreaks would indicate that in order to counteract the high multiplication rates, a large proportion of the population needs to be killed to prevent a plague from developing. Swarm control restricts the area to be treated when compared to hopper control and is therefore more effective. However, mobility of swarms and the narrow time frame available for control increases the risk of swarms escaping control efforts. A number of technical and organisational constraints severely limit the feasibility of control operations. Locust control is a learning process. Each control action needs careful evaluation in order to assess its impact on the prevention of plagues. Criteria need to be established whether and when to control.

Résumé. Durant des siècles, les peuples d'Afrique ont capturé des locustes non seulement pour protéger leurs cultures, mais aussi pour s'en nourrir. Au début de ce siècle, des méthodes de lutte mécanique ont été employées contre les locustes. Lorsque des insecticides persistants et des techniques avancées d'application sont devenues disponibles, on a voulu réduire les populations acridiennes de façon globale. Les trois stratégies étudiées sont déterminées par le moment choisi pour intervenir durant l'évolution du fléau acridien: prévention des pullulations, élimination des pullulations et élimination du fléau. Elles sont déterminées également par les moyens techniques disponibles. La dieldrine a joué un rôle capital dans la stratégie de lutte préventive. Les applications en ULV semble plus efficaces pour la stratégie d'élimination des pullulations, étant donné que la pulvérisation dans des secteurs délimités est plus efficiente quand la plus grande partie de la population acridienne est en phase grégaire. Les interventions d'élimination du fléau consistent à supprimer les essaims et les bandes larvaires partout et quand cela est possible. Des calculs théoriques sur l'impact de la lutte chimique pendant les invasions semblent indiquer que pour contrecarrer les taux de multiplication élevés, une grande partie de la population acridienne doit être tuée afin d'éviter une extension du fléau. La lutte contre les essaims permet de réduire la zone à traiter par rapport à celle traitée dans la lutte contre les bandes larvaires et est donc plus efficiente. Toutefois, la mobilité des essaims et le peu de temps dont on dispose pour les attaquer augmente le risque de les voir échapper aux efforts de lutte. Un certain nombre de contraintes techniques et organizationnelles limite sérieusement la faisabilité des interventions. La lutte antiacridienne est un apprentissage toujours renouvelé. Chaque opération requiert une évaluation précise afin d'estimer son impact sur la prévention des fléaux. Il importe de définir des critères sur l'opportunité des interventions et sur le moment approprié pour déclencher les opérations de lutte.

History of locust control

In historical records the first insect to be recognized as a tropical pest was the desert locust. At Seqqara in upper Egypt there are carvings of locusts on tombs dating from 2470 to 2220 BC. The book of Exodus (ca. 1300 BC.) records the catastrophic damage caused by desert locust swarms (Jones 1973). However, locusts were not only considered to be a nuisance. Bodenheimer (1951) cites a number of references from the 18th and 19th centuries indicating that people from different parts of Africa enjoyed the agreeable flavour of the locust dish. But eating locusts also allowed them to take revenge for the destruction caused to their crops. Some tribes even welcomed the approach of locusts because it saved them from hunger. So the effort of physically killing locusts was not only aimed at protecting crops from being attacked but also to catch them for food. However, when advanced control techniques became available, including the use of synthetic insecticides and spray aircraft, the emphasis was shifted towards plague prevention through an overall reduction in the locust population.

In the beginning of this century mechanical means to kill invading locusts were employed, such as destruction of eggs, collection of hoppers by catching machines, burning by (among other methods) flame-throwers, catching hopper bands in deep ditches, and burying or crushing hoppers which were captured by erected barriers. Chemical means involved mineral oils, kerosene, soap, kerosene-soap emulsions and arsenic compounds. These were applied by spraying, baiting or dusting (Uvarov 1928).

Since the 1950s the organochlorine insecticide dieldrin was crucial in obtaining cheap and effective population reductions, and the product was extensively used (Gunn 1979). It is not excreted from or detoxified in the insect's body when a sub-lethal dose is ingested, but accumulates until a lethal level is reached and the insect dies. It was used in barrier spraying for hopper control. Vast tracts of land could be sprayed with limited amounts of dieldrin (10–20 g active ingredient per hectare) in a short time from the air, using tracks as far as 5 km apart. It had the additional advantage that individual bands did not need to be found before spraying, although the area within which hopper bands were present had to be identified. Since 1985 dieldrin has been progressively withdrawn from the market for locust control because of its persistence and bio-accumulation.

With dieldrin no longer available, contact insecticides have to be used. For logistical reasons, this is mainly carried out with vehicles and aircraft by treating bands and settled swarms with concentrated ultra low volume (ULV) formulations, using wide overlapping swathes.

Control strategies

Strategies were evaluated during a seminar in Wageningen in December 1993 (van Huis 1994a). The three strategies considered in locust control are related to the moment of human intervention during the development of a locust plague which lies on the continuum outbreaks – upsurges – plague (for definitions, see Magor 1994):

- *Upsurge or outbreak prevention* is generally considered to consist of delimiting potential breeding areas by aerial survey, satellite imagery, weather reports and information from scouts and/or nomads, in order to control any gregarizing population found in this area.
- When the inconspicuous early stages are not detected in time, or access is difficult for logistical or security reasons, gregarization occurs unnoticed. Hopper bands or swarms become larger and increasingly cohesive, and more of the population occurs in gregarious units. *Upsurge elimination, suppression or containment* aims at tracing and controlling these hopper bands and swarms wherever and whenever possible. However, it is not clear at which population densities and degrees of gregarization upsurge prevention ends and upsurge elimination begins.
- The upsurge elimination strategy may fail, partly because there may be insufficient time available for organising adequate control. In that case the strategy changes to *plague elimination*. All bands and swarms are destroyed wherever and whenever they are found.

Strategies have to be designed according to the objectives put forward and have to deal with criteria as to whether and when to control locusts. Further, they should be adjusted according to the means available to detect and kill locusts. With dieldrin *outbreak prevention* was relatively easy, since one application in a potential breeding area would suffice for several months. However, with contact insecticides the procedure becomes much more difficult and may be even impossible, because gregarizing locusts have to be found and sprayed. Continuous vigilance is necessary in potential breeding areas, and locusts may have to be detected and possibly treated several times in the same area during one season.

During outbreaks or the early stages of an upsurge only a certain proportion of the population behaves gregariously, and numerous small gregarious hopper bands are scattered over a large area. Simulation exercises indicate that in potential breeding areas only a very small percentage of these locust infestations would be found, despite intensive searching (van Huis 1994a). During the development of an upsurge, bands and swarms become progressively larger and more cohesive, and the area infested diminishes. This can be illustrated from the development of the 1968 plague. Locust numbers during two generations increased from 2 billion to 30 billion, while the gross area infested decreased from over 100,000 km^2 to about 5000 km^2 (Bennett 1976).

Impact of chemical control

Contact insecticides can be applied by treating individual bands by vehicle or on foot. However, this is a very time-consuming exercise. Besides, probably only a small proportion can be treated, since resources (for control) are usually limited. The more common approach is to demarcate blocks with a high percentage of band infestation. However, this is also a difficult procedure, as criteria have to be established in order to decide which bands should be considered inside or outside the demarcated blocks. Because of the smaller area involved and the size and cohesiveness of bands and swarms, it will be easier to use contact insecticides in upsurge elimination than in upsurge prevention. That is why in India upsurge elimination is the favoured strategy (S. Chandra, personal communication).

Theoretical calculations indicate that plague prevention is only possible when insecticides can kill more than 80% of the population (van Huis 1994b). This is because of high multiplication rates observed during outbreaks, and figures as high as 16 have been mentioned (Roffey 1994). An 80% kill assumes that all hopper bands should be sprayed as well as scattered hoppers during early upsurge breeding. It has been argued that such coverage is practically impossible (Gruys 1991). Chemical control at high multiplication rates of desert locust would then only slow the development of a plague rather than suppress it.

Based on circumstantial evidence, it has been claimed that the upsurge prevention strategy has been successful, as plague severity has diminished since the sixties. However, the generally dry conditions during that period have been mentioned by others as a possible cause. Also, it could be argued that the availability of dieldrin was responsible for the presumed success, as locust outbreaks and upsurges have occurred more frequently since its abolishment.

Outbreak prevention conducted simultaneously over the whole desert locust distribution area has probably never been implemented, for a number of reasons: security problems in some countries limiting control to protection of cultivated areas in countries like the Sudan because of the huge area involved (van Huis 1994a); a late start of control operations; insufficient and inappropriate equipment; and a lack of trained personnel.

Swarm versus hopper control

Swarm spraying has been argued to be more efficient than hopper control (Courshee 1990; Symmons 1992). These authors even claim that it is the only feasible method of achieving general population reduction. Symmons (1992) calculated that to prevent formation of a medium-sized swarm covering 40 km², about 1000 km² would have to be sprayed at the hopper stage. These calculations are based on the assumption that in blocks for ULV treatment no more than 2% is covered by bands and that 1 km² of band gives rise to 2 km² of swarm. Despite this, most campaigns concentrate on hopper control. This is unavoidable in the early stages of an upsurge when swarms are small and perhaps transitory. In late upsurges, swarm control is theoretically attractive. However, swarms may escape control because of their mobility and the limited time available. Control of swarms requires timely action and excellent organisational and logistic capabilities.

Doubt is also cast on efficiency rates of pesticide treatments in locust control. The standard method for the treatment of hoppers using ULV techniques is often poorly understood and may seldom be applied correctly.

Conclusion

The desert locust has an amazing capability to respond to environmentally favourable conditions. Locust-affected countries and the international donor community are normally slow in their response to a rapidly developing locust plague. Most of these countries are only able to maintain a very low capacity of survey and control. In plague situations they rely on donor assistance for vehicles, aircraft, pesticides, fuel, communication equipment and so forth. Operators who have to carry out locust control operations are often poorly trained. The large number of countries involved makes international coordination difficult. During locust recession periods, national locust control capabilities decline. Regional locust organisations face similar problems, since they depend on contributions from member states. The main constraints to preventing upsurges can be summarised as follows:

Technical constraints
- Lack of criteria whether and when to control;
- excessive resources necessary to effectively monitor and control early upsurges;
- monitoring not possible due to inaccessibility or insecurity;
- low detection rates of gregarious and gregarizing locusts at the start of an upsurge;
- lack of insecticides that are persistent and accumulate in the insect body;
- lack of immediately available resources or backup capacity to quickly respond to developing upsurges.

Organisational and other constraints

- Monitoring and control operations are organised on a country basis, making international coordination complex;
- organising campaigns which require donor assistance is difficult (delays often occur);
- trained manpower is lacking;
- locust-affected countries and donors often lose interest during recession periods.

Synthetic pesticides are still the only option controlling locusts. However, we do not have a proven strategy for using these products. Although techniques are improving to better identify areas suitable for breeding, gregarizing or gregarious locusts still have to be located and controlled in large and remote breeding areas. More thought should be given to the strategy required. Should survey in some countries in the recession area of the desert locust be more intensive because of higher risk of gregarization? What is the most effective time of human intervention during the development of the plague, and under which conditions can swarm control be favoured over hopper control? How can pesticides be used such that considerable impact on the population is obtained while pollution of the environment is kept to a minimum?

It is in the interest of both locust-affected countries and the donor community to learn from locust control operations, and thus we should carefully evaluate the impact of our control activities on locust populations. That is the only way to know whether we can improve our efforts and whether we will really be able to prevent desert locust plagues.

References

Bennett LV (1976) The development and termination of the 1968 plague of the desert locust, *Schistocerca gregaria* (Forskål) (Orthoptera, Acrididae). Bulletin of Entomological Research 66: 511–552

Bodenheimer FS (1951) Insects as human food: a chapter on the ecology of man. The Hague: Dr. W. Junk, 352 pp

Courshee RJ (1990) Desert locusts and their control. Int Pest Control 32: 206–212

Gunn DL (1979) Systems and management. Phil Trans R Soc Lond B 287: 375–386

Gruys P (1991) Grasshopper and locust campaigns 1986–1989 and FAO's role: a review. Unpublished report, FAO-AGPP

Jones DP (1973) Agricultural entomology. Pages 307–332 in Smith RF, Mitttler TE, Smith CN (eds) History of entomology . Palo Alto: Annual Reviews Inc, 571 pp

Magor JI (1994) Locust glossary. Pages 119–127 in Huis A van (ed) Desert locust control with existing techniques: an evaluation of strategies. Wageningen: Wageningen Agricultural University, 132 pp

Roffey J (1994) The characteristics of early desert locust upsurges. Pages 55–61 in Huis A van (ed) Desert locust control with existing techniques: an evaluation of strategies. Wageningen: Wageningen Agricultural University, 132 pp

Symmons PM (1992) Strategies to combat the desert locust. Crop Protection 11: 206–212

Uvarov BP (1928) Locusts and grasshoppers: a handbook for their study and control. London: The Imperial Bureau of Entomology, 352 pp

van Huis A (ed) (1994a) Desert locust control with existing techniques: an evaluation of strategies. Wageningen: Wageningen Agricultural University, 132 pp van Huis A (1994b) Can we combat the desert locust succussfully? Pages 11 – 17 in van Huis A (ed) Desert locust control with existing techniques: an evaluation of strategies. Wageningen: Wageningen Agricultural University ,132 pp

Proaction: strategic framework for today's reality

A.T. Showler

Senior Technical Advisor, Africa Emergency Locust/Grasshopper Assistance (AELGA) Project, Disaster Response Coordination Office, Africa Bureau USAID*, Washington, DC 20523-0089, USA
* The views herein are those of the author and not necessarily those of USAID

Summary. Models for estimating locust damage during plagues tend to oversimplify potential losses; there is also a tendency to focus on the development of possible survey and control tactics with little attention to inter-facing them with coherent strategies. Further, discussions on strategies often center upon perceptions of what cannot be done without offering positive options. This chapter identifies salient challenges to locust control and the limited arsenal of available tools. Preventive, proactive and reactive approaches to desert locust control are summarised, and proaction is identified as being most practical and acceptable modality for now. It is cautioned that strategies should not rely upon simplistic or rigid assumptions, and that available tools and tactics should be appropriately integrated within a flexible proactive framework.

Résumé. Les modèles construits pour estimer les dommages provoqués par les invasions de locustes ont tendance à simplifier exagérément les pertes potentielles et les stratégies de surveillance et de lutte mises au point sont souvent loin d'être cohérentes. De plus, les discussions sur les stratégies mettent souvent plus l'accent sur ce qui ne peut être fait que sur ce qui peut l'être. Cet article présente les stratégies de lutte anti-acridienne les plus marquantes et l'arsenal des quelques moyens disponibles. Il décrit succinctement les approches préventives, proac-tives et réactives de la lutte contre le Criquet pèlerin, la «proaction» étant considérée à l'heure actuelle comme la méthode de lutte la plus pratique et la plus satisfaisante. Il importe que les stratégies ne reposent pas sur des hypothèses simplistes ou rigides et que les outils et tactiques employés soient intégrés de façon appropriée dans un cadre souple de lutte proactive.

A major acridid problem in North America was successfully tackled through integrated use of safe chemical tactics; collection and analysis of relevant environmental factors; and application of rational intervention thresholds (US Department of Agriculture, 1996). But nothing, even in the United States, replaced systematic visual monitoring. Although it is tempting to compare successes of some programs, such as the grasshopper management program in the United States, with failures of others, such contrasts risk being highly contrived and inappropriate. Desert locust (and other species in Africa and Asia) biology and behavior differs from those of American acridids. African and Asian locust habitats are markedly dissimilar, and the resources with which to control locusts there are, for the most part, considerably more scarce (there is a need to rely upon donors for substantial assistance [Office of Technology Assessment 1990]). This paper summarises realities inherent to locust control operations in Africa and Asia and proposes that early interventions can aim to avert full-blown plagues and their associated emergency control, crop loss and environmental costs.

Devising locust control strategies will necessitate cost-benefit analyses of interventions in affected ecozones and of various campaign scenarios. Some studies, centered strictly on monetary crop value, suggest that locusts may not be a serious economic problem (Krall 1995). Locust plagues, on the other hand, occur in some of the world's most famine-prone areas and thus generate great concern within both economic and humanitarian contexts.

I have heard much debate suggesting that, even during plague years, locusts cause too little overall damage to warrant control efforts. Evidence suggests that this is not universally true (Steedman 1988; PANOS Institute 1993), but even if it were, locusts are capable of causing total crop loss, within hours, at the local level. Denial of requests for donor assistance (especially when made as disaster declarations) can be viewed as being morally and politically unacceptable for regions where crop production is vital to the survival of farmers, and sometimes governments (Potter and Showler 1990). Analysis of cash economics of locust control is incomplete without reflecting upon the inestimable value of the subsistence farmer and the subsistence agrarian society, ramifications of damage to pastureland and fodder (e.g. tree locust defoliation of fodder trees), and expense of additional food aid from donors (Showler 1995a). Care must also be taken to avoid separating the cost of locust damage from other factors that are often associated with, or even linked to, locust-inflicted injury. Such factors (e.g. drought, *Striga*, stalkborers, grasshoppers and quelea) compound the damage caused by locusts.

At international fora we tend to focus upon potential tactics with scant attention to how they will interface within a strategy. Computer models, economic analyses, empirical intervention thresholds, forecasting technologies, biological control agents and semiochemicals are all worthy of discussion, but the most imminent question remains unaddressed: What do we do now?

We have been faced during the last decade with challenges to locust control that we never had to surmount in the United States, Europe or Australia. The following examples should help to put African locust control into better perspective.

- There are multiple locust outbreak species with overlapping recession and plague distributions. This is compounded by the possibility of simultaneous grasshopper outbreaks near cropping areas.
- The area is vast; many of the regions requiring survey are remote and rugged, and infrastructure is generally weak.
- There has been a Tuareg rebellion in northern Mali/Niger (in 1994, five Malian military escorts were killed while helping with locust survey). Polisario guerrilla activity in Western Sahara has stopped survey and control (in 1988, two US C-130 spray aircraft en route to Morocco from Senegal were hit with rockets; one C-130 crashed, killing the entire crew). There has been armed conflict and displacement of people in Somalia. Until 1992, a 30-year war for independence raged in Eritrea; this prevented early intervention there in 1986–1987.

Parts of northern Eritrea are still mined. Early interventions in 1986–1987 in Sudan were similarly precluded, and parts of northern Mauritania are mined.
- Sufficient funding seems to be a consistent shortcoming, and slow bureaucratic mechanisms by which funds are made available can be a severe constraint.

Despite the challenges, survey and control are carried out, albeit with a limited array of tools. Weather data is collected from satellites and by local synoptic means. Combined with other environmental information, these data can be assimilated for making forecasts. Several institutions, some sophisticated and relatively well funded, are involved in forecasting; but nothing replaces visual monitoring. Field scouting can be roughly guided by greenness maps (Tappan et al. 1988), but the discovery of locust bands and swarms is accomplished through the use of vehicles (terrestrial and aerial) that carry human eyes mounted in human heads. Furthermore, the only available control tactic is insecticides. While there is much discussion about developing tactics, a strategy that will incorporate such new technologies with an aim to avert plagues has yet to be devised.

How do we best apply available tools (accounting for pervasive funding constraints)? Within the context of what strategy? Basically, there are three approaches to locust control: preventive, proactive and reactive (Showler 1995b).

Preventive. Ideally, locust control should occur at or prior to the onset of gregarious behavior when locusts have amassed in small patches no more than several square metres in diameter in breeding areas. Success would likely require that a critical, though as yet undetermined, proportion of these patches be controlled with the ultimate aim of holding locust populations in the recession phase indefinitely (Showler and Potter 1991). Unfortunately, we have not yet developed this capability.

Reactive. The 1986–1989 desert locust campaign exemplifies the reactive approach, but it is generally not adopted by choice. In 1986–1989, an inability to effect early control in key breeding areas along the Red Sea coast permitted large-scale swarm development, migration and breeding in other regions without disruption until a full-blown plague had developed. Rapidity of the initial outbreak's evolution toward plague status and the subsequent magnitude of the plague overwhelmed local crop protection capabilities. Though emergency operations began in the latter half of 1987 to protect threatened croplands, deployment of limited resources to protect agriculture precluded operations in remote Sahelian breeding areas (Showler and Potter 1991).

Proactive. The word *proactive* means early intervention to mitigate or avert further development of a problem. In the context of locusts, proaction entails intervention against localised outbreaks before plague status is reached (Showler 1995b). Proaction relies on early detection of bands and swarms, preferably in breeding areas, and strategic prepositioning of resources.

Without empirical intervention threshold levels, timing of intervention is determined through a blend of estimated gregarizing locust populations, local capacity for control, experience, intuition, gestalt and political pressure. Empirically rational intervention decisions should be determined through an improved understanding of the impacts of control measures applied against gregarizing locusts.

Reliance on a single control strategy, as is sometimes suggested at international fora, is pedestrian and unrealistic. An appropriate approach would consist of a range of proactive options that can be adopted on a flexible, dynamic basis in anticipation of various permutations of locust outbreak scenarios. In other words, specific strategies should be selected on a situational basis. Adherence to a single modality is not a strategy, it is a regimen.

Conclusions drawn from international discussions on locust control strategies tend to be couched in negative terms. Many Africans and Asians will probably agree that they are too often told what cannot be done rather than what can be done. Proaction offers a positive option that can be both flexible and realistic.

The impacts of interventions during the 1986–1989 and 1992–1994 desert locust campaigns should be compared. Both campaigns relied on relatively nonpersistent insecticides, and both outbreaks originated along the Red Sea coast. In the 1992–1994 campaign, control operations began on the Red Sea coast in early 1993. Though the outbreak spread to Mauritania, Senegal and the India/Pakistan border (with lesser infestations elsewhere), these infestations were contained to varying degrees, and massive breeding failed to occur in the Sahel's interior breeding areas (Showler 1995b). Though the intrinsic impact of interventions in 1993–1994 is unclear, it was generally believed that countries in the desert locust's plague distribution should prepare for a prolonged campaign unless interventions were rapid and effective. Partly because of a subsidence of armed conflict along the Red Sea coast, it is conceivable that early interventions played a crucial role in mitigating a potentially explosive magnification of the outbreak. As a possible result, the number of hectares treated and the cost of the 1992–1994 campaign (4 million hectares, $19 million from donors) were notably less than those of the 1986–1989 campaign (25 million hectares, $300 million from donors) (Showler 1995b).

Serious consideration of the EMPRES program (Abate et al. 1994), centered quite appropriately in the central region of the desert locust distribution area, has begun. Though EMPRES is an acronym for Emergency Prevention System, it will actually facilitate, coordinate and catalyze proactive desert locust control until such time, if ever, true outbreak prevention can be achieved. For now, proactive control is the only practical strategic framework available; exploration for tactics should aim at safely, effectively and efficiently locating and controlling locusts within a dynamic and flexible program tailored to meet diverse scenarios.

Proaction, if given committed support by locust-affected countries, donors and international organisations – and if false expectations do not cause premature disenchantment – should help to alleviate the locust threat to crop production, and ultimately contribute toward the reduction of localised crop failure in regions chronically beset with drought, poverty, pestilence and famine.

References

Abate L, McCulloch L, Spendjian G (1994) Formulation mission report on Emergency Prevention System (EMPRES) for desert locust. Food and Agriculture Organization, Rome, Italy, 58 pp

Krall, S (1995) Desert locusts in Africa – a disaster? Disasters 19: 1–7

Office of Technology Assessment (1990) A plague of locusts. US Congress, Washington, DC, 129 pp

PANOS Institute (1993) Grasshoppers and locusts: the plague of the Sahel. PANOS Institute, London, 114 pp

Potter CS, Showler AT (1990) The desert locust: agricultural and environmental impacts. Pages 153–165 in Zartman IW (ed) Tunisia: the political economy of reform. London: Lynne Rienner Publishers

Showler AT (1995a) Desert locust control, public health and environmental sustainability in North Africa. In Bencherifa A, Swearingen W (eds) The North African environment at risk. Boulder, Colorado, USA: Westview Press

Showler AT (1995b) Locust (Orthoptera: Acrididae) outbreak in Africa and Asia, 1992–1994: an overview. American Entomologist 41: 179–185

Showler AT, Potter CS (1991) Synopsis of the 1986–1989 desert locust (Orthoptera: Acrididae) plague and the concept of strategic control. American Entomologist 37: 106–110

Steedman A (ed) (1988) The locust handbook. Overseas Development Natural Resources Institute, London, 180 pp

Tappan GG, Loveland TR, Orr DG, Moore DG, Howard SM, Tyler DJ (1988) Pilot project for seasonal vegetation monitoring in support of locust and grasshopper control in West Africa. EROS Data Center, US Geological Survey, Sioux Falls, USA Geological Survey, 72 pp

US Department of Agriculture (1996) Grasshopper program manual. US Department of Agriculture, Washington, DC

New Strategies in Locust Control
S. Krall, R. Peveling and D. Ba Diallo (eds)
© 1997 Birkhäuser Verlag Basel/Switzerland

Towards an integrated strategy for the control of the desert locust

M. Lecoq, J.-F. Duranton and T. Rachadi

CIRAD-GERDAT-PRIFAS, B.P. 5035, F-34032 Montpellier Cedex 1, France

Summary. The present strategy to prevent desert locust outbreaks and plagues is the result of long field experience and of research conducted since the beginning of the century. However, this strategy can no longer be assumed to be completely effective. It is proposed to create a new integrated strategy incorporating preventive, curative and palliative levels and associating action plans for each of these levels.

Résumé. La stratégie actuelle de prévention des pullulations et des invasions de Criquet pèlerin résulte d'une longue série de recherches conduites depuis le début de ce siècle. Elle est fondée scientifiquement et a été perfectionnée par une longue pratique de terrain. Toutefois, cette stratégie ne peut plus être considérée comme pleinement efficace. Une nouvelle stratégie intégrée incorporant les différents niveaux stratégiques possibles d'intervention – préventif, curatif et palliatif – est proposée en leur associant des plans d'action clairement définis.

Introduction

The strategy for the control of the desert locust is currently the subject of an extensive debate which predates the last resurgence in 1987–1988. This debate has been kept alive by the present situation after the major reproduction of 1993 and 1994. After years of confident complacency, it appears that nothing is now certain. The notion of a preventive strategy in particular is being brought into the discussion, especially its economic viability. The questions are manifold: Does any strategy exist? Is it possible to apply it? What prospects are offered by research in progress? Is the era of classical pesticides, much criticised for their impact on the environment, really over? Some people even go so far as to pose the question whether the desert locust is still a pest of major economic importance.

The strategy of preventive control of the desert locust

To claim that there is no strategy – or no longer is any – is to dismiss a bit too hastily the experience of the past, and the research conducted throughout this century, which has led precisely to the strategy of preventive control which was applied in the 1960s, in particular in West Africa by the OCLALAV (Organisation Commune de Lutte Antiacridienne et de Lutte Antiaviaire) and by the countries of the Maghreb. This strategy was the result of 70 years of research which led to the discovery of the theory of phases gregarisation areas, to a better comprehension of the dynamics of solitary as well as gregarious populations, and to the development of a specific locust control technology.

We will not review the principles of this strategy of preventive control, which have already been taken up by others (FAO 1969; Hemming et al. 1979; Magor 1994). Its scientific validity can scarcely be doubted. Its efficacy might be debated and one could, in particular, establish a correlation with the climatic change (increasing aridity) which occurred since the beginning of the 1960s. We should, however, note that there was a clear relation between the implementation of this strategy and the relative quietness of the years 1960 to 1985, compared to the catastrophic situation of the preceding years, when one invasion followed another almost without interruption. Incidentally, it was precisely when the administrative, economic and political problems (appearing successively, as well as simultaneously) were posed regarding the correct application of the strategy that badly controlled outbreaks were experienced. This is certainly more than a coincidence. One can reasonably assume that preventive control has played a positive role in preventing the return of major invasions of locusts since it was first put into practice in the 1960s.

The key point of preventive strategy is early localisation of the first signs of active gregarisation. For a long time all efforts have revolved around this point, with good reason. The utilisation of classical meteorological data, satellite data, the effort to develop a geographic information system (GIS) specifically for the desert locust, efforts towards modelling – all these are part of a coherent approach with one common objective: to identify areas to be surveyed and treated in time. Situations have to be anticipated as far as possible, for experience of the past shows that the less anticipation, the greater the risk of being overwhelmed by swarms of this extremely mobile locust. The time factor is of paramount importance, which is why operators in the field give priority to hopper band control if possible before the formation of dispersing swarms, which are more difficult to follow and to contain with insecticides.

Current problems

This preventive strategy has encountered a number of obstacles in recent years. These problems – which have largely contributed to the failure to contain the last outbreaks at an early stage – have, for the most part, already been mentioned by others: the banning of dieldrin, regional security problems, weakening of control organisms, late initiation of control operations (Lecoq 1991; van Huis 1994; Gruys 1994).

It should be stressed that what is being called into question is not the strategy per se, but the impossibility of implementing it correctly. We must now determine whether the problems which have arisen in the last decade can be resolved, and if it is possible to return to an efficient preventive strategy.

First of all, it is likely that the problem posed by the banning of dieldrin can be resolved with the advent of new molecules. The preventive strategy relied to a great extent on the use of chlorinated hydrocarbons, the strong persistence of which permitted successful barrier treatment. This type of treatment allows to be treated rapidly in the case of an outbreak, vast areas, a crucial point in face of the rapid reproduction and dispersal of the desert locust. It should be noted that the treatments were, by definition, performed with partial coverage and at sub-lethal dose rates, despite the noxiousness of the product, a positive factor in terms of environmental protection. At present, products like insect growth regulators (IGRs) and the new family of phenylpyrazoles (e.g. fipronil) constitute one of the best products for reviving the technique of barrier treatments. These molecules have a persistence comparable to dieldrin, but do not share most of its disadvantages. IGRs have already been tested as barrier sprays against the African migratory locust in Madagascar (Scherer and Rakotonandrasana 1993). Recent evidence confirms that fipronil can be equally well utilised in this manner (Rachadi et al. 1995). It is more toxic to the environment, but offers the chance, unlike IGRs, of treating hoppers and adults at the same time. In both cases more extensive, complementary experimentation is still necessary, but these compounds offer, for the first time in 10 years, a realistic prospect of overcoming one of the constraints to the implementation of an effective preventive strategy.

Most of the other problems affecting preventive control in recent years can also be resolved, with one exception, but an important one – the problem of security, which evidently cannot be solved by ourselves. This is an issue of fundamental importance (Kitenda 1992). A large proportion of the gregarisation areas of the desert locust are now situated in unstable zones. These problems may also be overcome, but we should not entertain too many illusions given the current African political context. Moreover, elsewhere new zones of conflict may emerge. With the preventive strategy it is those gregarisation areas which should be permanently surveyed in order to detect and treat populations at the onset of gregarisation. It is clear that this task is difficult at present and that it is likely to be so in future.

Doubt has been cast on the economic justification of preventive control and the true economic impact of the desert locust. These questions were never really raised 20 or 30 years ago, when the evidence of damage was still flagrant. But now a more rational approach to this subject can be taken. Reproduction in recent years leaves little room for doubt that the desert locust will again become an important menace. On the other hand, has the real extent of damage not been exaggerated in the past under the aura of mystery surrounding this insect (Krall 1994)? Here again, it seems as if a century of experience should be swept away, though definitely in a provocative sense. Of course, it must be conceded that the question deserves to be raised, and that the problem is complex. Allowing for an invasion to develop as a real-world experiment "just to see" what happens would be absurd. But a serious economic study has become indispensable. The single most important factor, however, is to distinguish short-term viability of control measures and the viability of the preventive control strategy at global level. The latter can only be evaluated within the scope of a simulation, rather than estimating the damage caused by desert locusts in the course of a full-scale invasion. In the course of the last few years desert locust density has not exceeded upsurge thresholds. During a "true" invasion, however, dispersal of totally gregarious populations can easily cover regions of intensive agriculture, and the damage inflicted can be much more significant. One such study on the potential damage by the desert locust was started 30 years ago (Bullen 1969). It should be brought up to date, emphasising that cash crops should not be treated on an equal footing with food crops.

Nevertheless, the problem is not only the economic viability of control operations. The question of viability becomes less clear-cut if we also take into account the human, social and environmental problems associated with an invasion. To reduce locust invasions to financial terms is an abstract, reductionist and even a bit egoistical viewpoint of donor countries which do not have to endure plagues and which are increasingly facing budget cuts. Ultimately, above and beyond the strict financial aspects, the control of the desert locust is, most certainly, a social necessity.

Is there another way?

It has been proposed that no treatments be carried out, and that we grant food aid instead, or that we underwrite anti-locust insurance. This latter solution appears to be completely unrealistic, given the economic, social and cultural context of the countries concerned. We must also consider the nature of the problem. The desert locust is a migratory pest, and those who took out insurance (as far as insurance of this sort is conceivable) would no longer carry out any control operations thereby harming those who do not have the financial means to cover themselves with insurance.

Similarly, it has been proposed that we wait until swarms have formed, because they are seen as easier targets to deal with in practical and economic terms (Symmons 1992). This solution is all the more tempting since donors disburse credits more readily for emergency aid. It is more spectacular, and it can be more immediately "economically viable". But this is a dangerous line of argument. It should not be forgotten that in the case of an outbreak – and a fortiori of an invasion – can very quickly be overtaken by events. To pretend the contrary is to make a very dangerous bet about the future, about our actual capacity to combat the swarms and, similarly, to ignore several decades of experience of the operators in the field in the control of the desert locust. This experience has led them to prefer precisely such preventive control, at the earliest possible stage, and the control of hoppers, the most easily organisable measure from a logistical point of view. The longer we wait, the more serious the problem becomes. It seems that the last outbreaks, not having been contained at an early stage, could not have been stopped so rapidly in 1988–1989 (to the surprise of all concerned) had it not been for a fortunate constellation of natural circumstances (although, of course, control efforts helped). Nonetheless, in view of the problems of security and the slowness in the transmission of information, the longer we wait, the greater the risk that we will be seriously overwhelmed. The problems associated with preventive control will in fact increase within the framework of a "wait and see" strategy in the case of outbreaks.

Preventive control is a necessity, and the problem is to know when to apply it and if it will succeed. Here, too, we must take into account past events. Again, technologically, we have the means to resume preventive control. New, persistent products are on the market, information on locusts is better collected and analysed than ever before. The potential of forecasting will without doubt improve in the years to come (GIS, models, satellite information). But experience shows that problems will continue to arise. They were numerous in the past, and some have still not been resolved and continue to weigh heavily on the chances of preventive control. And other, new ones have appeared. There is thus no guarantee of 100% success with this strategy of preventive control, especially when it is applied in a patchwork fashion. Conclusions have to be drawn, but conclusion is not to lay down arms and abandon this strategy, since it is probably the best and the most solidly founded both technically and according to the experience of the field staff in charge. It should be promoted to take advantage of acquired experience, which has clearly highlighted the pros and cons of this method. Poorly controlled outbreaks can return to haunt us. We should not rush into action, giving the impression that everything has to be invented again. We should not be so narrow-minded as to oppose the "pure and tough" preventive control strategy, on the one hand, and the strategy of "wait and see" during outbreaks, on the other. Possible faults of either system should be integrated into a global strategy which can be progressively implemented in relation to the accessibility of sites.

Towards an integrated strategy for control of the desert locust

This global strategy or "integrated control strategy" should first of all take into account the different possible strategic levels – preventive, curative and palliative – on the basis of a typology clearly defining ecological zones and locust situations. These situations can be characterised by the geographic distribution of locusts, their density and their phase status. This solution would appear to offer the chance of avoiding numerous misunderstandings, since the same concepts and definitions do not necessarily stand for the same thing for every partner based on personal experience. This means, in fact, completing the concept of preventive control, with plans of action of primary and secondary urgency, corresponding to the consequences of possible failures and predictions of the outcomes of this preventive control. These plans could be drawn up country by country. The most urgent plans would correspond to the curative level and to interventions in case of an outbreak, and the plans of secondary urgency to the palliative level and to interventions in the case of onset of an invasion.

This strategy should thereafter incorporate the various inputs available and propose standard solutions, corresponding to a sort of typology of inputs to be utilised in a given situation. This is the philosophy of "standard control systems", already proposed by Haskell (1993), which seems extremely pertinent and urgent in view of the current dispersion of inputs and the frequent lack of coherence of the control efforts undertaken.

Conclusions and perspectives

Given the strategic difficulties involved in controlling the desert locust, clarification is needed. It is imperative that we integrate preventive control in a more global strategy, benefiting from acquired experience. Alongside these problems – the real cause of the last resurgences – all others seem to be of secondary importance. In recent years much research work has been carried out, and many interesting perspectives for alternative control are now apparent. Utilising biopesticides against locusts is certainly one of the most spectacular possibilities. It seems nonetheless that none of the "biological" methods is currently in a position to take over entirely from chemical control, and the aim is not to replace chemical control but to achieve true complementarity, in line with the given situation, of low-pollution chemical control and other, more "natural", methods.

Yet all these recent achievements relate to methodologies rather than strategies, and – once again – the problems posed today by the desert locust are essentially strategic in nature, and it is these problems which must first be resolved. Otherwise, the problem of the desert locust will become a regular one in the form of emergency operations, more or less well improvised. We can only hope that the new control agents currently emerging will allow us to control locusts with less risk to the environment.

It is appropriate in conclusion to note that the causes of the last outbreaks and the current research priorities are out of synchronization. One category of research has been particularly neglected, although it has yielded a better understanding of the mechanism of invasions and has been the source of a strategy for preventive control, i.e., research into the dynamics of natural populations, in particular the dynamics of solitary and transient populations. Research activities in this field might help further improve strategic concepts.

References

Bullen FT (1969) The distribution of the damage potential of the desert locust (*Schistocerca gregaria* Forsk.). Anti-Locust Memoir 10. London, 44 pp

FAO (1969) Report of the Thirteenth Session of the FAO Desert Locust Control Committee, 6–10 October 1969. FAO Meeting Report no PL 1969/M/5. Rome, 53 pp

Gruys P (1994) Leçons à tirer du dernier fléau du Criquet pèlerin de 1986–1989. Pages 19–30 in van Huis A. (ed) Lutte contre le Criquet pèlerin par les techniques existantes: évaluation des stratégies. Compte-rendu du Séminaire de Wageningen, 6–11 December 1993. Wageningen (Netherlands): Université Agronomique

Haskell PT (1993) The need for development of "Recognized Control Systems". In Atelier international de la FAO sur la recherche et la planification en matière de lutte contre le Criquet pèlerin tenu à Marrakech (Maroc) du 24 au 28 mai 1993. Rome: FAO

Hemming CF, Popov GB, Roffey J, Waloff Z (1979) Characteristics of desert locust plague upsurges. Phil Trans R Soc Lond B 287: 375–386

Kitenda RA (1992) DLCOEA; pest control: the begging questions. Pages 41–43 in Lomer CJ, Prior C (eds) Biological control of locusts and grasshoppers. Oxon (Great Britain): CAB International

Krall S (1994) Importance of locusts and grasshoppers for African agriculture and methods for determining crop losses. Pages 7–22 in Krall S, Wilps H (eds) New trends in locust control: ecotoxicology, botanicals, pathogens, attractants, hormones, pheromones, remote sensing. Eschborn (Germany): Deutsche Gesellschaft für Technische Zusammenarbeit (GTZ) GmbH

Lecoq M (1991) Le Criquet pèlerin: enseignements de la dernière invasion et perspectives offertes par la biomodélisation. Pages 71–98 in ESSAID A (ed) La lutte anti-acridienne. Paris: AUPELF-UREF, John Libbey Eurotext

Magor J (1994) Le Criquet pèlerin: dynamique des populations. Pages 31–56 in van Huis A (ed) Lutte contre le Criquet pèlerin par les techniques existantes: évaluation des stratégies. Compte-rendu du Séminaire de Wageningen, 6–11 December 1993. Wageningen (Netherlands): Université Agronomique

Rachadi T, Balança G, Duranton JF and Foucart A (1995) Les effets du fipronil sur les acridiens *Schistocerca gregaria* (Forskål, 1775) et *Aiolopus simulatrix simulatrix* (Walker, 1870) et la faune non-cible en place. Montpellier (France): CIRAD-GERDAT-PRIFAS

Scherer R and Rakotonandrasana MA (1993) Barrier treatment with a benzoyl urea insect growth regulator against *Locusta migratoria capito* (Sauss) hopper bands in Madagascar. International Journal of Pest Management 39(4): 411–417

Symmons PM (1992) Strategies to combat the desert locust. Crop Protection 11: 206–212

van Huis A (1994) Peut-on réussir la lutte contre le Criquet pèlerin? Pages 11–18 in van Huis A (ed) Lutte contre le Criquet pèlerin par les techniques existantes: évaluation des stratégies. Compte-rendu du Séminaire de Wageningen, 6–11 December 1993. Wageningen (Netherlands): Université Agronomique

New Strategies in Locust Control
S. Krall, R. Peveling and D. Ba Diallo (eds)
© 1997 Birkhäuser Verlag Basel/Switzerland

Control of the desert locust: strategy, organisation and means

B. Chara

Institut National de la Protection des Végétaux, B.P. 80 El Harrach, Algiers (Algeria)

Summary. The desert locust (*Schistocerca gregaria* Forskål) is the insect most feared by farmers in the countries affected. These locusts can nullify many years of work by farmers, put a heavy strain on the budgets of countries affected and sometimes cause enormous environmental damage. In the course of the last decade, two locust invasions occurred, three years apart, which is a very short interval compared with the long remission period which preceded the 1985–1989 invasion. This chain of events made necessary the rapid implementation of a locust control strategy capable of ensuring freedom from this pest in the long term. This chapter, while seeking to point out the different factors which have favoured the locust outbreaks, will propose a global strategy to control the desert locust, integrating both operational and structural approaches. In addition, several activities will be suggested, which are intended to establish the strategy proposed (preventive control) and to make it effective.

Résumé. Le criquet pèlerin (*Schistocerca gregaria* Forskål) est l'insecte le plus redouté par les agriculteurs des pays soumis aux invasions qu'il provoque. Celles-ci peuvent en effet réduire à néant les efforts que fournissent les paysans durant plusieurs années, grever considérablement les budgets des pays envahis et causer parfois un préjudice énorme à l'environnement. Au cours de la dernière décennie, deux invasions acridiennes se sont produites, à trois années d'intervalle, ce qui est très court comparativement à la longue période de rémission qui a précédé l'invasion de 1985–1989 et impose la nécessité de la mise en oeuvre rapide d'une stratégie de lutte capable de maintenir un calme acridien durable. La présente communication, tout en essayant de cerner les différents facteurs qui ont favorisé ces recrudescences acridiennes, tentera de proposer une stratégie globale de lutte contre le criquet pèlerin intégrant des dispositifs opérationnels et structurels. En outre, elle suggère certaines dispositions destinées à asseoir la stratégie de lutte préconisée (lutte préventive) et à la rendre efficace.

Introduction

In the course of the last decade, two locust invasions took place, the first from 1985 to 1989. The second started in 1992. Thus only three years elapsed in between, which is a very short time, compared with the recession period of 25 years which preceded the 1985–1989 invasion. This situation shows how necessary it is to define a global control strategy for the control of the desert locust.

Why are invasions of the desert locust occurring more and more frequently?

The 25 locust-free years from 1960 to 1985 were not a matter of chance, but a result of monitoring efforts and early-warning measures against the desert locust undertaken by the countries concerned, regional and international organisations, and certain donor countries. It was this sustained monitoring of and intervention against *Schistocerca gregaria* which helped to prevent the outbreaks observed, some on a large-scale, notably in 1972–1973 (Karrar 1974), 1974 (Skaf 1978), 1980 (Castel 1982) and 1981.

The last two locust invasions could not be avoided mainly because of:

- the relaxing of monitoring of the gregarisation areas and of control measures against desert locust due to:
- the weakening of the regional organisations charged with monitoring and control in the Sahelian countries of West Africa;
- the insecurity which has reigned for a number of years in the principal gregarisation areas of East and West Africa (Chara 1988; Skaf et al. 1990) and which rendered them inaccessible for monitoring and early control;
- the poor exchange of information about the locusts among countries which are the permanent habitat of the desert locust, which is the vital factor in the success of the whole locust control programme;
- the quality of the information on locusts coming from the field, which is often incomplete and imprecise and does not, therefore, allow reliable forecasts to be made on the evolution of the locust situation in the short and medium term;
- the inadequacy of the resources mobilised for control in the majority of the countries affected by locust plagues, some of which are among the poorest in the world. This situation results in interventions which are more often than not too late and involve means not commensurate with the task in hand;
- the insufficient involvement of donors with regard to strengthening early control of the desert locust;
- the diversion in certain countries of physical and human resources intended for control activities against the desert locust to other activities, particularly during a recession period;
- the feeble efforts to date in the realm of operational research.

Some people also believe that the failure of preventive control is principally due to the unavailability of dieldrin (van Huis 1994; Skaf 1988), even if other factors play a part, in particular, the non-detection, at an early stage, of locust breeding.

Which control strategy should be adopted to avoid invasions of the desert locust and provide for a long recession period?

Control measures against the desert locust can be based on two possible strategies; the first consists of avoiding the outbreak of invasions, i.e., preventive control; the second is based on control measures against the invading swarms, i.e., reactive or direct control.

Reactive control requires considerable materials and funds not available in the majority of the affected countries. And since by that stage action generally has to cover several millions of infested hectares, enormous quantities of pesticides are needed which destabilise ecosystems and contaminate the environment, particularly when the techniques of treatment are not properly mastered and when highly toxic pesticides are used.

Direct control also requires the availability of a large number of qualified personnel who cannot be kept on the payroll permanently solely for this purpose. Thus, countries subject to locust plagues, when confronted with invasions, utilise, in addition to all the personnel of the plant protection service, other agricultural workers to the detriment of their primary activity. It should be noted that these recruited groups more often than not do not master the surveying and treatment techniques, which further prolongs the period of invasion and results in heavy expense until the necessary skills have been acquired.

Countries with a major agricultural potential to protect (e.g. Algeria, India, Morocco and Pakistan) maintain considerable quantities of equipment on stand-by during recession periods, including vehicles for surveying and control operations, application and camping equipment, spare parts, aircraft and insecticides, so that they are ready to tackle any invasion. This financial effort cuts enormously into the budgets of the countries concerned and constitutes a double-edged sword, considering the fact that certain materials, pesticides in particular, become obsolete during a long recession period. This causes serious environmental problems, since these products cannot be destroyed locally. Moreover, control operations during an invasion cannot prevent all locust damage to crops, pastures and forests; they can only minimise damage.

In contrast, preventive control entails permanent monitoring of the potential gregarisation areas and the rapid destruction of primary targets, if possible, before gregarisation begins. Any locust population with a density of the order of 1000 individuals per hectare can be considered a primary target, since gregarisation takes place at this density (Roffey 1994).

The effectiveness of the preventive strategy has been largely demonstrated. Since it was adopted by the DLCC (FAO Desert Locust Control Committee) during its 13th session held in 1969, and put into practice wherever possible, even in areas far from cultivated land, this strategy permitted control of numerous outbreaks which could have developed into major plagues.

Thus in 1980 and 1981, the OCLALAV (Organisation Commune de Lutte Antiacridienne et de Lutte Antiaviaire) and Algeria treated 177,000 hectares in zones of summer breeding (Northern Mali, Northern Niger and the far South of Algeria). This intervention considerably reduced locust populations, which migrated later to the zones of winter-spring breeding in the Algerian Central Sahara. Indeed only a few locust formations were able to migrate to the north and reach the Tadmaït plateau (Algerian Central Sahara), where 13,000 hectares with adults and hoppers were treated between March and May 1981. The success of this campaign was due to the two-pronged attack targeting two complementary breeding regions (summer and winter-spring) at an early stage.

Such early interventions in small areas also:

- considerably reduce the cost to the affected countries and the international community of controlling the desert locust during an invasion; the 1986–1989 invasion cost the international community US$315 million, besides the resources mobilised by the countries affected (van Huis 1994);
- avoid damage to crops, pastures and forests;
- allow other agricultural activities to continue without disruption when staff are drafted to perform monitoring and control work during an invasion;
- protect the environment from the harmful effects of an intensive, widespread use of pesticides: 16 million litres of liquid insecticides and 14 million kilograms of insecticides as powder were used in 1986–1989 (Shulten 1990), often in regions with fragile ecosystems.

The arguments against the strategy of preventing locust outbreaks do not appear sufficiently convincing to call into question its effectiveness and efficiency. Bennet (1976) raised three objections to preventive control:

- the inability of field teams to tackle additional infestations where control is not implemented during an outbreak. It must be emphasised that, logically, prevention measures should be carried out well before the outbreaks begin. Consequently, by assuring an adequate coverage of the gregarisation areas with qualified personnel and equipment suitable for the rough terrain, at the beginning of a favourable period it should be possible to control any outbreak of locusts.
- monitoring is more expensive than control, since the reduction, accompanying gregarisation, of the areas to treat does not necessarily imply a reduction of the area needed to be surveyed. It should be noted that locust populations, initially sparse, need before they gregarise to concentrate and multiply in the corridor zones and zones of accumulation of rainwater, where ecological conditions favourable to breeding persist for the longest. These environments, in the beds of wadis and meanders, are found in the vicinity of the mountain

massifs of the Sahara. They are a minute part of the permanent habitat of the desert locust. Expert scouts, having a perfect knowledge of the terrain and of the bioecology of the desert locust, should be able to direct their surveys towards the zones most favourable for gregarisation. Thus, monitoring requires few physical and human resources and is certain to be effective. Algeria spends, on average, US$335,000 per annum during a recession period; in contrast, in 1988, a year of invasion, it spent US$47.3 million for control activities (Chara 1994), of which US$7.3 million was provided by the international community (Anonymous 1989).

• the practical difficulties which can arise from preventive control. No problem is insurmountable, especially if the technical and scientific data available on the subject are sufficiently accurate; this is currently the case for the desert locust. Nevertheless, certain difficulties may continue, but they should not hamper a preventive control strategy, which must be the ultimate goal (Magor 1994). One of these constraints is the insecurity in certain regions favourable for the multiplication and gregarisation of *Schistocerca gregaria*, which hinders early control in breeding areas.

This constraint could be overcome, for the moment, by implementing rigorous control actions, on a reasonable scale, in the regions complementary to those where insecurity exists. They would aim to intercept and destroy groups of transient individuals and at the same time avoid the development of a second generation. Such an intervention should help to break the evolution towards gregarisation. Thus in West Africa, from the beginning of October every year, a calculated number of survey and control teams would have to be assigned in the central Sahara and central Algeria and in the centre and east of Mauritania in order to tackle any developments originating in northern Mali or northern Niger. This strategy could be very effective, because invasions occur only if the air currents and the rains reach a sufficient level on a certain space timescale. In an outbreak situation locusts might reach a complementary breeding area and continue to breed and gregarise for at least one to two generations (Wallof 1966).

Symmons (cited in Gruys 1994) does not think that at the present time any satisfactory technique exists for effective control of the desert locust at the beginning of an outbreak, when the populations are not sufficiently gregarious. All the experience of the last 30 years has proved the contrary. Moreover, it is not easy to conceive of a technique of control which would be effective against populations at higher concentrations and not be effective against locust formations of lower densities, and to accept a thesis based on the fact of an insecticide killing a gregarious insect and being ineffective against a solitary one.

Thus, the problem of the desert locust can only be mastered at minimum cost and without causing injury to the environment if a preventive control strategy is applied strictly, within reasonable time and with appropriate means.

What organisation needs to be set up to make preventive control effective?

The implementation of an effective preventive control requires a simultaneous reorganisation of control measures and of networks for collecting and disseminating locust information.

Control organisation

During the recession period from 1960 to 1985, preventive control was undertaken either by the countries affected (in North-West Africa, East Africa, the Middle East, and South-West Asia), or by OCLALAV, a regional organisation covering 10 West African countries, which planned and conducted surveys and control in the gregarisation areas, across the borders of member states. In the wake of financial difficulties, and since they thought that the long recession period meant that the problem of the desert locust had been resolved once and for all, member states stopped paying their regular contributions at the start of the 1980s. This made operations extremely difficult, and the organisation was forced to discontinue some of its monitoring and control activities.

At present, monitoring and control are the responsibility of the countries, most of which do not have the financial and material resources to ensure permanent monitoring of the gregarisation areas and rapid intervention against the primary target. Since preventive control is not carried out, substantial populations of desert locust may survive. Given favourable rainfall, these are sufficient to initiate an intensive breeding and gregarisation over vast areas, which occurred regularly over the last 10 years.

Aware of the need to carry out early control in the western region and to counteract the lack of resources available in the countries of the Sahel that are home to the gregarisation areas, in November 1989 the countries of North-West Africa created a task force to back up national efforts, particularly in Mali, Mauritania and Niger.

This task force, called the *Force Maghrébine d'Intervention* (FMI), implements the annual programmes worked out by the executive committee of the *Commission de Lutte Contre le Criquet Pèlerin en Afrique du Nord-Ouest* (CLCCPANO). These take into consideration the ecological characteristics of the gregarisation areas of the western region. The financing to maintain this force and the work programmes are guaranteed by the budget of the CLCCPANO, donations from member states, and contributions from FAO and the international community.

The actions undertaken by the FMI since its creation, involving numerous survey and control operations, are carried out with the countries concerned: Niger, Mali and especially Mauritania, where a permanent monitoring of gregarisation areas was carried out from 1989 to 1994.

Despite the constraints which it has faced, notably the lack of sufficient funds at the right time and difficulties of access to certain crucial regions, the FMI has made a substantial contribution to the evaluation of the locust situation in the western region (Zaidi 1993). It has also been able, on several occasions, to control primary targets in large and small areas in Mauritania from 1992 to 1994.

It was with FMI funds that Mauritania took the first steps to control swarms which invaded from East Africa in July 1993, and organised a large-scale control campaign in 1993–1994. This control of populations emanating from summer breeding also prevented the plague from becoming serious for the other countries of the western region in general and those of North-West Africa in particular which harbour the zones of winter-spring breeding.

Considering the above and the firm resolve of certain countries harbouring potential gregarisation areas to intervene against the outbreaks of the desert locust only when they constitute a direct menace to their agricultural production, it is indispensable that regional preventive capabilities be set up which can intervene at the right time, as and when the situation calls for it.

Regional intervention forces, unhampered by the constraints which the FMI has had to face since its beginning and intervening without respecting borders in potential gregarisation areas, would constitute an effective and appropriate means of preventive control.

Considering the size and complementarity of gregarisation areas found in each of the three principal permanent habitats of the desert locust, and the willingness of several countries to carry out preventive control in their territory with all necessary speed and effectiveness, a minimum of two regional forces are essential to take charge of surveying and controlling locust outbreaks in a recession period. These units should cover principal outbreak areas of desert locust, which are found on the Red Sea coast and the border region of India and Pakistan (Mahjoub 1988).

The administration and operation of these intervention forces could be the responsibility of regional organisations or commissions bringing together all the countries harbouring gregarisation areas. They would be in charge of coordinating and carrying out preventive control.

It is clear that all countries of the area invaded by the desert locust would benefit from the spin-offs of preventive control undertaken by these regional forces. Consequently, the procurement of materials and their maintenance, as well as the operational costs of these intervention units, should be financed by an international fund, answerable to the FAO, and sustained by contributions of countries subject to plagues, FAO and donor countries willing to get involved in the preventive control of desert locust.

Organisation of networks for collecting and disseminating information on locusts

Information about locusts determines the success of the whole control strategy. It is recognized that the current organisation is an obstacle which significantly delays locust information being provided to those who could use it, thus greatly detracting from its usefulness. Furthermore, the steps information has to pass through become at times filters which drastically distort its contents. To overcome these inadequacies, resituate the organisation of regional locust co-ordination and reduce the funds allocated for the operation of these structures, it is essential to rethink the existing organisation.

To this end, it is recommended that a body be set up which would favour groups of countries having complementary gregarisation areas. Thus, there should be a fusion, for the western region, of the OCLALAV and the CLCCPANO, and for the central region, of the DLCOEA (Desert Locust Control Organisation of East Africa) and the CLCCPMO, Commission de Lutte Contre le Criquet Pèlerin au Moyen Orient. For the eastern region, the CLCCPASO, Commission de Lutte Contre le Criquet Pèlerin en Asie du Sud-Ouest, should be made operational.

The structures emerging from this reform must not be top heavy and must gear their work to the collection and rapid transmission of locust information, the organisation and coordination of preventive action, the consolidation of preventive control by training staff and the encouragement applied research on the desert locust.

The operating costs of these structures could be financed by contributions of the member states and FAO. The donor countries will be able to participate by taking charge of the training programmes for staff involved in control and research.

Inputs needed for efficient preventive control

To be effective and economically viable, preventive control should be initiated at the right time and it should lie in the hands of qualified technical and support personnel. The material inputs should be suited to the rough conditions and the inhospitable terrain; the chemicals applied should be effective, with sufficient persistence, and they should have little negative impact on humans and the environment.

For the treatments, ULV equipment has proved most satisfactory, in view of the fact that control measures are carried out in regions where practically no water exists. Moreover, ULV treatments use very concentrated chemicals which can be applied at very low rates per hectare. Thus only small amounts of insecticides need to be transported to treat large infested areas.

Some of the spraying equipment currently in use is not used properly, and this often entails a significant waste of money and causes damage, sometimes considerable, to the environment. The exhaust nozzle sprayer (ENS), with which total coverage cannot be obtained with product volumes less than one litre per hectare, is being used with formulations at one-half litre per hectare. Symmons (1994) considered that the ENS is not a good sprayer for ULV treatments, given that the minimal output which can be obtained corresponds to a broad swathe, but gives overlapping drift and an uneven deposit. This effect is accentuated by the bad size distribution of the droplets, and most of the insecticide deposits close to the vehicle. This sprayer can, however, give good results with residual products if used in alternating strips. In contrast, for contact insecticides (organophosphates and synthetic pyrethroids), it is advised to use sprayers which produce sufficiently small droplets to be transported as drift and which will produce an even cover at a low volume rate. According to Rachadi (1991) and Symmons (1994), the best production of droplets is obtained with sprayers using a centrifugal mechanism with spinning cages or disks.

As for pesticides, those currently in use act mainly by contact and have low residual activity. But preventive control requires the use of chemicals which act mainly by ingestion and with a certain degree of residual activity, partly to ensure more cost-effective treatment of hopper bands. The IGRs (insect growth regulators) may be a solution to the problem posed here. In any case, additional research is required to improve the activity of these pesticides and define their impact on the environment.

Additionally, in order to avoid the problem of rapid acquisition of enormous quantities of insecticides, which is a huge financial burden for the countries and a menace to the environment, it would be better to keep stocks of insecticides at manufacturing companies, and to set up systems to make them available at the required time.

As regards monitoring, it is well known that major outbreaks are generally preceded by abundant rainfall (over 50 mm) over a wide area (several tens of thousands of square kilometres), followed by good rainfall at intervals of around two months, which favours the rapid development of several generations (Roffey 1994).

Consequently, the priority for monitoring should be in potential habitats where there has been sufficient rainfall to cause general, intensive and widespread breeding. To achieve this goal, it is imperative to have an adequately dense network of meteorological stations in these regions.

With the exception of India, Pakistan (Roffey 1994) and Algeria, the network of meteorological stations in the recession zones is not sufficient to provide quantitative and qualitative rainfall data, which requires the deployment of a large number of survey and control teams to cover a specific territory.

The use of remote sensing to estimate rainfall (Meteosat) or the state of the vegetation (NOAA/AVHRR) is still far from perfect for desert regions, although we can expect that progress will be made in the future.

It thus seems urgent to reinforce the network of meteorological stations of the principal gregarisation areas of West Africa, East Africa and the Middle East to the stage of development achieved in Algeria, with effective automatic stations which do not require the permanent presence of personnel in very remote and inhospitable locations.

At the human level, personnel engaged in locust control lack, for the most part, a thorough basic knowledge of locusts and are not skilled in spraying techniques. This leads most often to the following:

- The transmission of imprecise data from the field causes forecasts which do not reflect the reality in the field; at times, this has complicated the locust situation or has led some responsible parties in the countries affected to take decisions which subsequently proved to be inappropriate and extremely costly;
- Excessive or inadequate rates of insecticides, which can either make control measures ineffective or multiply costs of intervention and the level of pollution.

Consequently, to establish a better preventive control strategy, it is essential to set up specialised intervention teams with personnel completely familiar with the bioecology of the insect and the treatment techniques used, particularly ULV spraying with ground equipment.

In conclusion, a global strategy of control against the desert locust is needed more than ever. It should be implemented as soon as possible in order to avoid new invasions or limit their frequency. The FAO could act as a catalyst, and provides the ideal forum for deliberations that must lead to the adoption of a new strategy, with the final choice resting with the DLCC.

References

Anonymous (1989) Rapport sur les activités de lutte antiacridienne en Algérie. Bilan 1988 et préparation de la campagne 1989. INPV, Ministère de l'Agriculture, Algeria

Bennet LV (1976) The development and termination of the 1968 plague of the desert locust, *Schistocerca gregaria* (Forskål) (Orthoptera, Acrididae). Bull Entomol Res 66: 511–552

Castel JM (1982) La poussée du Criquet pèlerin en Afrique de l'Ouest en 1980. Field Research Station-Technical series FAO report no AGPP/DL/TS/23 75–107

Chara B (1988) Genèse de la situation acridienne actuelle. Publications de l'Académie Royale du Maroc. Collection "Sessions": Catastrophes naturelles et péril acridien. Rabat 28–30 November 1988, 211–220

Chara B (1994) Stratégie et moyens mobilisés pour la lutte contre le Criquet pèlerin en Algérie. Pages 73–75 in van Huis A (ed) Lutte contre le Criquet pèlerin par les techniques existantes: évaluation des stratégies. Compte rendu du Séminaire de Wageningen 6–11 December 1993. Wageningen (Netherlands): Université Agronomique

Gruys P (1994) Leçons à tirer du dernier fléau de Criquet pèlerin 1986–1989. Pages 19–30 in van Huis A (ed) Lutte contre le Criquet pèlerin par les techniques existantes: évaluation des stratégies. Compte rendu du Séminaire de Wageningen 6–11 December 1993. Wageningen (Netherlands): Université Agronomique

Karrar AM (1974) Study of the 1972–1973 upsurge of the desert locust (*Schistocerca gregaria* Forskål) and the effect of the control operations undertaken by national and international organisations. Working paper for the Eighteenth Session of the FAO Desert Locust Control Committee, Rome, 4–8 November 1974. FAO report no AGP: LCC/74/3, 29

Mahjoub N (1988) Le Problème du criquet pèlerin et les perspectives de sa solution. Nature et faune, Bureau région de la FAO - Accra (Ghana), 4(2): 16–20

Major J (1994) Le Criquet pèlerin: dynamique des populations. Pages 31–56 in van Huis A (ed) Lutte contre le Criquet pèlerin par les techniques existantes: évaluation des stratégies. Compte rendu du Séminaire de Wageningen 6–11 Décembre 1993. Wageningen (Netherlands): Université Agronomique

Rachadi T (1991) Précis de lutte antiacridienne: les pulvérisations d'insecticides. Ministère du Développement et de la Coopération: Paris/ CIRAD PRIFAS: Montpellier, 312 pp

Roffey J (1994) Caractéristiques des débuts de recrudescence du Criquet pèlerin. Pages 57–63 in van Huis A (ed) Lutte contre le Criquet pèlerin par les techniques existantes: évaluation des stratégies. Compte rendu du Séminaire de Wageningen 6–11 December 1993. Wageningen (Netherlands): Université Agronomique

Schulten GGM (1990) Needs and contraints of integrated pest management in development countries. Med Fac Landbouww Rijksuniv Gent, 55: 207–216

Skaf R (1978) Etude sur les cas de grégarisation du Criquet pèlerin en 1974 dans le Sud Ouest de la Mauritanie et dans le Tamesna Malien. Stations de Recherche Acridienne sur le terrain - Séries techniques. FAO Report No. AGP/DL/TS/17, 46 pp

Skaf R (1988) A story of a disaster: why locust plagues are still possible. Disasters 12: 122–126

Skaf R, Popov GB, Roffey J (1990) The desert locust: an international challenge. Phil Trans R Soc Lond B 328: 525–538

Symmons PM (1994) Les principes du traitement à ultra bas volume. Pages 65–70 in van Huis A (ed) Lutte contre le Criquet pèlerin par les techniques existantes: évaluation des stratégies. Compte rendu du Séminaire de Wageningen 6–11 December 1993. Wageningen (Netherlands): Université Agronomique

van Huis A (1993) Peut on réussir la lutte contre le criquet pèlerin? Pages 11–17 in van Huis A (ed) Lutte contre le Criquet pèlerin par les techniques existantes: évaluation des stratégies. Compte rendu du Séminaire de Wageningen 6–11 Décembre 1993. Wageningen (Pays Bas): Université Agronomique

Wallof Z (1966) The upsurges and recessions of the desert locust plague: an historical survey. Anti-Locust Memoir no 8, 111 p

Zaidi H (1993) La Force Magrébine d'Intervention (FMI) 1988–1993. Rapport de consultant. Commission FAO de Lutte Contre le Criquet Pèlerin en Afrique du Nord-Ouest Algiers (Algeria)

New Strategies in Locust Control
S. Krall, R. Peveling and D. Ba Diallo (eds)
© 1997 Birkhäuser Verlag Basel/Switzerland

Strategy for controlling the desert locust in Mauritania

M. Abdallahi Ould Babah

Centre de Lutte Antiacridienne c/o DRAP, Nouakchott, Mauritania

Summary. The quality of planning of the strategy to control the desert locust in Mauritania has been improved in the course of the most recent campaigns (1987 to 1995). This was due in part to selecting and retaining personnel more experienced in this area, and in part to support from partners for development. This strategy and its different forms are described in this article.

Résumé. Le niveau de conception de la stratégie de lutte contre le criquet pèlerin en Mauritanie s'est amélioré au cours de ces dernières campagnes de lutte (de 1987 à 1995). Cette amélioration est due d'une part à la sélection et le maintien du personnel le plus expérimenté dans ce domaine et, d'autre part, à l'appui des partenaires au développement. Cette stratégie et ses différentes formes sont décrites dans cette communication.

Introduction

Mauritania, in West Africa, covers an area of 1.1 million km^2 and represents an important area in which gregarisation takes place within the recession zone of the desert locust.

It serves as a base for both summer and winter-spring breeding of this pest and therefore constitutes a link between West Africa and the Maghreb.

Strategy to control the desert locust in Mauritania

The strategy is defined in general as investing inputs and resources, in line with appropriate methods, to attain well-defined objectives. In this context the following strategies should be mentioned:

- preventive: control of outbreaks
- curative: control of upsurges and plagues
- palliative: control in the vicinity of cultivated zones

Strategy of preventive control

The strategy of preventive control of the desert locust followed by OCLALAV (Organisation Commune de Lutte Antiacridienne et de Lutte Antiaviaire) since 1965 for the benefit of Mauritania and the other member countries was based on the experience of long years of research on gregarisation, breeding and swarm formation, which may occur in certain regions such as the Adrar and the Aftouts in Mauritania, where ecological conditions favour breeding and gregarisation.

Since 1989, and in the wake of OCLALAV's restructuring, Mauritania has resumed responsibility for monitoring and control activities with the assistance of the Commission de Lutte Contre le Criquet Pèlerin en Afrique du Nord-Ouest (CLCCPANO-FAO) and its other partners. This structure has permitted the country to maintain a preventive control strategy in close cooperation with national survey and control teams and the *Force Maghrébine d'Intervention* (FMI).

In the course of this cooperation six teams in the summer period for five to six months, and three teams for two to three months in the winter-spring period were operating. Their mission was to ensure monitoring and control of the first pockets of the desert locust before they disperse.

Strategy of curative control

The strategy of curative control is designed in general in the form of a plan of intervention based on:
- the situation of the desert locust as found in the gregarisation areas both in neighbouring countries and in Mauritania;
- ecological conditions;
- the biology and population dynamics of desert locust;
- the phytogeographic map of the country;
- passage corridors for the desert locust
- manpower and materials available;
- the delay before complementary measures can be taken;
- the physical environment, the infrastructure and logistics of the country;
- past experience.

Based on the ensemble of these points, a plan of intervention is worked out, taking into consideration three levels of risk:

- level 1: low probability;
- level 2: medium probability;
- level 3: high probability.

Each of these hypothetical risk situations is analysed with respect to the biology of the desert locust (probable breeding and traditional migration), and the equipment and preparations necessary for control (terrestrial, aerial, logistic etc.), quantified in terms of available resources and needs. The costs are calculated in local currency and in US$.

Schemes for the allocation of resources in time and space are mapped, indicating strategic corridors, after which organisational measures are implemented.

It should be noted, however, in view of the unpredictability of the desert locust, that no time must be lost in drawing up a plan of action, which has to be updated in the course of the campaign, depending on actual developments, at least every two months. The practical execution of the strategy follows the biological and epidemical evolution of the desert locust.

Oviposition sites

As soon as they have been identified, the location of zones of breeding and egg laying are noted and monitored carefully, with a view to immediately controlling hoppers when hatching occurs.

Hopper bands

The means of control are chosen depending on the terrain, whether crops are present or not, the size of the bands, the dominant larval stages, the activity of the bands (resting or migrating) and the ecological conditions.

Swarms

In case of swarm formation, one should proceed as follows:
- control on the spot before they disperse;
- block the nearest passage corridors;
- create a cordon around the zones where crops are located that are most at risk.

Strategy of palliative action

This consists of protecting cultivated zones to prevent damage to the crops by creating a 'safety belt".

A new approach for managing operations in the winter-spring zones: the 1995 invasion in northern Mauritania

In the winter-spring breeding zones, where logistics and infrastructure are not well developed (lack of water, bad road system, difficulties in fuel and pesticide supply etc.), the organisation and administration of a control campaign are difficult and costly.

For these reasons, and in view of past experience, the following model of operations management has proved best suited and most efficient for this zone. Its form and role are discussed below.

A team from the Poste Central de Commandement (PCC) was assigned to the heart of the infested zone in the northern part of the country (600 km east of Zoueratte). It was led by an operations coordinator, assisted by a technical repair crew comprising a radio technician, a pesticide application technician and a mechanic. A supply crew consisting of a crew chief, a liaison agent and a guard was based in Zoueratte along with three truck drivers and labourers.

This team was responsible for technical coordination between the ground crews and the air units; supervision of operations and logistics and maintenance of vehicles, radios and application equipment, while the repair crew also carried out calibration of sprayers and necessary checkups.

This team also requested the deployment of Poste Central de Commandement/Direction du Développement des Ressources Agro Pastorales PCC/DRAP teams and notified them of requirements for pesticides and other materials not available in Zoueratte.

This structure allowed to improve the efficiency of control in the following ways:
- By providing the logistic back-up for the teams, these could dedicate themselves entirely to survey and control for 30 days instead of 20 days per month (10 days were needed to provide the logistics for each team onwards from Zoueratte, the only supply point, within 600 km to 800 km from the zone of intervention);
- The delay before making a decision has been reduced from a few hours to a few minutes;
- A new survey method called "light camping" has improved the mobility of the teams and their effectiveness in controlling swarms arriving from outside the zone. In the course of the months of January and February 1995, out of 100 swarms located, 70 were treated.

The effectiveness of the team was also improved thanks to:

- the use of GPS (global positioning system), which has improved the accuracy of site location and marking the locust targets, without counting its usefulness in navigation on the ground.
- The use of aircraft (Canadian aircraft) equipped with the PICODAS system (a computer navigation system linked to the GPS) has facilitated and improved aerial treatments considerably. For example only a single marker is needed in one spray block. Moreover, application parameters such as swath width, track spacing and actual dosage can be determined (recorded) more rapidly and accurately.

Conclusion

The improved organisation for the control of the desert locust in Mauritania is due to the following factors:

- capitalising on lessons learned from past experience:
- maintaining skills between campaigns through permanent employment of reliable personnel, thanks to the financial support of Mauritania and the assistance of partners;
- maintenance of equipment;
- organisation of training courses for relevant personnel and reserve personnel during the off-season
- adoption of management and operation models in relation to the zones of reproduction of the desert locust;
- creation of a technical structure in which the PCC has responsibility for the management of all operations throughout the campaign. This structure is well suited to the management of an urgent situation thanks to its technical specificity and the specialisation of its members, as well as to the decision-making power it has been given.

Grasshopper control in Siberia: strategies and perspectives

A.V. Latchininsky

All-Russian Institute for Plant Protection (VIZR), 3 Podbelsky street, 189620 Saint-Petersburg, Pushkin, Russia
Current address: University of Wyoming, Dept. of Plant, Soil and Insect Sciences, P.O. Box 3354, Laramie WY 82071, USA

Summary. The area of potential grasshopper damage in Siberia covers a wide zone of meadow-steppe localised between 50° and 55°N, 68° and 132°E. Among some 40 grasshopper species inflicting damage to grasslands and crops, about half a dozen are regular pests. The strategy for their control is essentially curative: large-scale insecticide spraying in breeding areas soon after mass hatching of hoppers. The average surface of annual treatments is about 200,000 ha, exceeding 500,000 ha in the years of heavy outbreaks (e.g. 1994). The list of conventional insecticides registered for grasshopper control includes a dozen formulations, among which malathion (2–3 l/ha) and deltamethrin (0.4–0.5 l/ha) are most commonly utilised. Alternative strategies of grasshopper control involve the use of prospective natural enemies (e.g. fungus *Beauveria tenella*, nematode *Steinernema carpocapsae* and others). With the use of such biopesticides, we hope to shift the existing strategy of grasshopper control towards methods less hazardous to the environment.

Résumé. La région de Sibérie potentiellement menacée par les acridiens couvre une large bande de steppe-prairie s'étendant entre les 50e et 55e degrés de latitude Nord et les 68e et 132e degrés de longitude Est. Parmi les quelque 40 espèces d'acridiens provoquant des dommages aux herbages et cultures, environ une demi-douzaine constituent des fléaux réguliers. La stratégie de lutte employée est essentiellement curative: épandage d'insecticides à grande échelle dans les zones de reproduction peu de temps après l'éclosion en masse des oeufs. La surface moyenne traitée annuellement est d'environ 200 000 hectares, mais elle peut dépasser 500 000 hectares les années de forte infestation (par exemple en 1994). La liste des insecticides conventionnels homologués pour la lutte anti-acridienne comporte une douzaine de formulations, dont le malathion (2 à 3 l/ha) et la deltaméthrine (0,4 à 0,5 l/ha) sont les plus communément utilisées. Les stratégies alternatives employées sont basées sur l'emploi d'ennemis naturels potentiels (par exemple le champignon *Beauveria tenella*, le nématode *Steinernema carpocapsae*, etc.). L'usage de ces bio-insecticides devrait, nous l'espérons, permettre le passage à des méthodes de lutte moins déprédatrices de l'environnement.

Siberia, a territory of some 10 million km², occupies the vast north-eastern part of the Eurasian continent, between the Ural in the west and Pacific mountain chains in the east. From the shores of the Arctic Ocean in the north, it stretches south to the steppes of Kazakhstan and the Mongolian border. The zone of economic importance of grasshoppers in Siberia is localised in its southern part covering a wide area of wooded meadow-steppe, approximately between 50° and 55°N and 68° and 132°E (Fig.1). Topography, climate and vegetation vary greatly in South Siberia as it stretches east-west for 6000 km. In brief, most of the area is low lying but gradually rises towards the east (Transbaikalia), which is characterized by alternating plateaus and valleys. The climate is extremely continental, with long cold winters and short but hot summers. The range between the mean temperatures of January (−25 °C) and July (+18 °C) is about 40 °C, reaching almost 90 °C (−50 °C; +38 °C) for the extremes (data for Chita, Transbaikalia).

Precipitation is low, averaging annually about 300–350 mm, with maximum at the end of summer. The predominating short-grass vegetation is represented by the species of the widespread genera – *Stipa, Koeleria, Poa, Hordeum, Alopecurus, Festuca, Agropyron*, as well as by some endemics (e.g. *Puccinellia tenuiflora* in north-eastern part of Siberia named Yacutia). The unique Yacutian zone of grasshopper outbreaks is described by Latchininsky (1993; 1995).

Principal economic species

In the extensive Siberian plains, grasshoppers are serious pests of natural grasslands, competing with cattle for food. The complex of species damaging grassland and crops is numerous, including some 40, mostly graminicolous, grasshoppers. Most of these species are occasional pests,

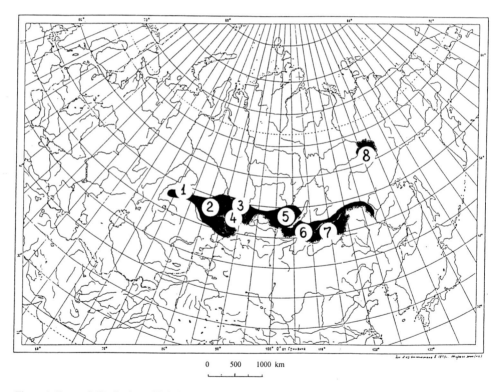

Figure 1. Zone of distribution of injurious grasshopper species in Siberia (1 - Omsk region; 2 - Novosibirsk region; 3 - Krasnoyarsk region; 4 - Khakassia; 5 - Irkutsk region; 6 - Buryatia; 7 - Chita region; 8 - Yacutia)

and only about half a dozen of them are regularly numerous enough to be regarded as serious: *Podisma pedestris* (L., 1758), *Calliptamus italicus* (L., 1758), *Chorthippus albomarginatus* (De Geer, 1773), *Stauroderus scalaris* (Fischer de Waldheim, 1846), *Dasyhippus barbipes* (Fischer de Waldheim, 1846), *Aëropus sibiricus* (L., 1767). With the exception of *Calliptamus italicus*, which can produce a gregarious phase at irregular intervals in West Siberia, all economic species are non-swarming grasshoppers, mostly gomphocerines.

Life cycle

All Siberian grasshoppers are univoltine, hibernating in the egg stage, which persists for the major part (sometimes, up to 9 or 10 months) of the year. A typical annual cycle of one of the most dangerous species, *Chorthippus albomarginatus*, is as follows. Hatching occurs at the beginning of June. Nymphal development comprises four instars and lasts 24–35 days. Hopper density can reach several thousands per square metre in the early instars and several hundred per square metre in the late instars. Adults appear at the end of June. After 4–9 days of sexual maturation, adults copulate, and 2–3 days after the first copulation females begin laying eggs. An egg pod contains 4–10, more frequently 8–10, eggs. A female lays an average of 8 (maximum 16) egg pods, for a total of some 60–120 eggs per female during the reproductive period, which lasts 30–40 days. It is interesting to note that most of the pest species (*Chorthippus albomarginatus, Aëropus sibiricus, Stauroderus scalaris*) hatch earlier than others. Thus, their active stages (hoppers and adults) can exploit the vegetative resources of the habitat for a prolonged period. The insects with such "early hatching" development appear to be more harmful to plants than "late hatching" species: the former attack the first, easily damageable, growing stages of plants, whereas the latter begin to feed on mature tissues, when the plants have already gained their vigour and strength (Tansky 1988).

Monitoring grasshopper populations

The system of grasshopper monitoring consists of four successive surveys during the growing season. They are executed by specialists of the Federal Plant Protection Service in cooperation with agronomists from collective farms and individual cultivators and ranchers. The *spring survey* begins at the onset of mass hatching of hoppers and is carried out until the majority of population reaches the third instar. During this survey, the sites of mass hatching are mapped and the infested areas are designated, if necessary, for control operations. The threshold for chemical intervention is an average hopper density exceeding 1–3 individuals per square metre for non-swarming grasshoppers and 200–300 individuals per hectare for locusts (Tsyplenkov 1979). The *summer survey* is carried out when grasshoppers reach the adult stage. It aims to locate areas of concentrated adults. The results of the summer survey serve as a basis for planning control campaigns the following year. The *autumn survey* of egg pods takes place late in the season, at the end of the adult period. It aims to establish the areas where the egg-pods were laid and to evaluate their densities. An additional *early spring survey* is carried out before hatching to establish the egg overwintering survival rate. The percentage of damaged or dead eggs is used to adjust the grasshopper forecast for the current season. As a rule, this survey is executed only after years of heavy outbreaks.

In Siberia, grasshopper survey is very costly, demanding immense human and logistic resources. For example, in 1994, the total area inspected during the summer survey in Siberia reached 1.1 million ha (total in Russia: 5.2 million ha) including about 400,000 ha in a single Irkutsk region. At present, the first steps are being made towards introducing phenological and population dynamics modelling for long-term forecasting of grasshopper outbreaks for better timing and siting of survey and control operations (Latchininsky and Launois-Luong 1992).

Control strategies

Chemical control

At present, the strategy of grasshopper control in Siberia is essentially curative, based on chemical treatments of the infested areas soon after mass hatching. Areas of hopper concentration, where densities exceed the action/treatment threshold, are determined during the spring survey and selected for treatment. Insecticides used include organophosphates and pyrethroids (Tab. 1) applied with ground or aerial equipment, at high or ultra low volumes (ULV). The areas treated in different geographical zones of Siberia in 1994 are shown in the Table 2. It is evident that the most dangerous situation remains in the Irkutsk region and in Transbaikalia (Buryatia, Chita region). The effectiveness of treatments (hopper mortality) is usually about 90%. Perspectives for improving chemical grasshopper control are connected with selecting appropriate acricides, optimizing application rates and introducing modern application techniques.

Table 1. Insecticide formulations officially authorized for use in Russia against locusts and grasshoppers on grasslands and cultures

N	Insecticide	Formulation	Application rate (l or kg/ha)
	Organophosphates		
1.	Malathion	50.0% emulsifiable concentrate	2.0–3.0
2.	Malathion	40.0% emulsifiable concentrate ULV	2.0–3.0
3.	Fenitrothion	50.0% emulsifiable concentrate	0.6–1.8
4.	Chlorpyriphos	40.8% emulsifiable concentrate	0.5–0.75
	Synthetic pyrethroids		
5.	Deltamethrin	2.5% emulsifiable concentrate	0.4–0.5
6.	Fenvalerate	20.0% emulsifiable concentrate	0.4–0.5
7.	Lambda cyhalothrin	5.0% emulsifiable concentrate	0.1–0.4
8.	Fluvalinate	25.0% emulsifiable concentrate	0.1

Authorized insecticides

In the beginning of 1990s, the authorized list was updated; highly toxic and persistent formulations were replaced by those less hazardous to non-target organisms and the environment. Thus, the dust of HCH (organochlorine) was very widely used in grasshopper and locust control in 1960s and 1980s, until banned in 1990 by environmental legislation. The less toxic synthetic pyrethroids (deltamethrin, fenvalerate) were introduced in the mid-1980s. After large-scale field

Table 2. Areas inspected, infested and treated by acridicides in Siberia in 1994

Region	Area (ha)		
	inspected	infested	treated
West Siberia			
Novosibirsk region	131,300	90,600	-
Omsk region	140,300	57,100	-
East Siberia			
Western zone			
Krasnoyarsk region	156,600	111,400	18,000
Khakassia	39,900	26,000	16,300
Eastern zone			
Irkutsk region (Cisbaikalia)	380,000	352,800	325,700
Chita region (Transbaikalia)	73,500	60,700	63,000
Buryatia (Transbaikalia)	186,000	162,000	106,600
Total	1,107,600	860,600	529,600

trials in 1994, the list of insecticides authorized for grasshopper control was supplemented by two more formulations, lambda cyhalothrin (Karate) and chlorpyriphos (Dursban). The former compound, a synthetic pyrethroid produced by Zeneca, has shown the best results (hopper mortality 91–100%) when applied at the rate of 0.15–0.2 l/ha. The latter compound, an organophosphate produced by DowElanco, applied at the rate of 0.5 l/ha by ground and aerial sprayers, caused high mortality (>90%) in both hoppers and adults.

Optimization of application rates

The aim is to use an acridicide at the rate sufficient to guarantee the protection of rangeland and crops with minimal side-effects for beneficial fauna. In this respect, in 1994, the field trials of fenitrothion (Sumithion, an organophosphate produced by Sumitomo) were intended to optimize its efficient application rate. We found that it was possible to lower this rate from 0.8–1.8 l/ha (registered earlier) down to 0.6 l/ha for non-swarming grasshoppers. Moreover, the results of these trials established, for the first time in locust and grasshopper control in Russia, rates of insecticide application specific for different species and life stages. The recommended doses are:

Fenitrothion:
- 0.6–0.8 l/ha for hoppers and adults of non-swarming grasshoppers;
- 0.8 l/ha for hoppers of first to third instars of locusts (e.g. *Calliptamus italicus*);
- 1.8 l/ha for late instar hoppers and imago of locusts.

Lambda cyhalothrin:
- 0.1–0.15 l/ha for hoppers and adults of non-swarming grasshoppers;
- 0.4 l/ha for locust hoppers.

The theoretical base for this differential approach to acridicide dosage was developed in the publications of VIZR specialists (Kurdyukov et al. 1983; Kurdyukov and Naumovich 1984).

The tests of a new acridicide named fipronil (Adonis), a phenyl pyrazole compound produced by Rhône-Poulenc began in 1995 (Latchininsky 1996). Given the moderate vertebrate toxicity of this compound (Anonymous 1996), its application at extremely low rates (about 4 g of a.i./ha) would represent a further step towards environmentally less hazardous grasshopper control. In the large-scale field trials in East Siberia in 1996, the aerial spraying of fipronil at the rate of 4.56 g of a.i./ha resulted in 90.4% hopper mortality 6 days after treatment, attaining a maximum of 98.6% mortality 2 weeks posttreatment (Latchininsky and Duranton 1996). Future plans include application of fipronil in the so-called barrier treatments, in which treated swaths are alternated with untreated intervals. The actual pesticide load in such treatments could be reduced to 1 g of a.i./*ptotected* ha, and the natural enemies and pathogens preserved in the untreated swaths could contribute significantly to the suppression of grasshopper populations. Such a strategy has yielded very promising results in locust control in many African countries (Rachadi et al. 1995). In light of the potential preservation of natural biological control agents, barrier treatments could be considered as an example of integrated pest management, based on the optimal use of the appropriate chemical product.

Introduction of modern application techniques
More broad utilisation of ULV, both ground and aerial, is vital during heavy grasshopper outbreaks when immense areas have to be treated in a limited span of time. The tests of an appropriate formulation of Dursban (22.5% ULV) sprayed from specially equipped Russian aircraft (ANTONOV 2), began in 1995.

The area of annual treatments against grasshoppers in Siberia usually does not exceed 200,000 ha. However, in years of heavy outbreaks usually associated with abnormal droughts, the surface of rangelands and crops subject to grasshopper depredation (and therefore needing to be treated) is much larger. Thus, in 1993, chemical treatments against these pests in Siberia were conducted on 380,000 ha, representing about 57% of the total area of grasshopper control in Russia. In 1994, the total area of chemical treatments against grasshoppers in Russia was lower than in 1993, but the proportion in Siberia has increased dramatically to 530,000 ha, or about 92% of the total.

Alternative control agents

In Siberia, the search for possible alternative agents (primarily microbiological natural enemies) that could be used in grasshopper control started almost 50 years ago (Vinokurov 1949). However, the rapid expansion of comparatively inexpensive and highly effective chemical agents diminished the interest in alternative control strategies until the 1980s, when interest was revived by growing environmental concern. Recently, the screening of native microbiological pathogens capable of eliciting grasshopper epizooties was accomplished in East Siberia by the specialists of VIZR (Leskov 1990; Latchininsky 1993). The protocols of laboratory and field testing of entomopathogens, and the methods of their identification, are outlined in Issi et al. (1993).

The microorganisms of four groups (fungi, nematodes, protozoans and bacteria) were selected for laboratory testing of their efficacy. Consequently, the following fungal pathogens were proposed for possible utilisation: *Entomophthora grylli* (Fres.) Nowak (*Entomophthorales*);

Cephalosporium lefroyi Horne, *Beauveria bassiana* (Bals.) Vuill., *Beauveria tenella* (Siem.) Delacr., *Metarhizium anisopliae* (Metsch.) Sorok., *Verticillium lecanii* Zimm. and *Paecilomyces farinosus* Brown. (*Deuteromycetes*). Among these, *Beauveria* spp. seem to be the most promising, as they cause high hopper mortality even under conditions of low relative humidity (RH). According to Nurzhanov (1989), *B. tenella* showed the maximum virulence when applied at temperatures ranging from 24 to 29 °C, and RH between 50 and 58%. Neither an increase of temperature (up to 33 °C) or humidity (up to 75%) caused a significant rise of the pathogen's effectiveness in laboratory and field trials of second instar *C. italicus*. The optimal application rate varied from 110 to 240 l of water suspension per hectare with 2 to 5 kg of active ingredient (5×10^7 spores/ml of *B. tenella*). The best results were obtained when the suspension was prepared 24 to 48 h before treatment. Gogolev (1990) reported 71.1% mortality of second instar hoppers of *C. albomarginatus* in small-scale (0.5 – 1 ha) field trials in Yacutia. This level of mortality was observed on the eighth day after treatment with a water suspension of *B. tenella* (4×10^7 spores/ml). The application rate was 2 kg of suspension in 400 l of water per hectare; the temperature at the soil surface was 16 – 28 °C and RH 45 – 95%. It should be noted that this strain of the pathogen (B85) was originally obtained by Nurzhanov (1989) from *Locusta migratoria migratoria* collected in Central Asia. A Central Asian strain (52 M) of the fungus *Beauveria bassiana*, obtained from the Moroccan locust, *Dociostaurus maroccanus*, was tested under laboratory conditions against the second instar hoppers of the Italian locust, *C. italicus*. The application of spores at the rate of 10^7/ml caused the complete mortality of insects 7 days after treatment. In these experiments, the insects were kept in cages at 28 °C and RH 60 – 65% (Nurzhanov and Shamuratov 1988). The same strain when applied at the rate of 5×10^7 spores/ml caused the mortality of 85.3% of hoppers of *C. albomarginatus* in Yacutia one week after treatment. In small-scale field trials in 1994 in the Volga region, the mortality of Italian locust hoppers reached 68.7%, 15 days after treatment by the spores of *B. bassiana* (B52) strain and 69.8%, 14 days after treatment by the spores of *M. anisopliae* (M200) strain. Earlier studies had found that *M. anisopliae*, applied at the rate of 10^8 spores/ml, caused 72.5% mortality of the Italian locust hoppers in small-scale (0.5 ha) field trials in Central Asia (Nurzhanov and Pavliushin 1990). These strains could be recommended for formulation of mycoinsecticides.

In the field experiments of Ogarkov (1990) in East Siberia, conducted in 2-ha plots on a complex of grasshopper species (*C. albomarginatus, A. sibiricus* and others) hopper mortality 11 days after treatment with dry spores of the local strain of *B. bassiana* varied from 47.2 to 84.8%.

With other entomopathogenic fungi, high mortality rates of Italian locust hoppers (68–70%) were reported 10 days after treatment by a water suspension of spores (10^8/ml) of *Aspergillus flavus* and *A. ochraceus* (Nurzhanov and Latchininsky 1987). However, because the metabolites of the *Aspergillus* fungi are highly toxic to plants and mammals, use of this fungi is prohibited by environmental legislation. As for *Entomophthora grylli*, which is known to cause spectacular epidemics in grasshopper populations in Siberia, concomitant with the decline of mass outbreaks (e.g. in 1995 in the Irkutsk region), it can produce infective stages only *in vivo*, which hampers its practical utilisation in grasshopper control.

Regarding nematodes, encouraging laboratory results were obtained by Danilov and Karpova (1990) who reported 96% mortality of hoppers of *C. albomarginatus* in Yacutia 3 days after application of a water suspension of the local race of *Steinernema carpocapsae* (at 20–22 °C; 90–100% RH). However, as in the case of most fungal pathogens, development of nematodes depends almost entirely on weather conditions, particularly humidity and wet soils, thereby posing serious problems for their use in grasshopper control.

Among protozoans, several different species of microsporidians of the genus *Nosema* were found in the Malpighian tubes of grasshoppers (Issi, VIZR, personal communication). Some of them, such as *N. maroccanus*, obtained from the Moroccan locust, appeared to be highly virulent – causing 100% mortality of infected hoppers in 14 days (Issi and Krylova 1987; Nurzhanov 1989). However, attempts to use this pathogen in a bait mixture under the field conditions in Yacutia failed. Cases of grasshopper infestations by other protozoans (e.g. gregarines and amoeba) were extremely rare.

As for bacteria, several strains of *Bacillus thuringiensis* which seemed to produce grasshopper bacterioses were selected in 1994, but their insecticidal activity must be reconfirmed in future experiments.

It should be emphasized that some microbiological agents could lead to the traditional, curative control strategy being replaced by a less environmentally hazardous preventive approach. In this respect, the creation of foci of heightened activity of microbiological natural enemies in the grasshopper outbreak centres by regular application of bioinsecticidal formulations of varied nature could open promising perspectives. However, to be realistic, one should admit that due to the current economical constraints in our country, such perspectives may only be realised in the distant future.

Acknowledgements
The author is indebted to Prof. Jeffrey A. Lockwood (University of Wyoming) and to an anonymous reviewer for their invaluable comments and suggestions on the paper.

References

Anonymous (1996) Fipronil. Worldwide Technical Bulletin. Rhône-Poulenc, Research-Triangle Parc, 20 pp

Danilov LG, Karpova EV (1990) Testing of entomopathogenic nematodes against locusts and grasshoppers. Zastchita Rastenii 7: 34–35 (in Russian)

Gogolev AN (1990) Possibility of utilisation of the entomopathogenic fungi of the genus *Beauveria* in the control of non-swarming grasshoppers in Central Yacutia. Page 220 in Proc Conf Ecological Problems of Plant Protection, VIZR, Leningrad (in Russian)

Issi IV, Krylova SV (1987) The Microsporidia of locusts. Pages 58–62 in Shumakov EM (ed) Locusts - Ecology and control methods. Trudy VIZR, Leningrad (in Russian with English summary)

Issi IV, Latchininsky AV, Gogolev AN (1993) Recommendations on the screening of microbiological agents and testing of their acridicidal properties. Russian Academy of Agricultural Sciences, Moscow, 22 pp (in Russian)

Kurdyukov VV, Latchininsky AV, Naumovich ON (1983) Utilisation of organophosphorous insecticides by means of ULV spraying against injurious locusts in the different zones of their range. Bull of VIZR 56: 21–26 (in Russian with English summary)

Kurdyukov VV, Naumovich ON (1984) Sensibility to insecticides in different locust species. Bull of VIZR 58: 7–12 (in Russian with English summary)

Latchininsky AV (1993) Grasshopper problem in Yacutia (Eastern Siberia, Russia) grasslands. Metaleptea 14(3): 13

Latchininsky AV (1993) Advances in utilisation of microbiological agents for grasshopper control in Russia. Metaleptea 14(3): 13–14

Latchininsky AV (1995) Grasshopper problems in Yacutia (Eastern Siberia, Russia) grasslands. J Orthoptera Res 4: 29–34

Latchininsky AV (1996) International studies of the newest acridicide: the future of fipronil. Proc. XX. International Congress of Entomology, Firenze 1996, 594

Latchininsky AV, Launois-Luong MH (1992) Le Criquet marocain, *Dociostaurus maroccanus* (Thunberg, 1815), dans la partie orientale de son aire de distribution. VIZR, St.-Pétersbourg/CIRAD-GERDAT-PRIFAS, Montpellier, XIX + 270 pp

Latchininsky AV, Duranton J-F (1996) Les effets du fipronil (en concentré emulsifiable) sur les sautériaux en Sibirie. D. 550 CIRAD-GERAT-PRIFAS/VIZR, Montpellier/Saint-Petersbourg, 47 pp

Leskov LI (1990) Entomopathogenic fungi of grasshoppers *Chorthippus albomarginatus* DeG. and *Gomphocerus sibiricus* L. in Central Yacutia. Pages 223–224 in Proc Conf Ecological Problems of Plant Protection, VIZR, Leningrad (in Russian)

Nurzhanov AA (1989) Entomopathogenic microorganisms of locusts in Uzbekistan and their prospective utilisation in the biological plant protection. Doctoral (candidate) thesis, VIZR, Leningrad, 18 pp (in Russian)

Nurzhanov AA, Latchininsky AV (1987) Pathogenic microorganisms of gregarious locusts in Uzbekistan. Pages 62–69 in Shumakov EM (ed) Locusts – ecology and control methods. Trudy VIZR, Leningrad (in Russian with English summary)

Nurzhanov AA, Pavliushin VA (1990) The virulence of the entomopathogenic fungi for Italian locust hoppers. Page 246 in Proc Conf Ecological Problems of Plant Protection, VIZR, Leningrad (in Russian)

Nurzhanov AA, Shamuratov G (1988) New data on the pathogens of the Moroccan locust in Uzbekistan. Pages 107–111 in Shamuratov G (ed) Crop protection from the principal pests and weeds in Karakalpakia. Karakalpakstan, Nukus (in Russian)

Ogarkov BN (1990) Biological background for creation of fungal insecticides and their utilisation in pest control. Doctoral thesis, VIZR, Leningrad, 36 pp (in Russian)

Rachadi T, Balança G, Duranton J-F, Foucart A, Amadou D, Ould Senhoury C (1995) Les effets du fipronil sur *Schistocerca gregaria* (Forskål, 1775), divers sauteriaux et la faune non-cible. D. 513 CIRAD-GERAT-PRIFAS, Montpellier, XII + 116 pp

Tansky VI (1988) Biological base of insect harmfulness. Agropromizdat, Moscow, 182 pp (in Russian)

Tsyplenkov EP (1979) Methodical instructions for locust and grasshopper control. Kolos, Moscow-Leningrad, 36 pp (in Russian)

Vinokurov GM (1949) Sterilisation of grasshoppers by microbiological formulations (preliminary report). Trudy Altayskoy Kraevoy Stantsii Zastchity Rastenii 1: 35–51 (in Russian)

Management strategies

Poster contribution

New Strategies in Locust Control
S. Krall, R. Peveling and D. Ba Diallo (eds)
© 1997 Birkhäuser Verlag Basel/Switzerland

A new approach to the control of *Rhammatocerus schistocercoides* (Rehn, 1906) in Brazil

M. Lecoq[1], E.E. de Miranda[2] and I. Pierozzi Jr.[2]

[1]*CIRAD-GERDAT-PRIFAS, B.P. 5035, 34032 Montpellier Cedex 1, France*
[2]*EMBRAPA-NMA, C.P. 491, 13001-970 Campinas SP, Brazil*

Important plagues of the locust *Rhammatocerus schistocercoides* (Rehn 1906) (Orthoptera, Acrididae, Gomphocerinae) have resulted in the major destruction of crops for more than 10 years in the states of Mato Grosso and Rondônia in Brazil. This was considered to be a new problem, linked to the intensified farming of these areas since the 1980s, together with the introduction of intensive mechanised agriculture.

A research programme, initiated in 1992, has shown that the hypothesis that the plagues are a consequence of the introduction of intensive mechanised agriculture into the border areas of the cerrados of central-west Brazil was not correct. This hypothesis, postulating an ecological disequilibrium and the development of new, favourable environments, was found to be untenable. It has been shown that the plagues of locusts in the Mato Grosso are not a new phenomenon, having occurred on a large-scale in the past (since the beginning of the century) and in exactly the same areas as now. What is new is the economic problems caused by locusts, beginning, clearly, with the introduction of intensive agriculture in the area in the 1980s and in precisely those areas where locusts have multiplied in the past. Furthermore, where agriculture has been established, it has been mainly away from the breeding areas of this locust (campo-cerrado areas on sandy soils), i.e., with breeding areas and agricultural areas in juxtaposition. Much original data has been collected on the biology and ecology of *R. schistocercoides*. This has shown that this species is in no sense migratory, as a superficial observation might suggest and as has been accepted up until now. The swarms can move over only a limited distance. This locust is only locally nomadic throughout the dry season, in areas of degraded cerrado and campo-cerrado of the Chapada dos Parecis (s.l.) in the Mato Grosso. The swarms are of no danger to any other states in Brazil. It is very probable that multiplication depends mainly on rainfall and its variability between years at certain key points of the life cycle. Biotopes of the locust have been identified, described and their locations determined. The relationships between agriculture, animal breeding and the biological cycle of the locust are now well understood. These relationships depend on the season, crop type, cultivation methods and the locust biotopes where agriculture has developed. These are complex relationships which sometimes interact in opposing directions.

These results are preliminary but are sufficient to enable a new control strategy for populations of this locust to be devised, a strategy based on a knowledge of the bio-ecology of the species and on an exact knowledge of the geographical location of its biotopes. The aim is to destroy hopper bands during the rainy season. This control method, in use in the past and then abandoned, is now once more seen as being valid, as a result of the data collected in this project. Joint control operations at the farmer's group level can significantly reduce locust population levels. The control methods can be enhanced by a detailed geographical location of the breeding areas, using satellite images (Landsat).

Management strategies

Working groups

New Strategies in Locust Control
S. Krall, R. Peveling and D. Ba Diallo (eds)
© 1997 Birkhäuser Verlag Basel/Switzerland

Results and recommendations of the working group *Management strategies*

Working group 1

Y. Mbodj (Chairman) and M. Lecoq (Secretary)

Economic estimates of problems caused by locusts

Whilst stressing the need for an economic approach to the locust problem, the group acknowledged the difficulties involved. It concluded that a simple cost-benefit ratio is not an adequate criterion for evaluating the impact of locusts, and desert locusts in particular, and commented that not only the economic impact but also the social and environmental costs should be weighed. Nevertheless, the development of an appropriate methodology for assessing the profitability of anti-locust campaigns should be encouraged, as none of the current approaches is deemed completely satisfactory. A study of this sort should be entrusted to a multi-disciplinary team, combining biologists, economists and sociologists, to consider the various aspects of the problem. A clear distinction must be drawn between the case of grasshoppers (where regular damage assessment makes sense) and that of desert locusts (where simulation studies alone should suffice to calculate of the potential risk posed by an uncontrolled invasion). It was felt that, at present, there are no viable methods other than eliminating plagues and developing preventive locust control strategies, and that other solutions proposed – especially insurance – are completely unrealistic in view of the nature of the problem (migratory insect pests) and given the economic, social and cultural circumstances in the countries involved.

Recommendations

⇒ The working group recommended developing a completely new methodology for assessing the economic impact of locusts and the profitability of control operations. This methodology should take account of the diversity of the problems caused by locusts and their various economic, social, cultural and environmental dimensions.

Locust control strategy

First of all, the working group stressed that there are as many anti-locust strategies as there are locust species, and that preventive control must be given priority whenever possible.

Desert locust

In the main, the studies under way show that new products are emerging which are more environmentally sound. None of these products is beyond the trial phase, and some as yet have only a very remote and highly theoretical possibility of being applied. Not one of the products yet gives grounds for expecting fundamental change in desert locust control strategy. Given the current state of research, insecticide spraying techniques will remain the only possibilities for use in the immediate future, at least as far as controlling large-scale plagues, renewed outbreaks and the beginning of invasions is concerned. Nevertheless, it should be noted that a few of these products (growth inhibitors, phenylpyrazoles) may make a return to the barrier zone method possible in the very near future. This would strengthen the effectiveness of preventive control, undermined as it was some years ago by the ban on dieldrin. Such products should be tested under operational conditions. As far as the control strategy to be adopted against the desert locust is concerned, preventive control must remain the absolute priority. The objective should be to locate and eliminate the first aggregations at an early stage in gregarisation areas. Whenever possible, control must be aimed at eliminating hopper bands in their earliest possible phase, as swarms remain more difficult to control. The preventive control strategy against the desert locust is the result of several decades of experience and has a firm scientific foundation. None of the data obtained from recent studies (economic approach, modelling control operations) provides grounds for questioning it. Although preventive control is the basic strategic level to which priority should be given, the experience of past years (showing that its effectiveness cannot be 100% guaranteed), leads to the conclusion that preventive control should be included in an overall strategy, with the aim of integrating all possible levels of intervention: preventive, curative and palliative. These levels should be clearly defined, particularly in terms of the geographical location, density and age of populations. There must be an exact typology of means to be implemented and precise action plans to suit each level. These action plans must make it possible to rationalise operations, present more coherent and credible requests to donors, and ensure that experience gained is not lost when staff changes occur.

An integrated strategy of this kind implies specific requirements at each level. First, the working group emphasised the need for international co-ordination of the response to the desert locust problem, stressing the fundamental role of the FAO in this respect. The need for regional solidarity between the countries affected and the fundamental role of regional co-operation was emphasised, e.g. the Maghreb and Sahel regions. It would be helpful if regional cooperation in the latter was much stronger. The FAO is strongly advised to make use of this regional potential. Problems in co-ordinating and integrating the two regions are to be expected.

Prevention level

As the strategy depends on the collection of information, it makes sense to give priority to means of collecting and processing information on the desert locust (increasing the network of meteorological stations, validating the use of satellite data, developing geographical information systems and modelling techniques, etc.). More particularly, the working group stressed the importance of the survey and control units within the gregarisation areas themselves that monitor, collect basic information and carry out initial control operations when aggregation occurs. These units play a key role in the action plan and must be revitalised. They should be permanent fixtures, assigned to the desert locust alone, and have their own resources. In addition they should be highly mobile, low cost and well integrated into the physical and human environment of the desert locust.

The working group touched on the various problems currently facing preventive control, but judged that none of them give grounds for questioning the strategy. Various problems were given special attention: budgets and working resources, the use of teams outside the locust season and during periods of recession, training and replacement of personnel, the need to maintain a permanent organisation etc. The problem of the inaccessibility of certain areas for security reasons was given particular attention. It was felt that it was appropriate to provide for "boundary-marking" strategies in combination with remote monitoring of these areas (for example by remote sensing methods), as well as increased monitoring of neighbouring regions. However, the importance of ground-level surveys must be stressed, as they are the only reliable source of information, and the feasibility of such surveys should be carefully examined in each case.

Curative and palliative levels

The first level, the curative level, relates to operations against populations essentially in the *transiens congregans* phase, outside gregarisation areas and already starting to invade some agricultural areas. Here, the aim of operations is not only to protect crops but also to stop the invasion. The second level, the palliative level, relates to operations against fully aggregated populations, when an invasion cycle is already well established. Experience has shown that at this level control operations can do no more than protect crops and probably have only a small effect on the overall dynamics of the invasion.

Particular emphasis was placed on the problem of regional solidarity between states and the need for international co-ordination (even more imperative at these levels than in the preventive control phase). For these control phases more and more resources are needed, reserve stocks of pesticides must be available, it should be possible to mobilise international aid more quickly, and an emergency operations fund should be set up. Environmental protection should be a constant concern when selecting products. Mention was also made of the problem of stocks of insecticides which have passed their expiry date or are unused. Finally, the working group stressed the magnitude of the resources needed to implement palliative control in the event of invasion.

Recommendations

⇒ The working group recommended taking all possible steps to facilitate the implementation of an integrated desert locust control strategy, in which the preventive level would be the primary element.

Attention should be given to
⇒ building up regional solidarity and especially the role of regional organisations, in terms of coordination, harmonisation of operations, information, relationships with donors and fund-raising;
⇒ revitalising detection and control teams and allocating the necessary resources;
⇒ formulating action plans for each intervention level: preventive, curative and palliative;
⇒ developing the means for collecting and processing information, both on the locusts themselves and on their environment;
⇒ increasing decision-makers' awareness of the problems of preventive control;
⇒ mobilising international aid more quickly;

⇒ researching and testing a product for barrier zone treatment, in real-life conditions;

⇒ developing an economic approach specific to the desert locust;

⇒ finding treatment equipment better suited to the difficult conditions of the desert environment;

⇒ setting up a bank of crop protection products;

⇒ setting up an emergency operation fund aimed at quickly countering new outbreaks which are out of control.

⇒ The working group also strongly recommended testing new products intended for locust control as quickly as possible on a large-scale in real-life control conditions. Research into new products must become less remote from the operational reality of locust control.

Grasshoppers

The working group acknowledged that these are chronic pests and that the strategy to be adopted is fundamentally different from that proposed for the desert locust. The strategy consists essentially of intense crop protection, and it was acknowledged that routine treatment outside cultivated areas should be avoided. It was generally recommended that operations be carried out with the simplest and most decentralised means possible, within each village community, enabling action to be taken early (also a form of prevention). The implementation of other prevention methods was also recommended whenever possible (seeking out laying areas in the dry season, using grasshopper development models, monitoring the environment on the ground and using satellite data etc.). The working group acknowledged that grasshopper control is now well organised and generally presents fewer problems than desert locust control. The working group noted with satisfaction that new products are appearing which offer valuable possibilities of replacing pesticides. It hoped, as in the case of the desert locust, that these products could be tested as quickly as possible on a large-scale under real-life control conditions. However, it was concerned about the time some of these products take to act, as such delays are incompatible with the need for rapid action in crop-growing areas. The working group hoped that target species and precise methods of application of these products would be clearly indicated.

In more general terms, the working group drew attention to the role of the CILSS in the monitoring and preventive control of desert locusts and grasshoppers through the AGRHYMET Centre, supplying a large amount of basic data for monitoring the locust biotope. In conclusion, the working group hoped that the possible introduction of any of the emerging new products would stay strictly in line with plant protection regulations and professional ethics.

New Strategies in Locust Control
S. Krall, R. Peveling and D. Ba Diallo (eds)
© 1997 Birkhäuser Verlag Basel/Switzerland

Results and recommendations of the working group *Management strategies*

Working group 2

H. Posamentier (Chairman) and J. Magor (Secretary)

The working group confined its deliberations to control strategies for the desert locust and to currently available control methods which use contact pesticides. The currently implemented strategy seeks to achieve plague prevention through population reduction by trying to eliminate the first gregarious populations appearing. These localised outbreaks occur during recessions or represent the beginning of a plague upsurge sequence (Fig. 1). Inaccessibility, lack of resources

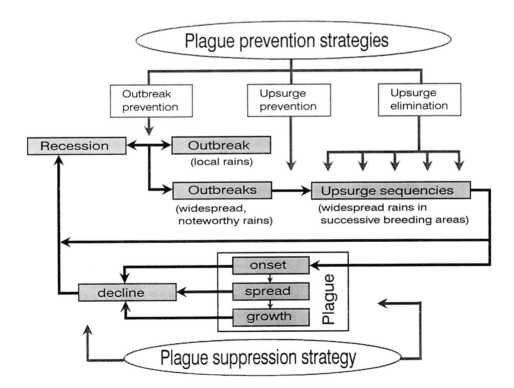

Figure 1. Desert locust cycle from recession to plagues with intervention strategies.

and slow, reactive responses, however, lead in practice to control activities throughout upsurges (upsurge elimination). The study of the development and control of the 1968 plague (Bennett 1976) suggests that a plague will not be prevented by eliminating the first outbreaks or those at the beginning of an upsurge, as an insufficient proportion of the population is in gregariously behaving targets suitable for control.

Indeed, to date there is no clear indication that the present strategy effectively prevents plagues, and the group identified some widely held concerns regarding this strategy:
⇒ outbreak prevention is not feasible;
⇒ upsurge prevention is not feasible at reasonable cost;
⇒ responses to serious infestations are reactive, often culminating in fighting swarms in the absence of proactive planning;
⇒ preventive operations are extremely expensive;
⇒ support of locust operations displaces other equally important plant protection activities;
⇒ many stakeholders vie for scarce funds and resources.

In formulating its recommendations, the working group considered four overall objectives:
⇒ to increase consensus among the stakeholders by clarifying costs and benefits of locust operations;
⇒ to increase preparedness by concentrating operational and control activities and suggesting contingency plans for the medium to long term;
⇒ to reduce pesticide problems;
⇒ to reduce direct and indirect economic, social and environmental costs.

The group identified two points which should be considered irrespective of any new strategy.

Economics. The group welcomed the FAO's initiative in holding a technical meeting on assessing the social and economic impact of locusts; besides professional socio-economists, it should include experts on locust biology and control. These findings should be complemented by studies monitoring control costs and environmental impacts to enable the evaluation of strategies. The group did not discuss details on implementing the above, but left it to the working groups on ecotoxicology and control methods.

Pesticide stockpiles. Donations of pesticides are specially tied to desert locust control. The working group recommends that in the future, pesticide banks should be implemented and donations should not come with strings attached. This would reduce stockpiles and thereby potential environmental contamination.

In view of the above and desert locust population dynamics, the group retained the idea of plague prevention, but in the long term considered it most efficient to concentrate on controlling swarms. It would:
⇒ lead to less use of pesticides and contaminate less land area, as is the case in treating the hoppers;
⇒ reduce overall costs, as surveying activities can be targeted towards swarm control and fewer pesticides are required;
⇒ free spare capacity for other urgent plant protection activities.
The strategy must be supplemented by controlling hoppers that threaten crops during upsurges. The working group realised that its strategy would fail unless the following components are agreed upon and soundly and sustainably financed. Recession area countries should maintain small, well organised locust units to ensure that the surveys required are carried out and to retain experienced campaign managers throughout recession periods. This would normally be the responsibility of the respective plant protection services, possibly assisted through multilateral or bilateral programmes designated to strengthen services overall. Rapid access to aircraft and pesticides must be assured through reserve funds and prearranged contracts. Assurance should be provided by invasion area countries and donors.

A central information centre should be established whose purpose would be to receive data from the entire desert locust area to assess inter-country and inter-regional risks by providing three types of warnings:
⇒ Rainfall data 1–2 years before a potential plague to allow long-term organisational and administrative processes to be put into place.
⇒ Confirmation or reduction of risk forwarded seasonally to finalise organisational requirements.
⇒ Warning of imminent danger and targeting of the intervention area and size.
This activity would be undertaken by the FAO and existing regional organisations. Change is contingent on achieving consensus among countries that are affected, specialists and donors. It is unlikely that different strategies will be able to be compared, which is in the nature of the problem. However, improving the information base on the biology and ecology of locusts, assessment of risks in swarms actually converging on valuable crops and the economics involved may facilitate more objective decisions by those involved. Once this objectivity is attained, a detailed contingency plan centred on proactive swarm control can be designed and implemented.

Reference

Bennett LV (1976). The development and termination of the 1968 plague of the desert locust *Schistocerca gregaria* (Forskål) (Orthoptera: Acrididae). Bull Entomol Res 66: 511–552

Subject index